Cancer

The Complete Recovery Guide

Everything that everyone should know about
cancer and how to recover from it

Jonathan Chamberlain

Dr. Joe Brown
Green Drink

Cancer: The Complete Recovery Guide

While the author has made every effort to provide accurate internet addresses at the time of publication, neither the publisher nor the author assume any responsibility for errors or for changes that may occur.

ISBN: 978-0-9545960-1-9.

Published by Long Island Press   www.fightingcancer.com

1. Cancer   2. Health & Healing   3. Alternative Medicine

4. Mind Body Spirit

Dedication

This book is dedicated to the memory of Bernadette, Sau-fong – for whom it was too late.

Acknowledgments

The original version of this book was *Fighting Cancer: A Survival Guide*. I would like to thank Pam Dix who agreed to be my agent and for finding me my first publisher, Hodder Headline. Without Pam's enthusiasm the book might very well have died an early death.

I also owe a profound debt to Vicky Parker who supplied detailed comments on the chapter on radiation and whose commentary enabled me to avoid many errors. Vicky was one of the leading activists of RAGE—an organisation founded by and for victims of radiation treatment. Sadly, this organization has ceased its activities as the radiation victims were physically unable to maintain their work.

In writing this book I have also been very fortunate in having the library resources of the Hong Kong Cancer Fund. Without access to these books it is unlikely I would have been able to start work on this project.

I wish also to acknowledge the invaluable help of Edith Segall, Annette Crisswell, Gary Oden, Hazel Thornton, Charles Ha, Alan & Martha Cheng, Louise Aylward, Chris Teo, Dr. Alan Greenberg, Jack Gontier, editor of the French edition, whose input has resulted in this new edition of the book being very much better than its predecessors; Leonard Rosenbaum, who combined editorial savvy with unbridled enthusiasm and support for this book; and to Dr. Shamim Daya and her staff at the Wholistic Health Centre in London, for reviewing this book and educating me in some of the latest testing modalities; to Pete Spurrier for facilitating the publication of the book and Margit Whitton, whose support on the home front was very much appreciated.

I would also like to acknowledge the input of the people whose stories appear at the end of this book who had the courage to follow the alternative route, solely or partly in their own cancer journey, and who have shared their stories in books or in emails to me personally. Some of their stories are told in the following pages. Thanks are also due to those contributors to various health Yahoogroups who provided many much needed discussion and information that has molded my own understanding. To them all, I would like to say thank you.

Disclaimer

Reviews and Responses

Leonard S. Rosenbaum

"First of all let me say: Congratulations on your superb book! Your book is…much more comprehensive and better balanced than the vast majority of other books on the topic. Also, it has much valuable material that I don't recall seeing in any other book. The tone is engaging and lively and will appeal to anyone sympathetic to alternative approaches to cancer. You have succeeded in making a complicated subject accessible."

Leonard S. Rosenbaum Dir., Alternative Cancer Information Resources;
Board of Dirs., Intl. Assn. of Cancer Victors & Friends (IACVF www.cancervictors.net); Board of Dirs., Washington Professionals for the Study of Psychoanalysis (WPSP; www.washpsp.org)

Annette Lynch

"Thanks for your brilliant Fighting Cancer website www.fightingcancer.com. I was diagnosed with lung cancer a week ago and my immediate reaction (after the shock) was to fight it every inch of the way. I came home and decided to see what I could learn from the internet and your site was the first one I found. I have found this immensely inspiring and helpful."

Mike Howell, in a review of internet resources for cancer patients published in the UK's Positive Health magazine (October 1998)

"If I wanted to search the web and learn about cancer, my starting point would be Jonathan Chamberlain's site located at www.fightingcancer.com"

Ron Crennell

"I recently bought your book *Fighting Cancer* because I have become very involved in the life of an old friend and the challenges she faces with a diagnosis of secondary liver cancer. We were both comforted and somewhat inspired by the broad sweep of your book."

Mrs. Nickie Bunyan

"I have found your book 'Fighting Cancer' one of the most useful I have come across - thank you for researching and writing it."

Rev. Bill Newbern, San Diego.

"This book tells me everything I want to know. Why didn't my doctor tell me this?"

Andrew Saul, PhD, DOCTOR YOURSELF WEBSITE (Vol. 4, No. 4 January 20, 2004)

"Jonathan Chamberlain's website has long been one of my favourites...Mr. Chamberlain has a voice that is at once humble and powerful. I like writers that cut to the chase, and then do not skimp on the practical details...and I really like his attitude. He speaks from the heart, but clearly wants you to use your head. Good combination."

Jim Cole

"Thank you for the organization of a fragmented body of information. This book is now *the* reference book on alternative treatments."

Richard Thompson

"Jonathan: You might remember me, as the guy with multiple myeloma that had trouble with downloading your book. I now can recommend your book to the people in my support group, as "the" book to read. You have covered just about everything that I have read, and it took me over twenty books and innumerable downloads to do it. The book is more precious than gold!"

Karl-Heinz Klaeser, Oslo

"Thank you for your most informative and educational book. What did I know about cancer? But now, because of your book, your work, I have an idea what is involved… Your book gave me an insight into the world of cancer and potential ways of fighting the disease."

Gerald White, Founder of Seeds of Joy Foundation, USA

"Your book is a masterpiece of both content and composition.…I have been impressed by the originality, persistence and quality of your work…. Your dedication to principle in the face of what must be overwhelming odds is most heartening. I could not help but notice that your work was in response to your loss of your wife. I know that you will never get over it but your wonderful work is a grand testimonial as to how you did, in fact, get through it and turn this personal tragedy to something of value to mankind. I admire you for that."

Mrs. Colleen Crim, San Mateo

"My husband of 30 years was initially diagnosed with a high-grade sarcoma in January, 2003, had his left foot amputated in March and was told in May that it had metastasized to his lungs, is incurable, is not treatable and he has 6-12 months to live. An incredible despair seized us and we couldn't see anything but hopelessness through our tears. Then I Googled "fighting +cancer" and the first link I went to was a chapter from your brilliant book. A spark of hope came back into my life. I quickly printed out the entire book and devoured the entire thing in one sitting. As I read hope grew and grew.

"My darling husband, still in the bottomless pit of despair, wouldn't read it, so I just began reading it aloud to him. He got up to leave the room but I followed him, reading aloud as he went from room to room and finally out into the garden. The part I choose to read was about Linus Pauling and Vitamin C. Suddenly he stopped, turned around and took the pages from my hands saying, "I had forgotten about Vitamin C". He sat down on the steps and began to read. He sat there for over two hours. When he was finished, he came in the house and said "Let's go find some sodium ascorbate and all that other stuff on Linus' list. We have a path now." So off we went.

"I just wanted to say thank you from the bottom of my heart. You gave us hope when all we could see was despair and you gave us a path when we thought all was lost."

FOREWORD

This book will tell you more about cancer than you ever thought you would know: The two ways of conceptualizing cancer, the causes, the diagnostic tests, the problems with the orthodox treatments and the enormous range of alternative approaches that there are. You will also learn about the business of cancer and cancer research. But before we go any further we need to pause a moment.

There is a famous Chinese saying:

Know yourself.
Know your enemy
One hundred fights
One hundred victories

Read that first line carefully: Know yourself. In order to be victorious you need first of all to understand, not your enemy (in this case cancer), but your own self.

I know from experience that it is no good simply hoping that the information you will read in this book will help you. You come to this book with a world view and a whole bag full of prejudices. These have been formed by your reading, the newspapers, television. And almost all your prejudices, thoughts and ideas about cancer are almost certainly wrong. But it may be that my telling you this has merely served to make you defensive: How do you know that what I know is wrong? Who are you to…? Etc.

Let's just say that I've been there. Goethe put it succinctly: "The half-known hinders knowing. Since all our knowing is only half, our knowing always hinders our knowing." In short, what we think we know gets in the way of our learning something new.

There is a lot of information in this book. In fact there may be too much. If you start feeling that this book is just too much then I would recommend to you that you read the companion book: **Cancer Recovery Guide: 15 Alternative and Complementary Strategies for Restoring Health** (Clairview Books, 2008) - www.clairviewbooks.com.

That book is the short overview. This volume is a more detailed resource. Together they go hand in hand. The short book was written to provide a quick orientation designed to help you make quick decisions. This book provides a much more detailed discussion of the options and the arguments—and is therefore organized in a different way. Together, it is my hope, these two books will provide you with the confidence to make decisions that suit you and will, I hope, lead to you becoming well again without having to undergo damaging treatments.

In this brief preface, I'm going to suppose that you fall into one of three groups of people and I'd like to say something to each of you.

1. You Have Just Recently Discovered That You Have Cancer.

You are, I imagine, suddenly very scared. Life that seemed so firmly based has now become very precarious. You have to a certain extent closed yourself off from the world. You are locked into your own head. Your fears are echoing around the empty chambers of your mind. You are trying to strengthen your grip on things by saying to yourself: "I will do whatever is necessary to get through this thing!" You know that it is going to be fearfully damaging and painful. But you're going to do it. Yes, you are! And you will ignore all obstacles in the way. You are going to grit your teeth and…STOP!

Yes, please stop this line of thinking. I am going to tell you two things. One will scare you a little more and one will reassure you (I hope!).

The Scare:

The minute you heard that you had cancer, your cancer almost certainly started to become just a little more aggressive. The problem is stress and anxiety. The biochemistry of these emotional states is actually provoking the tumour to grow faster. Your doctor probably didn't tell you that – he thought it would just make matters worse. And perhaps it would make matters worse if I left it there. But by knowing this fact you can now start working to change this stress to a state of relaxation, even calm acceptance perhaps: Meditate, swim, go for long walks, book yourself an aromatherapy massage, take up singing, listen to Javanese gamelan music or the hypnotic Indian dulcimer music of Shiv Kumar Sharma.

Yes, go and do it now. This will, hopefully, have the reverse effect of slowing the growth of the tumour. Also, get the amino acid supplement L-Theanine. This is widely available on the internet and is a proven, quick acting and totally safe anxiety eliminator.

If you do not have access to the internet - for whatever reason - then find someone who does. Or go down to the library and find out how you can learn. This is a vital resource for many of the products recommended in this book.

The Reassurance:

Cancer can be beaten—there are dozens of cures in this book. No matter what your cancer, these will work. It's true that none are 100 percent certain but several have extremely good track records – and you will be relieved to know that most of them are pain-free. If one therapy – or one combination of therapies - doesn't work, you can move on to another. There is time.

Also I would like you to tell yourself the following message: Say to yourself these important words: **I am not going to do anything until I have read this book. I want any decision I make to be truly informed. I want to know something more about cancer. I will spend the next few days reading. Maybe I will get a copy for a close friend to read at the same time so that I can talk about it. Then I will be in control. Above all I am not going to undertake a treatment just because the doctor or my wife, husband or mother says that's what I should do.**

It may also be helpful if, before you start reading this book from the beginning, to read the last chapter of this book. This is about decision-making. Do it now to get some further ideas of how you can think about your options. Read also the personal stories at the back of this book. These people cured themselves of their cancers – you can too. Good luck.

2. You Have Undergone Cancer Treatment But Now You Want to Learn More About the Options Just in Case It Returns.

When you first got cancer you probably went along with what your doctors advised. Why wouldn't you? The doctors have 'science' on their side. Well, now maybe you are prepared to reconsider that position. I hope so. The problem is that there are large areas of health-related information and expertise that doctors know nothing about – certainly they are not taught about them during their medical studies: diet, supplements, herbs, electromagnetic interventions and a great deal more. In many places – the USA, for example – doctors are in fact forbidden by their medical boards from discussing these subjects. If they insist on doing so they can find themselves struck off the medical register. So if there is any value in these areas you will not learn about them from your doctor — which is a great pity.

Also, if you are wise you will already have come to understand that you can't treat cancer as a disease that you can 'cure' and then forget about. Your cancer hasn't come from Mars. Cancer is the result of a natural process which is almost certainly connected with the way you choose to live your life. If you don't change your way of life then you can probably expect the cancer to return at some stage. But what do you need to do to avoid this happening? I hope this book will help you find answers that you can happily incorporate into your life.

Good luck.

3. You Are Helping Someone Who Has Cancer

You have a very difficult job. You want to help but you're not sure how. As someone who has been in this position let me tell you some of the conclusions I have come to.

a) Not Everyone Wants Information

Recently I met Peter. On our first meeting he told me that he had liver cancer. It had been treated but had returned. "Well, this is your lucky day," I said to him. "I happen to know what you can do." But Peter waved me away. "Oh don't tell me anything. I just have to live with it as long as I can." "Really," I assured him. "I know something you can do. It's cheap and people say it has a 90 percent chance of working." "No," he said. "I don't want to know." So I smiled and we talked about something else.

The truth is denial does have some survival value – it stops people getting overstressed (and stress exacerbates cancer) and if that's how he wanted to deal with it, fine. I just had to accept it.

b) You May Disagree About What to Do.

This is particularly difficult if you are living with someone who is making decisions that you think are wrong. Perhaps they want to do chemo and radiation while you think the Budwig approach (see p. 153) is best. Or they want to see a spiritual healer while you think surgery is the only sensible thing to do. Well, here is what you have to do: say your piece - once, twice or even three times – and then shut up. The person who has cancer is the person whose decision counts. I can tell you this is not an easy thing to do. But it is important because…

c) Your Relationship Is Vital

The person you are caring for is utterly vulnerable. Your relationship may be one of the things that is making the present bearable. Do everything you can to nurture it. This is not a time for you to impose your feelings on the relationship. Instead, it is a time for you to listen and to quietly be of help. Again this is often not easy but I assure you it is important. If you feel frustrated take your frustrations elsewhere.

d) Is Your Relationship Part of the Problem?

This is a hard question to ask and an even harder one to answer. If there are problems between you and the person you are caring for then this is the time to confront them. Nagging emotional obstacles can hinder healing. Healing the emotions can release very profound energies. Perhaps counseling—for both of you—would be beneficial.

e) Take Care of Yourself

You are not perfect. You can't do everything. There will come a time when you, yourself, will need the support of others. From time to time you will need to put your own needs first. Give yourself treats. Nurture yourself.

And good luck.

Jonathan Chamberlain
Brighton
May 2008

Table of Contents

Introduction

Why Did I Write This Book ?

This book arose out of my own personal encounter with cancer — not as a patient but as the often inadequate husband of a cancer patient.

My wife, Bernadette, was diagnosed with cervical cancer in 1993. She underwent surgical investigation, radiation and chemotherapy and was dead almost exactly a year later. Looking back, if I were to summarize my experience, I would say the biggest mistake we made was to do what the doctors advised. Bernadette could not have died sooner if we had done nothing.

In addition, that year - the year of her illness - caused us a great deal of seemingly unavoidable, painful relationship difficulties as we responded to her illness in very different ways. Yet, how could we have avoided these difficulties? If only we'd had a book that could lead us through the whole field from an intelligent non-ideological point of view.

Eventually I was to read close to two hundred books and still I could not find the book I was looking for. Most of the books were selling single cures. Others talked about a range of alternative cures but gave no rationale for choosing this route over the orthodox route. Many others vilified anyone who suggested anything other than surgery, radiation and chemotherapy, accusing them of being victims of quacks and charlatans. What was the truth?

Throughout my ordeal I found myself reading book after book recommending diets, herbs, supplements and other interventions. But when I raised these ideas with the doctors they poured scorn on them. Vitamin C? They laughed. Coffee enemas? 'What a joke,' they said. And Bernadette too dismissed these suggestions. 'Are you a doctor?' She asked me. 'Do you know more than the doctors?'

This was how I discovered the war of medical ideologies that is out there. What I needed was a sane, personal, intelligent and critical voice that could lead me through these contending beliefs; that could put both sides of the case and point up the limitations of any arguments there might be. But I never found this voice. So, I have taken it upon myself to provide this voice for others. This then is the book I wish I had had at hand when Bern was diagnosed with cancer.

After Bern died, I nearly despaired. But then I realized that if I did not persevere with my reading then it was likely that the same fate would befall me—for I had discovered that I, along with everyone else in North America and Western Europe, had a 40-50 percent likelihood of getting cancer myself. If I did get cancer, what would I do? I needed to create for myself a strategy that I would have faith in, based on all the facts. I needed to build up a complete picture of all the therapies that were recommended in the case of cancer and to look at these with a very critical eye: What was the rationale? What was the risk involved? What was the cost?

Only when I had a global picture of cancer would I be in a position to make a decision. And what went for me went for everybody. I was writing this book not just for myself but for everyone who did not wish to be panicked into doing what the doctors advised.

It was not my intention to write a book telling people what they should do. There are already too many books screaming propaganda of one sort or another, both the virulently pro-orthodox and the equally virulently pro-alternative. What was needed was a book that took a cool look at the whole world of cancer. I have left it to you, the reader, to make up your own mind as to which strategies you believe will work best for you.

In the more than twelve years that I have been running an informal cancer advice website, I have come to realize that we bring very different psychological profiles to the party. What makes sense to you may seem madness to me. But I need to respect your point of view and you need to respect mine.

This book is based very much on what experts have said in their own field for the world of cancer is so large that there are no general cancer experts. But the book I have written is no bland summary. It is deeply engaged and it draws conclusions. I now believe that the search for a cure for cancer is a waste of time. We already have the cure – or rather the cures. There isn't just one cure for cancer, I believe, there are dozens.

Am I Qualified to Write This Book?

This is a good question. But the more I have thought about it the more I have realized that no one is qualified to write this book. When Socrates asked the Oracle at Delphi if he was the wisest person in the world the Oracle replied: "There is no one wiser than you." Socrates was wise enough not to boast for he understood his own ignorance. Although he did not feel that he was wise, he knew only that no one was wiser. That is how I feel. I may not be particularly well qualified, but the truth is that no one is more qualified.

I am not a doctor, but doctors have to placate professional colleagues and bend to professional pressures. They are also subject, as we shall see, to powerful temptations placed in their way by the pharmaceutical companies. I am not a complementary therapist so I am not professionally biased in the opposite direction. I am not a cancer patient myself and so I am not obsessed by the specifics of my own particular cancer. I have no particular professional or personal axe to grind and I have no financial interest in any of the therapies mentioned in this book. All these qualifications may, at first sight, appear to be negative but nevertheless they make me almost unique. In this matter I have a pure heart.

However, I do have one positive qualification. I am powered - as a result of the traumatic experience of my wife's agony - by an urgent need to know the truth. The neurologist, Antonio Damasio, in his book *Descartes' Error* (Putnam 1994), has shown how vital it is to have emotional engagement. Without this engagement, using only objective reason, we will always make profound errors of judgment. To arrive at sensible decisions we need to engage both intellect and the emotions. And experts, for all their virtues, do not tend to be emotionally engaged.

To those who say only a medical professional should write about cancer, I say this: Do you have to be Portuguese to write a travel guide to Portugal? In some ways, being Portuguese could be seen as a disqualification. What is needed is an impartial but committed critical mind. That is what I bring to the party. This book should be seen as a travel guide to the strange country of Cancer.

So, to summarize, my qualification is simply this: I have a powerful need to know the answers. I need the answers for myself so that I will not make the same mistake we made in my wife's case. What I have written I have written for myself first of all. However, I willingly share the fruits of this pursuit with you or anyone else who is interested but, and this is also important, you and they are responsible for making whatever decisions you or they do make on the basis of this information.

And I am pleased to say that my book has been of benefit to people who have read it. The comment that puts the key point most succinctly is this from a San Diego pastor who had just been told his cancer was terminal: "This book tells me everything I want to know. Why didn't my doctor tell me this?" Sadly, for him, the information came too late.

I offer this book to you in the hope that it helps you clarify for yourself how you wish to approach the treating of the cancer you (or perhaps someone close to you) have been diagnosed with or the cancer that you would like to prevent in advance.

Why Should You Read This Book?

If you have cancer, then the answer is clear. This book will help you understand the range of options you have. These are real choices and many hold out the very real hope of a cure, no matter what stage your cancer is at, no matter if the doctors have written you off. Yes, even so-called 'terminal' cancer patients, who in the opinion of their doctors are only weeks away from death, have been cured, have gone on to live for decades longer. Some, like Anne Frahm and Beata Bishop, have written books telling their stories.

If you don't already have cancer then it is equally important for you to read this book. Why? Because it is 100 percent certain that you - or someone close to you - will get cancer. This is an absolute certainty. Imagine you are on a narrow road and a huge truck is bearing down on you at a great speed. You can either close your eyes and keep your fingers crossed, or you can keep your eyes fixed on the danger and think about how you can avoid being hit. I think we can all agree the second strategy is best. Also, a book like this is a good starting place for a couple, say, to discuss which options might make sense – a discussion that will pave the way for mutual understanding and so lessen the risk of frustration and lonely, unvoiced despair.

The Importance of Being Prepared

Imagine the doctor were to tell you today that you had cancer. How would you react?

Many people have had the following experience. One day a doctor does a test and the result comes back positive. Oh my God! It's CANCER!!!! The doctor puts on a very grave face and says he has to put you in hospital. He recommends surgery followed by radiotherapy and chemotherapy. There's no time to think. The doctor recommends the greatest urgency: "The quicker we open you up, the quicker we can deal with this thing before it gets too big, before it spreads." Oh my God!!! It's going to spread!!! Panic! There's no time to think. There's no time to make a reasoned assessment of all the options. There's no time to even think up the questions you know you should be asking. And anyway the doctor knows what's best. And before you know it you've been cut open and you've been blasted with so many rads and your hair has fallen out - maybe half your rectum has been cut off and you have to carry a plastic bag around with you – possibly for the rest of your life - and then, only then, you come across this book. Only then do you see the range of options that are available. And yes, it seems that for some cancers established medicine does seem to have made good progress. And yes, a number of alternative therapies do seem to offer attractive - and viable - alternatives. The fact is, you need to know what you're going to do, and the best time to make that decision is *before* you get cancer. If you don't, you may find that things are done to you that, in retrospect, you would rather, hadn't been.

Some Interesting Statistics

The incidence of cancer is rising inexorably as the following statistics show:

Early 1800s: one in 50
1900: One in 27
1920: One in 10
1930: One in 12
1940: One in nine
1950: One in seven

1960:   "According to present government statistics, one out of every six persons in our population will die of cancer. It will not be long before the entire population will have to decide whether we will all die of cancer or change fundamentally all our living and nutritional conditions." (Max Gerson [1958] author of *A Cancer Therapy*)

1980   "If the present trend continues, at least one in four of us will contract cancer. One in five will die of the disease."

1993   "Cancer may be the most feared disease of our time. It is second only to heart disease as a leading cause of cancer in the United States, and it is estimated that one in every three Americans will develop cancer at some point in their lives." Geoffrey Cooper (1993) author of `The Cancer Book'

2002   "Today, one of every two men and one of every three women in the United States alone will confront cancer over the course of their lives" (Andrew von Eschenbach M.D. Director of the National Cancer Institute–preface to *Everyone's Guide to Cancer Therapy*, 2002).

(Unless otherwise stated, these figures are from Ralph Moss's excellent book 'The Cancer Syndrome' - reprinted as 'The Cancer Industry' 1982)

I hope those figures got your attention because they certainly got mine. Decade after decade cancer incidence has risen inexorably. However, some have suggested that in 2004-6 these figures may have peaked, others have pointed out that the post-war baby boomer generation are just beginning to hit the age when cancer incidence rises markedly so the apparent flattening out of the curve may be a very temporary phenomenon. For some these figures are merely impersonal abstractions that have little immediate personal relevance. But there are those whose experience of cancer's seemingly insistent onward march is more traumatic.

> "Cancer, and cancer, and cancer. My mother, my father, my wife.
> I wonder who is next in the queue?" - C.S. Lewis

Cancer is now the cause of a third of all deaths in Western industrialized countries – up from about 20 percent not much more than a decade ago. And it is not just because people are living longer. Actually, they - we - aren't! The life expectancy of a 45 year old person hasn't changed significantly in the last 100 years. In 1870, the 45-year-old person could expect to live to the age of 70 to 75. Now, he or she can expect to live to somewhere between 75 and 80 or more. If average life expectancy appears to have increased by great leaps in that time it is because there are fewer diseases decimating children - and fewer women are dying in childbirth. So the argument that there's more cancer because people are living longer is not a very good one. The fact is, overall cancer incidence is increasing at every age level. In 2000, for example, more women of 40 had breast cancer than they did in 1950.

Until recently, cancer was almost a taboo word. Fortunately, it has now come out of the closet. It is no longer seen to be an automatic death sentence. The good news is the fact that people with cancer are, according to statistics, living longer and that 40-50 percent of people diagnosed with cancer do not die of the disease. The bad news is that the statistics cannot be trusted for reasons that will be explained later in this book.

The fact is, more and more people are developing cancer. While, death rates for most cancers have not changed in decades, some have declined (often for reasons unknown), while some are increasing at an enormous rate: lung cancer being the prime example. With the possible exception of breast cancer (where there may (I stress 'may') have been a slight improvement in survival rates in recent years), the orthodox methods of treating cancer – surgery, radiation and chemotherapy – have not had a clear impact on death rates. Many people have therefore taken the view that alternative ways of treating cancer hold out more hope. These alternative ways include dietary regimes, the taking of vitamin and herbal supplements–and a host of other approaches from copper coils to magnetic beds, from acidophilus to visualization - which I have listed in the last section of this book.

The problem for the patient is that doctors, generally speaking, are very hostile to these alternative approaches. It is not excessive to describe the present state of affairs as a war of ideas. Anyone wishing to make reasoned decisions in this battlefield needs to understand where the battle lines are drawn. I have discussed these issues in the chapters on cancer politics.

Can We Avoid Getting Cancer?

For those of us who do not (yet?) have cancer, two questions pose themselves.

1. Is there any way that we can reduce our chances of getting cancer?

2. If we do get cancer, what is the best way to making sure that we are among the 40-50 percent who do not die from the disease within 5 years - perhaps even one of the 25-30 percent who do not die of the disease at all?

So, How Can We Improve Our Chances Of Not Getting Cancer?

The quick answer is to stop smoking - one in two smokers dies from a smoking related disease - and to reduce dietary fat to not more than 30 percent of total calories, but note that very-low-fat diets are also associated with some cancer risks. A medium-fat diet is optimal—and make sure the fats are good fats! Avoid transfats and hydrogenated fats like the plague.), eat more fibre, get more exercise, avoid burnt and barbecued foods, and avoid drinking alcohol in liver damaging quantities. Alcohol in reasonable quantities does not appear to be measurably carcinogenic on its own, but evidence suggests that it can speed the passage of other carcinogens into the cells. For heavy-drinking heavy smokers, this is bad news. You should also avoid chemical pollutants and excessive radiation.

But cancer-prevention is not simply about avoiding cancer-causing substances. A more pro-active regime will involve increasing exposure to the sun (for the vitamin D), changing one's diet to one that includes lots of apples, oranges, carrots, cabbage and other dark green vegetables — preferably organic (pesticides have been linked to breast cancer). It may also involve taking vitamin and herbal supplements. More information on these can be found in the second half of this book. You are going to have to change the way you live to maximize your chances of living a longer cancer-free life. That's your responsibility, no one else's.

Being Prepared for Cancer

Let's look back at the statistics. These demonstrate beyond a shadow of doubt that something very frightening is happening. It is not exploding as fast as AIDS, maybe, but the cancer spectre is much larger and affects many more people. And dying of cancer is a painful, debilitating, traumatic and traumatizing experience. To give you an indication of how great the problem is, imagine eight fully loaded jumbo 747s crashing every day with no survivors: That is the number of people dying of cancer everyday in North America and Western Europe combined. That's right. Eight jumbo jets today, another eight tomorrow, eight more the day after that and so on. Double that and you have an idea of what is happening globally.

For myself, confronted with my wife's newly diagnosed illness, I discovered that I knew nothing at all about cancer. Cancer was just a word. I talked to my friends, who were supposedly bright, literate, and highly educated. None of them knew anything worth a damn about cancer or its treatments. Here is a disease that is going to kill one in two of us within the foreseeable future and we knew nothing about it. We weren't doing anything about it either. We had simply blinkered ourselves to reality. We didn't do it consciously but we were doing it. We were heading like lambs to the slaughter. If the situation is that bad, why isn't everyone panicking?

I think part of the reason is that it is all happening so slowly. There is an experiment that went as follows. A number of frogs were put into a shallow pan containing scalding hot water. Without exception they immediately leapt out. A number of other frogs were placed in a similar pan containing water at room temperature. This water was ever so gradually heated. The water heated up but the frogs didn't move. They all eventually died of heat shock.

The moral of this experiment is that when something is gradual, it slips under our genetically primed warning systems that are geared to protect us against sudden or gross changes in our environment. We become habituated. The slow creeping increase in cancer and heart disease has slipped through more or less unannounced. Oh yes, there have been stories in the press. But the sense of urgency is entirely missing. We may be able to perceive it intellectually. But we are not emotionally alerted. Our fight or flight systems are not switched on. There's no adrenalin. There's no panic. We continue to live as we have always lived. One of the purposes of this book is to trigger a little adrenalin.

You Have the Choice of Being or Not Being a Victim.

Let me state this bluntly: If you don't inform yourself about cancer, you will significantly increase your chances of being a victim. Why do I say this? Because when confronted with a diagnosis of cancer, you may make choices that you will possibly regret later. You need to be informed that there is a medical war out there. There are major disagreements as to how cancer should be treated. You need to know what the issues are. You need to understand what is happening in the world of cancer, what the arguments are, what the options are. You need to read this while your mind is clear and unworried. Imagine the doctor were to tell you today that you had cancer. How would you react? What decisions would you make? Remember, it is your decision. You, and you alone, are responsible for making whatever treatment decisions that are made - not your doctor.

Here is the opinion of a qualified doctor, Dr. Eugene D. Robin: "The doctor's opinion is not infallible... you, the patient, have the highest stake in the decision - the most to gain and the most to lose. You, the patient, are the one to decide what constitutes a happy and productive life. Don't let your doctor, however well intentioned, usurp this right."

Dr. Eugene Robin is saying here that if you don't want an operation because you don't want to live with the consequences of the operation then it is your right not to have the operation.

To make any decision, you need to understand the range of options that are available. That is what this book aims to provide.

We can define a victim as someone to whom damaging things are done without him or her having any say in the matter. A non-victim is someone who makes the decisions about what is done, who takes responsibility.

What Is The Right Decision?

The right choice is simply the choice each patient makes for him-or-herself based on the best information at hand, and based on each person's world view, given the circumstances that each person finds her-or-himself in.

Over the last decade or more in which I have been giving advice through my website, it has become very clear to me that there cannot be one set of right answers that cover all situations. Not only are the specific situations unique – but so too are the people who find themselves faced with cancer. Some are fearful, others are aggressive; some want to take control, others want control to be taken away from them – still others just don't want to know. I have therefore summarized the options that people can take as follows:

1. Follow the orthodox regime only. Do what the doctor advises. Avoid anything unorthodox.

2. Follow a regime of a combination of alternative therapies only. Do not consider any of the orthodox regimes.

3. Follow doctor's orders first and if that doesn't work then try the alternative route later.

4. Follow the alternative approaches first and if they don't succeed, fall back on the orthodox treatments

5. Combine orthodox and alternative therapies together from the start.

6. Do nothing.

It is possible to make out a sensible case for each one of these options – even the last one. How do we decide? For some, the decision will be made on essentially emotional grounds. Others will want to base their decisions on hard evidence. Some people will insist that there must be proof that a treatment works before they will do it. Others will accept that there are many types of evidence and that low quality evidence (a friend of a friend told me…) need not necessarily be rejected out of hand. In this case, a risk-benefit analysis may be more appropriate. If the risk is low and the potential benefit high then this might be an adequate reason for choosing a course of action.

Each person facing a diagnosis of cancer needs to consider the options coolly. Read this book. Then keep it on your shelf so that when you, or a member of your family, or a friend, or a colleague, or a neighbour, gets cancer - as they assuredly will - then you will have immediate access to advice.

Introduction

Your decision to read this book means that you have elected to take responsibility for your own health. Putting into effect what you learn in these pages could help you (and your loved ones) to live longer and avoid a great deal of pain. For I believe there isn't just one cure for cancer – there are dozens. People who take responsibility for their health are healthier and happier.

It may be useful at this point to say a few words about what I mean by 'cure'. I do not believe that there is one approach, one therapy, one supplement or chemical that will cure all types of cancer in 100 percent of the people taking it. However, I do think there are approaches that come close to that ideal. But let's say Approach A has a 70 percent success rate and Approach B has a 60 percent success rate and Approach C has a 50 percent success rate then out of a hundred patients following these approaches in this order until they found something that worked, 70 would find the first approach all that they need. Of the remaining 30, 18 would be cured by Approach B, leaving twelve. Of these twelve, six would benefit from Approach C, leaving only 6 out of the original 100 who still hadn't found a cure. A 94 percent success rate over all. And then there are still Approaches D, E, F…Z to go.

I appreciate that this is a bit simplistic - after all, we haven't defined what we mean by a cure - but it does indicate that if the approaches dealt with in this book are beneficial as many people claim then working your way through them one or more at a time is likely to result in a greatly enhanced life span – both in terms of quantity of years and quality of life experience and the pleasure of living each day.

I wish you the best of luck in your own search for the answers that make sense to you.

Section 1: The Basic Facts

What is Cancer?

Doctors and other health professionals usually give one of two answers. One answer is that cancer is not one disease but a general name for a group of over two hundred (possibly two thousand) diseases all of which are characterized by rapid and irregular cell growth. Another characteristic is the spread of the disease from one site to another. That, in brief, is the first answer. The other answer is that cancer is really a disease of the whole body, one of the symptoms of which is rapid and irregular cell growth in one or more sites.

At first sight there doesn't appear to be much difference between these two answers. But there is a crucial difference. Is the area of rapidly dividing cells the disease itself or only a symptom of the disease? Is it one disease or two hundred or more? Dr. Salomon, a French oncologist at the National Center for Scientific Research, stated the matter in the following words: "The notion that cancer is a localized disease which tends to spread and become general may be opposed by the idea that cancer is a general disease which results in a local tumor."

It is very important that we answer this question correctly. How we define the disease affects how we treat the disease. So we must ask ourselves: is the tumour the disease or is it a symptom of the disease? Do we concentrate on attacking the tumour or do we try to heal the body?

Orthodox modern Western medicine, generally speaking, considers the cancerous tumour to be the disease itself. How or why it arose they have no idea. But having arisen, it must be attacked. It must be surgically removed. Or it must be irradiated. Or it must be killed with highly toxic chemicals. Or it must be defeated with the aid of some sort of immunological vaccine. Or some combination of these.

So-called 'holistic' medicine, on the other hand, posits that the tumour-symptom will disappear once the root cause disappears. And the root cause, they say, is the fact that the body as a whole has been poisoned and is not getting the right kind of nutritional and/or natural support.

To put it another way, there are those who believe that cancer cells have something wrong with them, that they are deviant cells and because they are deviant they must be destroyed. The other view is that cancer cells are essentially normal cells forced to live in, and accommodate themselves to, an abnormal tissue environment. The problem is not the cells themselves but the surrounding environment.

Who is right?

We are so used to right-wrong polarities that it seems easy to ask this question. But potential patients - and we are all potential patients - must be very wary of taking a 100 percent position. Perhaps we need to embrace the question with both hands and suggest that there may be an element of right on both sides.

It is certainly true that some people have been diagnosed with cancer, have undergone surgery with or without radiation and chemotherapy and have gone on to live long and happy lives.

This was true of my own mother who had breast cancer and who had no further problem with cancer after having had surgery and radiation treatment. It is also true that what appears to work for one type of cancer will not work for another - and therefore it makes sense to talk of different types of tumour. So, on these grounds, we have to accept that the orthodox medical approach has some merit.

It is also undoubtedly true that some people have utterly rejected these therapies and have cured themselves of cancer by doing no more than drinking or taking a particular substance, or even by simply mentally rejecting the cancer. One case is that of Dr. Benjamin Spock, the "world's best known paediatrician" who in his early eighties was reportedly diagnosed as having a bone cancer in his spine. Being so old he had no desire to undertake any burdensome treatment. He knew in any case that cancers grow slowly in elderly people. He decided therefore simply to refuse to believe he had the cancer. A few years later tests showed that he no longer did have any cancer.

What often happens in cases like this is that sceptics call into question the original diagnosis of cancer. How can we know that he really did have cancer? They ask. But they don't call into question the cases that respond to their orthodox treatments.

So the answer we choose for ourselves to the question "What is cancer?" depends on the model - or paradigm - of medicine that we choose to follow. What is important is that we know there is a question and that there is no simple black and white answer.

About 90 percent of cancers are solid-tumor cancers and 10 percent "soft" cancers such as leukaemias and lymphomas.

One point that does need to be made clear is that cancer cells were once normal cells that have become abnormal. This change can be reversed. It is possible to turn a cancer cell back into a normal cell. This fact has enormous implications as we shall see.

At a metabolic level there is a key difference between normal and cancer cells as to how they get their energy. The normal cell satisfies its energy needs using oxygen that is processed by mitochondria, which are rod like structures within the cell. These mitochondria are also responsible for controlling normal cell death. In a cancer cell, the cell, unable to get its energy in the normal way because there is a lack of oxygen in the surrounding tissue environment, is forced to use a whole-cell energy-production process that requires a large amount of sugar. This process has been likened to fermentation. One of the consequences of making this change – or perhaps a necessary pre-condition - is that the mitochondria are switched off. The cancer cells now cannot die because the cell-death controlling mechanism has been switched off. The cells have become immortal. They keep dividing and dividing until they take over the system. Fortunately this process is reversible and the mitochondria can be switched on again. *hmmm.....I've heard this can happen. What do other books say?*

Basic Cancer Terms

Before proceeding with the discussion of cancer treatments it is best to describe some basic facts.

A tumour is a growth that contains both normal and abnormal cells. The abnormal cells divide faster than the normal cells. The rate of division varies. Some tumours grow very slowly while others are more aggressive. Tumours are not always cancerous. The classic division is between tumours that are benign and those that are malignant.

A benign tumour generally has limited growth potential and does not destroy normal cells while they are growing. It does not metastasize (another way of saying: "spread to other parts of the body") and remains localized in one site. It grows in an orderly fashion and does not produce serious side effects unless it is pressing against an organ like the brain in a limited space.

By contrast, **a malignant tumour** will keep on growing relentlessly and is capable of sending particles away from the main tumour which can then travel to distant parts of the body to develop other tumours. This process is called **metastasis**. Frighteningly, this can happen up to many years later.

Tumours Are Classified According to the Type of Tissue Involved:

Carcinomas: The most common form of cancer. This arises in the tissue that divides most often: the surface cells of organs or the cells that form the linings of the body and its organs (e.g., skin, lung, intestinal, uterine and breast cancers).

Sarcomas: These arise in the muscle and connective tissue, such as bone and muscle.

Myelomas: These attack the blood plasma cells in the bone marrow.

Lymphomas: Lymph is a water-like fluid that bathes and cleanses all the cells of the body. Lymph originates in small bean-sized nodes and glands. Lymphomas arise in the lymph organs.

Leukaemia: Cancer of the bloodforming tissue and blood cells, characterized by the over-production of white blood cells.

Cancers are also classified according to the stage of their development

> **Stage 1**: small tumour with no signs of spread
> **Stage 2**: some local spreading has occurred
> **Stage 3**: more widespread local metastasis is detected
> **Stage 4**: the cancer has spread to different sites

It is also very important that patients understand the words that doctors use to describe the success of treatment and to understand what they mean by these words. Here are the key words and their real meaning.

Response rate: This indicates the portion of patients for whom the cancer shrank more than 50 percent after treatment. But tumours that have shrunk can quickly return. This measure usually has relatively little meaning for patients. Response rate does not always correlate with survival.

1-3-5-10 year survival rate: This means what it says. Short- and medium-term survival rates are highly suspect, as they are skewed by improvements in diagnosis. If cancers are found earlier, the survival rates will apparently go up without any actual improvement in treatment.

Disease-free survival: How long the patient survives without any signs of the tumour. Length of life may not be increased in any way even with increased disease free survival. The tumour, when it returns, may grow with aggressive speed.

Regression/Partial Remission: The tumour has grown smaller. Again this is meaningless, though it may give rise to some short-term hope. Chemotherapy, for example, often makes tumours grow smaller—but when they grow back they do so faster than they previously did. The end result is usually little or no improvement in life expectancy despite the often horrendous pain of the treatment.

Complete remission: Complete disappearance of cancer tumours for a significant period.

Cure: If a doctor uses this word, ask what is meant by it. It often means five-year survival.

What Are the Symptoms of Cancer?

The development of most tumours usually goes unnoticed. They are painless and do not have an obvious negative impact on health. Generally speaking, only tumours that are located on the surface of the body are likely to be detected by chance or by means of precautionary examination. Deeply located tumours such as tumours of the brain, stomach, intestines, kidneys or lungs are hardly ever discovered early. So, unfortunately, it is rare for any symptoms to become evident before a cancer has reached a fairly advanced stage. The American Cancer Society issues the following warning signs:

* Unusual bleeding or discharge from any orifice.
* A solid lump
* A sore that doesn't heal.
* Changes in bowel or bladder habits
* Persistent hoarseness or coughing
* Indigestion or difficulty in swallowing
* Any change in a wart or mole
* Sudden unexplained weight loss.

Cancer Doesn't Necessarily Kill

It is not inevitable that a cancer left untreated will proceed to a terminal stage — some cancers grow very slowly (e.g., most prostate cancers), and some simply disappear of their own accord or remain in a stable state. This is sometimes associated with some deep seated change in the emotional life of the patient, but may be associated with what doctors would call placebo cures, or dietary changes that are assumed to have no therapeutic effect. Or it may simply be because that is their natural progression.

Other patients appear to be able to live in a static, symbiotic relationship with their cancer — the tumour growing neither bigger nor smaller. One woman with breast lumps described how they tended to harden when she was stressed and so acted as a warning signal. They would then soften when she was more at ease with herself.

Then there is the fact that some cancers are known not to be fatal. Professor Michael Baum of King's College Hospital, London estimates that 30 percent of all breast cancers are self-limiting - and therefore need no treatment at all.

Cancer and Pain

Cancer is generally painless - but if you feel pain, don't accept your doctor's opinion that it can't be cancer. If a tumour presses against a nerve or other healthy tissue it may indeed cause pain, and cancer does cause pain when it reaches a terminal stage. This pain is extreme and it is managed - if that is the word - often with morphine. This is when the tumour takes over the body's energy generating system for the purpose of its own energy requirements that the patient feels pain. This is the pain of the body's own tissues dying.

There are other ways of managing pain apart from morphine, and anyone suffering chronic pain should investigate the books generally available on the subject.

One of the most effective pain relievers is the enzyme serrapeptase. Not only is it pain relieving but it may help fight the cancer tumour by helping to digest the fibrin coating that cancer tumours produce to protect themselves against the body's immune system. There are a number of products available — high-dose, enteric-coated capsules or tablets are best. Inholtra, a natural pain relief product designed for arthritis sufferers, has also been advised by David Walker, a bio-physicist who cured himself of cancer.

According to Dr. Earl Mindell, author of *The Vitamin Bible*, DL-Phenylalanine is as effective if not more effective, in relieving pain than morphine and other opiates, and does not have the dangerous side effects that more potent analgesics have. It also has the ability to potentiate opiates so that if you are taking morphine you can boost its effectiveness by also taking DL-Phenylalanine. Cough suppressants containing dextromethorphan (DMX) also have this boosting effect. Of course, you must check all medication combinations with your doctor.

Some herbs that have pain killing qualities are white willow bark and cayenne. Some herbal cures are also associated with pain relief: Essiac and pau d'arco, among others. Cabbage leaves also appear to have powerful pain-relieving qualities. I was told of one cancer patient in extreme pain who could find relief only by lying naked on a bed of cabbage leaves. Hydrazine sulphate (see p. 246) also rapidly brings about relief from pain. The reason it does so is that it stops cachexia. MGN-3 and pycnogenol have also had the same pain-relieving effects, according to anecdotal reports.

Some people are also making claims for a static-electricity approach to pain relief. The theory is that static electricity helps to normalise the body's own intercellular electrical currents. Get a pair of gloves such as a painter would wear and a one-foot section of PVC pipe. Rub the pipe vigorously with the gloved hand and then—when it is charged—sweep the pipe over the painful area. Pass the pipe down from the head to the tow about half an inch from the skin and keep repeating for three or four minutes—keep recharging the pipe every three passes. It is claimed that pain relief can be speedy and dramatic.

There are a number of energy machines that claim to be very effective in relieving pain. One is the Quantronic Resonance System which is a pulsed magnetic field therapy developed in Germany. Another is the Skenar, or S-K-E-N-A-R, developed by Russian scientists for use by cosmonauts in space. It has been described as a Star Trek-like device as it receives and sends back energy waves. Both these devices are available on the internet and health claims are made for both machines beyond simply providing pain relief.

Linus Pauling discovered that megadoses of vitamin C given to terminal cancer patients not only increased longevity but also enhanced personal well-being. The lengthy pain-filled weeks of the normal terminal cancer patient were almost totally eliminated. Instead, patients on high vitamin C regimes tended to have a very sudden, speedy and virtually painless end after an extended period of well-being. This occurred using only 10 grams a day of sodium ascorbate. What might have happened if they had taken 20 or 30 grams a day?

Hydrazine sulphate, cesium chloride, laetrile, Willard water, colloidal gold and organic germanium are also considered to be effective relievers of the pain of terminal cancer. One person has reported adding MSM to the Budwig Protocol and finding that this substantially reduced pain levels.

For a pain relieving bath, one recipe is to run a hot bath (as hot as is bearable) and add 3 cups of Epsom salts, 16 oz. of hydrogen peroxide (6 percent solution) and the contents of a small container of baking soda. Enjoy.

What Causes Cancer?

This is the question everyone wants an answer to and which the experts duck to avoid. The truth is that there is no one generally accepted answer. However, there is an answer that is widely accepted among those who favour the alternative approaches. In their view, a primary cause of cancer – and indeed the cause of all diseases – is a low-oxygen environment within the body's tissues. Many things can cause this low oxygen environment, such as toxic chemicals. This low-oxygen environment forces cells to get their energy through a fermentation process which creates an environment suited to cancer. Otto Warburg, a Nobel-prize winning scientist, explains the situation with extreme clarity: "Cancer, above all other diseases, has countless secondary causes, but there is only one prime cause...The prime cause of cancer is the replacement of the normal oxygen respiration of body cells by an anaerobic cell respiration."

Having said this, some people fear that a search for single causes obscures the reality of cancer and at the same time leads to too much focus on research to discover single intervention 'cures'. Instead, they suggest, we should talk about contributing factors.

The Major Contributory Factors.

Smoking: We all know that smoking causes lung cancer. Smokers die of lung cancer in much larger numbers than non-smokers.

Dietary Fats and Sugars: Not all fats or sugars are unhealthy. The baddies are the hydrogenated fats and refined sugars. Although a high intake of fats is implicated in a number of cancers - very-low-fat diets are also implicated in some forms of cancer. A medium fat intake is best. Omega 3 oils are very important for fighting cancers while Omega 6 oils tend to promote cancer. Flaxseed oil is a very good oil.

Sugar is very directly correlated with tumour growth as it supplies the fuel tumours need for their anaerobic metabolism—as well as stimulating the release of cancer-promoting hormones. While simple sugars should be avoided, fruits, vegetables, grains, and legumes, which are complex carbohydrates, are important cancer fighters and are very definitely OK. Also OK is the natural sweetener, Stevia. (Organic stevia green leaf powder is available from www.healthherbs.com). Aspartame, on the other hand, is definitely not OK. It has, among other things, been fingered as a trigger for brain cancers, the incidence of which is rising. In general, foods that are low on the glycaemic index are preferred and are healthier than those that are high on the index.

There are also good sugars—known as glyconutrients—which play an important role in fighting cancer. *Other book by Blaylock says eliminate fruit or limit to ½ c. of certain types while fighting cancer.*

Dietary Fibre: Low fibre diets are strongly correlated with high incidences of cancer of the colon and rectum.

Obesity: Body size, large waist measurements and high body mass index (BMI) are associated with an up to 500 percent increase in the risk of developing myeloid leukemia, a malignant disease of the white blood cells, from which more than 9,000 people die each year in the U.S. alone.

It has been suggested that obesity may significantly impair immune function and that the chronic hyperinsulinemia (the persistent elevatation of insulin levels in the blood) that commonly accompanies obesity may be associated with increased levels of insulin-like growth factor (IGF-1). IGF-1, which is also present in dairy products, has been shown to increase the rate of cell division and has been linked to the development of a number of cancers.

Nitrites in Processed Foods: Pickled, smoked and cured foods are associated with stomach cancer. They contain large amounts of nitrites which can be easily converted to a class of highly potent carcinogenic chemicals called nitrosamines. Vitamin C is known to interfere with the formation of these compounds.

Burnt and Chargrilled Foods: Foods that are burnt, especially barbecued foods, have been found to be carcinogenic.

Stress and Reduced Immunity: Stress is a well-known precursor of illness, particularly cancer. Stress is known to result in a lowered immune response. If the lowered immunity is allowed to remain for any length of time then the chances of serious illness occurring rise sharply.

However, the connection between cancer incidence and lowered immune systems is not absolutely proven. For example, people with AIDS, whose immune systems have completely collapsed do not have a higher incidence of most cancers. They do have a higher incidence of Karposi's sarcoma, an otherwise rare cancer, lymphomas and cancers of the anal-genital area which are known to have a viral cause.

Stress is, however, believed to release corticosteroids which have the effect of making any existing cancer more aggressive and invasive. This may mean that simply receiving a diagnosis of cancer will make a cancer worse. The herb Gingko biloba has demonstrated an ability to interfere with this process. Conversely, relaxation and release from stress, especially emotional conflicts (anger, the desire for revenge, etc.), have been notable parts of many healing stories. Many have stressed that their healing seemed to start with a fit of crying despair or from a sincere act of forgiveness.

Anxiety attacks can be eliminated or reduced with the help of the amino acid L-Theanine. Other useful natural interventions include: lavender essential oil, evening primrose oil, valerian herb, St. John's wort, Bach's Rescue Remedy. If anxiety attacks are acute and continuing, it may be useful to have thyroid functioning checked.

Fungal Infections: There is increasing and very much belated recognition that fungal infections may be a major cause of cancer. A number of doctors have noted that in the case of leukemia, the co-presence of a severe fungal infection is extremely common. Intriguingly, treatment with an anti-fungal drug has also been associated with a number of remissions from cancer. Patrick Quillin, in his book *Beating Cancer with Nutrition* quotes the story of a well-known oil magnate, 'Doc' Pennington, who was diagnosed with advanced colon cancer in 1972. He got his doctor to prescribe Griseofulvin, an antifungal drug, and three months later his cancer had disappeared. He went on to live another 22 years, dying at age 92 in 1994. He founded the Pennington Biomedical Centre to study the link between yeast, nutrition and cancer. Research that he funded has shown the Griseofulvin causes cell death in cancer cells in test tubes.

An Italian doctor, Dr. Tullio Simoncini, bases his radical approach on this assumption that cancer is caused by fungus (specifically *Candida albicans*) and treats his patients, with seeming success, with 5 percent solution of sodium bicarbonate injected close to the site of the tumour. For more detailed discussion of his treatment go to www.curenaturalicancro.com.

In 1999, Meinolf Karthaus, M.D., reported that he had seen three children with leukemia suddenly go into remission upon receiving a triple antifungal drug cocktail for their "secondary" fungal infections. This was echoed by the experience of another doctor, Dr. Doug A. Kaufman. "[A] young lady phoned into my syndicated radio talk show. Her three-year-old daughter was diagnosed last year with leukemia. She believes antifungal drugs and natural immune system therapy has been responsible for saving her daughter's life. She is now telling others with cancer about her daughter's case. After hearing her story, a friend of hers with bone cancer asked her doctor for a prescriptive antifungal drug. To her delight, this medication, meant to eradicate fungus, was also eradicating her cancer…When she could no longer get the antifungal medication, the cancer immediately grew back" (reported by Dr. Mark Sircus in an email 2007) hmm m - - - - - -

Viruses and microbes: As many as a third of cancers are believed to be caused by viruses of one sort or another. One minority view is that all cancers are caused by microbes which can change shape so that sometimes they appear to be viruses and at other times appear to be bacteria.

Campylobacter pylori, recently discovered to be the cause of stomach ulcers, has also been implicated as a cause of colon cancer. Cervical cancers are now known to be caused by Human Papilloma virus. More recently, researchers at Tulane Medical School have identified a virus that is present in 90 percent of breast cancer cases, known as human mammary tumour virus (HMTV). This appears to be present in the blood of 15 percent of otherwise healthy women and men. wow .

Chronic viral and bacterial infections and Chronic Inflammation (especially of the gums): The body's normal response to inflammation is to flood the area with stem calls and various growth factors to aid healing. Where the inflammation, for whatever reason, persists (perhaps because an irritant persists or because of low immune function) then these growth factors can transform the stem cells into malignant cells.

Bacterial and viral infections that cause inflammation that is not speedily resolved can result in cancer. The teeth, for example, have long been seen as a potential source of such problems and some doctors in the past have recommended removal of infected teeth—or teeth with root canals - for this reason. The other side of the coin is that anti-inflammatory drugs and herbs will tend to be useful in the fight against cancer. Note, however, that pregnancy and cancer are closely related in metabolic terms and anything that is effective against cancer is likely to lead to a miscarriage of a foetus.

Free radicals: Free radicals are highly reactive molecular fragments that are hungry for oxygen. If left uncontrolled they would quickly destroy every living creature as they scavenge for oxygen in the cell walls - so damaging the cells. They cause mutations to the cell's DNA and this can result in cancer. Very little, if anything, is mentioned about them in orthodox medical cancer books. One reason for this is that the main orthodox anti-cancer weapons create free radicals and the best known means of controlling or minimizing their effects are through the use of antioxidant vitamins (vitamins A, C and E). Since the use of vitamins has been very generally vilified by propo-nents of orthodox medicine, the whole area of free radicals was for many years an intellectual 'no go' area in some scientific circles.

It should be noted that there are situations in which free radicals are beneficial—such as when the body is fighting acute bacterial infections.

Trauma: Another cause of cancer appears to be physical or emotional trauma. This is why some people disapprove of mammograms, which require the breasts to be squeezed and therefore traumatized. Some studies have indicated that breast cancer is more common among women who have annual mammograms than among women who don't.

Toxic chemicals: There are now around 30,000 chemicals in everyday use. The safety of these chemicals on their own has been established only in a rough and ready way. However, what happens when any of these chemicals combines with one or more of the other chemicals? It is impossible to test all the possible combinations. We are living guinea pigs in an enormous experiment.

Rough and ready estimates for safe levels of these compounds assume a simple linear reality in which higher doses always lead to worse results. But the truth is infinitely more complex. Sometimes an organism may be unaffected by relatively high doses but seriously disrupted by low level doses. Also, organisms are not static. At various stages in their life cycle they may be extremely vulnerable to extremely slight biochemical aspects of their environment. It is believed that hormone disruption during the foetal stage is the main cause of testicular cancer and falling sperm counts.

And of course many chemicals do not break down easily. Every one of us is carrying chemical residues in our fat layers. Various studies have found that the average person is carrying residues of 40 or more potentially toxic chemicals – and that even animals in remote habitats (polar bears and arctic seals) are polluted chemically in the same way. What effects are all these chemicals having? Who knows?

It is well known that sudden exposure to large doses of any pollutant for a limited period of time is unlikely to lead to cancer. But even low doses of a pollutant over a long period of time may result in cancerous growths as the tissue attempts to adapt to the change in its environment. New carpets that have been treated with a variety of chemicals have been implicated as a cancer cause. There are studies that show long-term exposure to vehicle exhaust is a definite risk factor. Benzene and vinyl chloride are known to be dangerous to chemical workers. These occupational carcinogens are now found in drinking water!

Almost every pesticide used today is recognised by one or more regulatory agencies in Europe or America as being disruptive to our endocrine system—which controls and regulates every gland and every hormone in the body.

Plastic containers release dioxins, a family of chemicals that are known to be carcinogenic, into the fats of the food it contains—especially when microwaved. This also applies to the plastic wrap used to cover foods that are being microwaved. Also, dioxins are released into water when plastic bottles are put in the freezer.

Some pharmaceutical drugs have been associated with cancer– if you are taking any drug, check the small print of cautions.

EMFs: Electromagnetic fields have also been implicated as a major cause of cancer–; the evidence is mounting. One study conducted by the University of North Carolina School of Public Health found that children of mothers who slept under electric blankets developed 250 percent more brain tumours, 70 percent more leukaemia and 30 percent more cancers than those who didn't.

One of the earliest reports on the dangers of EMFs appeared in the *Journal of Occupational Medicine* in 1985. This article reported that deaths in Maryland from various cancers were up to 3 times higher among electricians, electrical engineers and linesmen than any other occupation. Since World War II, we have filled the air with electromagnetic waves. They beam down on our houses through telephone wires, television satellite dishes, AM and FM radio receivers. Add to this beepers, cell phones, CB radios and other radios. Add to this the overhead power lines and we see how dependent we are on EMF producing equipment. Dr. Robert Becker, a world expert in this field is in no doubt: "At this time the scientific evidence is absolutely conclusive: 60 cycle magnetic fields cause human cancer cells to permanently increase their rate of growth by as much as 1600 percent and to develop more malignant characteristics."

It's not just cancer. EM fields have now been linked with suicides, nervous system disorders, sexual dysfunction, reproductive hazards, abnormal foetal development and heart disease. Mobile phones are also being investigated as possible causes of brain, and more recently of mouth, cancers.

The new vogue for digital phones has also increased the threat of harmful frequencies in the home – the base units in particular are at fault. These frequencies can be detected with electro-smog detectors. For further details, see www.electrosmog.org.uk and www.lessemf.com.

Oestrogen (Estrogen): Excessive oestrogen in the body is a cancer causing factor–as are the intermediary metabolites of oestrogen created as oestrogen is broken down in order to be eliminated from the body. If there are problems relating to this process so that these metabolites cannot be further broken down then they can remain in the body and are potentially even more carcinogenic than the original oestrogen. This is particularly so if we have a high sodium and high glucose levels while at the same time we have low potassium and magnesium levels in the tissues. The combined effect is to cause havoc in normal cells - potentially making them malignant.

This is not just a concern for women. Unfortunately there are a lot of estrogen mimicking chemicals in our environment–the chief of which is Bisphenol A, a chemical used in plastics and food packaging. Bisphenol A has been shown to have biological effects at levels 200,000 times lower than the presumed safety level. The lubricants on condoms are also estrogen mimics.

One of the side effects of excessive estrogen is an increase in body weight. The large size of many Americans may reflect their estrogen levels as much as their food intake.

Overexposure to the sun's rays: It has recently become a mantra that the sun's rays are bad for us–certainly it is true that the relatively benign form of skin cancer is associated with over-exposure to the sun. But there is also strong evidence that sunlight is good for us – and that people who spend a large part of their lives outdoors under the hot sun have significantly lower incidences of most cancers.

Genes and Oncogenes: Some genes appear to provoke the onset of cancer. Such genes are referred to as oncogenes. In some cases these oncogenes are triggered by a genetic predisposition. The result is that there are families with high incidences of certain cancers. However, it has been estimated that this genetic cause accounts for less than 5 percent of cancers.

Alcohol: There appears to be, if taken in excessive quantities, and in association with other pollutants, a measurable tendency for alcohol to exacerbate a cancer risk in cases of cancers of the lips, tongue and other areas in the mouth and throat. Against this, it is now generally accepted that alcohol in smaller quantities has a beneficial effect on health. The divisive question is this: at what level of intake does alcohol cease to be beneficial? And alcohol's main benefits relate not to cancer but to heart disease. So it is possible that a slight cancer risk is outweighed by greater heart disease benefits.

Certainly, rural Greeks who like to drink a glass of red wine with their meals have one of the highest life expectancies in the world. But French men, who are not abstemious, have one of the world's highest cancer rates for men (fifth) - more than double that of French women who have a far lower incidence (35th).

Bras: Many women wear poorly fitting bras. In fact, some experts have suggested that as many as 85 percent of women are wearing the wrong size bra. This is not just a problem of fashion or even comfort. Bras cause breast cancer according to a Harvard University study (Hsieh, C.C. and D. Trichopoulos, *Eur. J. Cancer* 27:131-5, 1991). It's not the fabric of the bras, it seems, but the fact that they constrict lymphatic drainage and, at the same time, have a negative impact on melatonin secretion. Women who wore their bras 24 hours per day (!) had a 3 out of 4 chance of developing breast cancer; wearing a bra for more than 12 hours a day resulted in a 1 in 7 risk while wearing a bra for less than 12 hours a day brought the risk down to 1 in 152– very close to the risk factor for women who never wore bras (1 in 168). A number of other studies have supported this conclusion (see www.breathing.com/articles/brassieres.htm for details).

Others: Almost everyday it seems that some new cancer cause is announced. Some fear chemicals in shampoos, others talcum powder. The latter certainly does seem to worth avoiding, especially near female genital areas. It has been likened to asbestos. Similarly, fears have been expressed about underarm deodorants – especially in relation to breast cancer. Fingers have also been pointed vociferously at the mercury laden dental amalgams that dentists have used for fillings. Some people are so convinced of this threat that they have all their fillings replaced with non-toxic materials. However, the process of doing this replacement is likely to release large amounts of heavy metals into the bloodstream if special measures are not taken to prevent this from happening.

The problem each of us faces is what to do in the face of these suggested threats. Should we maintain a very high level of scrutiny on every product we buy or should we just shrug our shoulders and carry on regardless, taking the view that life cannot be lived entirely without risk?

Causes Don't Always Lead to Results

Some people argue that carcinogenic substances cannot adequately explain the cause of cancer because in most cases of exposure to a carcinogen, there are some, usually a minority, who will get cancer - the others won't. That suggests that the physical and mental health of the person exposed to the carcinogen is a key factor. There is no doubt that the terrain of the body has a key say in whether the seeds of cancer will be able to take root and thrive.

For us, the key question that arises from this is whether we are going to spend our lives examining the external world checking it obsessively for things to avoid – pesticides, chemicals in shampoos and so on – the so-called 'defensive shopping syndrome' – or whether it is enough to focus on our own physical, mental and spiritual health. This is the crux of a scientific schism that split 19th-century France and which has had repercussions ever since. Is disease caused primarily by the alien germs and environmental poisons that attack us or is it caused by the weakened soil of our bodies. Is it the toxin or is it the terrain? Where do we place the emphasis? If poor soil causes diseased plants, can we cure the plants by just treating the plant, or must we treat the ailments of the plant by focusing on the soil?

A sensible strategy, it seems to me, is to minimize as far as possible the chemical impacts on the body while at the same time not being too over-concerned about occasional lapses. At the same time, we need to make sure that the food we eat, the supplements we take and the daily habits we follow are adequate to maintain good health.

The latin motto *Mens sana in corpore sano* - A healthy mind in a healthy body - has got it right. This is the prescription for happiness and longevity.

Incidence of Cancer

Epidemiological studies show that cancer incidence varies greatly from country to country, being low in the third world and increasingly high in the west. Interestingly, those who argue that cancer is also a disease of the spirit and psyche need only point to the case of Hungary – the country with the world's highest cancer rate is also the country with the world's highest suicide rate. Does this mean health and depression are caused by Hungarian genes or by the Hungarian diet?

Cancer incidence also varies enormously from one area to another within a single country. And the closer we look the stranger the facts. In Cumbria, an area in the North of England, the incidence of malignant melanoma is fifty percent higher than average among the women of this area, while for men the incidence is thirty percent lower than average. How can we explain these variations?

"The difference is far too big to be explained by genes. We have to look at diet, at excess calories. It may be that diet is linked in a very complicated way" (Dr. Gordon McVie, scientific director of the Cancer Research Campaign – quoted in The Independent [25 March 1994]).

This kind of epidemiological research reveals that 70-90 percent of cancers relate to lifestyle and environmental factors, and only 5-10 percent is gene-related. Such research is clearly valuable because prevention is better than cure.

Some Problems with Cancer Statistics

If you want to look on the bright side of things it is possible to conjure up figures that show that there has been significant progress in the battle against cancer. The National Cancer Institute publishes a chart of five-year relative survival rates. These figures show clear improvement. But statistics are meaningful only when they are accurate. One source if inaccuracy is exposed by the following personal testimony: "[M]y husband recently died of pancreatic cancer and he was listed as death by heart attack because he was in the end stages of his cancer and his heart gave out. Statistics can be whatever the people keeping the results want them to be." (quoted in Ralph Moss's newsletter 1st February 2007)

Another problem is that five-year survival rates, while seeming to represent increased survival, may actually measure only improvements in diagnosis.

The incidence of cancer depends upon accurate diagnosis. Improved screening programmes tend to raise incidence figures because they lead to the detection of many 'early cancers' which are either not cancers, or they find cancers which would resolve themselves without treatment, or they find cancers earlier than they would otherwise.

Even with no improvement in treatment these will have a major impact on official survival figures as we can see from the following example: Take two identical twins, age 65, both of whom have prostate cancer. One, Man A, is diagnosed with prostate cancer and starts treatment. The other, Man B, also has prostate cancer but is not diagnosed until he is 70. Let us imagine that Man B's cancer, when it is eventually diagnosed, is now too advanced, and so no treatment is given. Now, let us assume that Man A's treatment has no effect at all and does not help to extend Man A's life – and neither does it have a negative impact that shortens his life. Let us further assume that both men die of their prostate cancer at the age of 72.

For the statistician, Man A was diagnosed early, received treatment and lived seven years. Man B, on the other hand, was diagnosed late and lived only two years. Early diagnosis followed by treatment appears to have allowed Man A to have lived three and a half times longer than Man B. So, the statistics appear to demonstrate huge benefits for early diagnosis – but in fact these huge benefits are in this case entirely illusory.

It may be that the apparent slight improvement in prognosis for women with breast cancer is not a result of improved chemotherapy but may be a result of improvements in diagnosis and the consequent impact on survival statistics. Or, of course, it may be due to the fact that women are much more aware of the range of alternatives and are taking more vitamins, etc. Who knows?

Another Problem with Statistics.

Statistics give us figures for a population or a group – but they cannot tell us anything useful about any specific individual. If we discover that we have a cancer for which there is a 50 percent chance that we will die within five years, some people will become very depressed, while others will interpret this to mean that there is a 50 percent chance that they will live longer than 5 years. Both are correct but the second patient has the better prognosis. Imagine a group where half the people died before 6 months and the other half lived ten years. The doctors would say you have only a 50 percent chance of living for 6 months! A much gloomier picture than we would get from saying, equally correctly, you have a 50 percent chance of living 10 years.

Even if the 5-year survival rate is only 10 percent, the positive patient will see that ten percent of the population survives somehow. Statistics demonstrate this clearly. How do these people do it? Sadly, very little research is done on survival.

It is also important to know what is meant when you read that the average life expectancy for a particular form of treatment is 5 years, say. Most people think that this means you add up all the life spans of a particular group and divide by the number in the group. But that is unlikely to be the case. The Harvard biologist, Stephen Jay Gould wrote an essay on the subject that is a must-read. You can find it at Steve Dunn's excellent Cancer Guides website at www.cancerguide.org

The key point he makes is that, put very simply, scientists are most likely to measure the 'average' life expectancy as that point at which half the sample have died. This figure says nothing of value about the life expectancy of those who live longer.

Yet Another Problem With Statistics

Every so often the newspapers erupt with news of a new wonder drug. The result is cancer patients become desperate to get their hands on this new drug that according to the newspapers will give them a 30 percent or 50 percent or 70 percent better chance of being cured. Sadly, these people are victims of innumerate newspaper reporters who are doing little more than rewriting press releases issued by the pharmaceutical companies. It's not that the drug companies are lying. They are telling a sort of truth – but it is a highly inaccurate truth as you will see.

Let us imagine that out of a group of 100 women with stage 4 cancer, ninety eight are expected to die of their disease within 5 years. These women are given a drug (drug X) and after five years it is found that only ninety-six died. In this case two were expected to live but four actually did live. This is a 100 percent improvement. We can say there is a relative benefit of 100 percent. The newspapers will carry headlines saying that drug X doubles your chances of living for five years; they may even say it doubles their chances of being cured.

But we can see that in fact only two of the group actually benefited. There is, in this case, an absolute benefit of only 2 percent. This is not a figure that will sell many newspapers. We must be very aware of the difference between these two terms 'relative benefit' and 'absolute benefit'. Add these terms to your vocabulary and you are less likely to be taken in by drug company propaganda.

Cures for Cancer?

The word 'cure' carries with it such a lot of implicit baggage that it is worth looking at more closely. First of all, to talk of cures implies a situation where there is a clear-cut opposition between a state of health and a state of illness. You either have cancer or you don't have it - as though cancer is a thing in itself separate from the body in which the cancer is present and that it is there or, preferably, not there. If it was there before and now no longer is there then you say there has been a cure.

But how real is this image? Are there not intermediate stages between having and not having cancer? And similarly, if you get rid of a cancer tumour but make no change to the bodily environment that produced the cancer tumour, how long is the state of not having a tumour going to last? What causes a cancer to appear in the first place? What is being done to correct this situation?

If these two questions are not addressed, as they usually aren't in orthodox clinical settings, then to talk of cures, even in the absence of a tumour for an extended period of time is probably inappropriate.

Some cancers are fast growing others are slow growing. Some stop of their own accord. Others stop after some form of treatment and others still resist all forms of treatment.

The hard reality is that between 1930 and 1990, in the USA, for men, only two cancers have actually declined in incidence: stomach cancer has dropped from 38 to 7 per 100,000 men and liver cancer has dropped by 50-65 percent and now kills only about 5 per 100,000 men per annum. For women there have been significant improvements in cancer of the uterus, stomach, liver and some improvement in colorectal cancer.

The problem for orthodox medicine is that none of these improvements are recent, and for many cancers there has been either no change at all or a slow but steady increase in death rates. Prostate deaths have nearly doubled - as have deaths from cancer of the pancreas and leukaemia. And lung cancer deaths have just gone through the roof. One possible exception is with breast cancer. There does appear to have been a recent improvement in death rate figures. The problem is that there has not been any change in treatment to account for this improvement. Could it be that more and more women are following alternative treatments that are having an impact?

But there is another way to look at the subject. Cancers are never "cured" - even when they appear to have gone. The potential for cancer is always there lurking in the microscopic depths of the body. Hazel Thornton, who was diagnosed in 1991 with breast cancer, wrote this to me: "Whilst I believe that attitude is crucially important in coming to terms with a life threatening disease so that one may live one's life fruitfully and in tranquility, I cannot accept that one can say, at any given moment, that one has 'beaten' the illness...I hope that I am in a state of truce with my body's inefficiencies, rather than waging war with it." (Personal communication, Dec. 1995).

Making Decisions

This book was written to help you make your decision as to what you should do if you get cancer. I have surveyed the orthodox anticancer weapons with a critical eye and I have listed the alternative approaches – of which there are a great many. But the final act must be yours, and yours alone. You must look through the options provided and make the choices that seem most sensible to you. Your choices will be different from my choices. We are different and we must respect those differences.

This is one of the most difficult things to do when you and a loved one take divergent views as to what to do. I have been through this and know the damage it can do to couples. So let me repeat my advice: It is for the person with the cancer to make the final decisions about what therapies to follow and those who are in a supporting role should support these decisions as far as they can — putting the need to give loving support over all other considerations. That doesn't mean that you cannot revisit that decision and offer the patient opportunities to review the decision — but at all times you are best advised to be respectful and supportive of the patient's own wishes. I have written elsewhere about how difficult this is. But there is no other option. For those of you who are supporting someone who has decided to treat their cancer in a way that you personally do not approve of – or worse, which you actively disapprove of — you have my deepest sympathy. Nevertheless you need to put your caveats aside and support your loved one with the therapies they have selected.

This, then, has been a quick overview of the subject. It is now time to turn to the treatments. In the next section I will review the orthodox approach to cancer.

Section 2: The Orthodox Approach to Treating Cancer

CANCER TESTING

The first step in any approach to cancer - as with any disease - is diagnosis. Initial suspicions of cancer may arise from a regular health check up or, more likely, as the result of noticing some bodily changes.

There are a number of ways in which these suspicions can be confirmed or ruled out. However, there are also a number of dangers associated with testing and you should be aware of these dangers before proceeding.

First let's look at the kind of tests that are available.

Blood Tests

Most blood tests are non-specific - hat is, they can indicate the presence of a health problem but not clearly specify the exact cause. The blood test may show, for example, that you are anaemic but there are many possible reasons, including cancer, for why you might be anaemic.

There are also a number of specific blood tests that look for chemical markers produced by specific cancers. For example, breast, lung and bowel tumours produce a protein called carcino-embryonic antigen (CEA). If a very high CEA level is found, then a tumour is assumed to be present until proved otherwise. Cancers of the prostate, testicles and ovaries also produce known chemical markers that can be tested for.

Markers	Cancer
CEA	Colon, Rectum, Lung, Breast, Pancreas
CA-125	Ovaries, Uterus
CA 15-3	Breast
C 19-9	Colon, Pancreas, Stomach, Liver
PSA	Prostate
PAP	Prostate

Blood tests can also directly indicate blood related cancers. The presence of blood itself, in the stool, for example, may itself be an indicator of cancer. Sometimes, blood in the stool is not obvious and thus has to be tested for. This test is known as the "faecal occult blood test' ("Occult" in medical matters—and particularly in relation to cancer - means "hidden," not clearly visible).

Imaging Techniques

Doctors have access to a number of imaging techniques that help them to see into the body: X-rays, CT scans, MRI scans, ultrasound, PET scans and so on. While these may be helpful in determining the presence and location of cancer tumours, none is 100 percent effective. Most of these imaging techniques provide ill-defined results – as one doctor describes it: they show that "something is taking up space." The PET scan is significantly more likely to pick up metastases than other types of scan, but still picks up on average less than 90 percent of metastatic lymph nodes. Even so, neither the PET scan nor any of the others can distinguish between cancer and benign lumps. Also, with a number of these scans, a problem for the patient is the extent of exposure to radiation. One new technology, Electron Beam Tomography, uses very low doses of radiation.

Endoscopy

In addition, there are a number of ways of achieving direct visual access to parts of the body with specially constructed telescopes. The general name for these kinds of tests is endoscopy - which is Latin for "looking at the insides." Specific terms relate to the part of the body they are looking at: colonoscopy takes a look at the colon, bronchoscopy looks at the lungs, and so on. In all cases, this involves feeding a fibre optic tube with a camera at the end into the body, usually through the nearest major orifice.

Cytology (biopsies)

Finally, there are the cytological tests which study the cells that have been removed from the body. Usually the cells are obtained by physically cutting them out of the body. With **excisional biopsies** the tumour is removed in its entirety. This is best. Alternatively, an **incisional biopsy** may be performed. This involves the cutting out of part of the tumour or, in the case of **needle biopsies**, the removal of cells from the interior of a tumour using a needle. Lymph nodes surrounding a tumour may also be removed at this stage for analysis to see whether there has been any spread.

Problems with Tests
False Results

The first problem associated with any test is that of reliability. The perfect test would be one where a positive result would always mean 'yes' and a negative result would always mean 'no'. Unfortunately, by this standard, almost all tests are unreliable.

The first risk of any test is the so-called 'false positive' result. That is, the test indicates the presence of cancer when there is no cancer in fact. The problem for people with false positives is that they may undergo cancer treatment: surgery, radiation and chemotherapy unnecessarily. They may suffer permanently from this treatment, and they may even die from it.

The opposite problem is the 'false negative,' where the patient gets a negative result when in fact cancer does exist.

These are not rare problems. Almost every test has a failure rate, and sometimes this can be as high as 20-30 percent. It is always therefore worth asking what the reliability rate of any test is – and it is worth getting re-tested if you have any concerns. For example, if you have worrying symptoms but the test comes back negative, it is probably worth repeating the test.

Safety

Another problem relates to the safety of the test. For example, some tests require the inspection or removal of tissue in an operating theatre - all such tests have what professionals refer to as a morbidity factor - a possibility of causing permanent injury. Incisional biopsies particularly should be avoided where possible for two reasons. One is the high risk of releasing cancer cells into the bloodstream. The second reason is that the tumour can be provoked into becoming aggressive when it may previously been slow growing. Dr. Vincent Gammill has reported: "I have seen lesions that have been quiescent for years become aggressively malignant and apparently metastatic after a biopsy." However, he dismisses the suggestion that exposure to oxygen can cause a cancer to become more malignant.

But excisional biopsies, and indeed surgical removal of a tumour, may also raise other safety issues. There is the curious fact that a primary tumour is known to be able to inhibit the growth of distant, microscopic metastases by releasing two substances, angiostatin and endostatin, into the blood stream. These prevent the growth of the blood supply (known as angiogenesis) that the metastases need to develop into full-blown tumours. Once the primary tumour has been removed, so too has this constraint on growth. The result of surgical removal of one tumour therefore has a catastrophic impact on the body by stimulating the unrestrained growth of these metastases. The surgery itself requires that the body initiate healing activities that also have the unfortunate side effect of helping to stimulate the growth of cancer tumours. This caution against surgical removal of a tumour applies particularly to cases of node positive breast cancer in premenopausal women, where the oestrogen-rich environment also promotes the dissemination of cancerous cells.

Long-Term Impact

The removal of lymph nodes may make you susceptible to oedema. This is the very painful swelling of a limb as a result of lymph being unable to drain away. It is a problem that cannot be completely corrected, only ameliorated with the aid of pressure bandages or by manual lymphatic drainage procedures. One school of lymphatic drainage, the Dr. Vodder School of North America, is specifically recommended. There is a worldwide list of qualified practitioners at their main site, www.vodderschool.com . There are also a number of lymph drainage remedies that are claimed to be effective. A homoeopath can advise if this is a problem – or do a web search for 'lymph drainage remedies'. See also www.jovipak.com for various lymphodema products.

Finally, anyone experiencing problems with lymphatic drainage or, more seriously, lymphoedema, should investigate the use of a light beam generator (for more details go to www.lightbeamgenerator.com) or a microcurrent electrical device (for more information go towww.trivedigroup.com/btcpl/dat-products.html).

Usefulness of the Test

Again, a test should be done only if it is likely to lead to a treatment. There is no point in discovering that something exists for which there is no known treatment. This is well illustrated by the following personal story. I know a man whose chest X-ray indicated that there was a possibility something was seriously wrong with his lungs. "These shadows could be old tubercular scars, in which case there's no problem, or it could mean lung cancer," the doctor told him. "If it's cancer, it has spread throughout your lungs and I can only give you a few weeks or months to live. The only way I'll know for sure is by going in and having a look." Amazingly, my friend opted for a visual inspection and the result was painful and expensive surgery that showed there was no problem. I had to laugh when I heard this. "Why didn't you just wait to see if you were still alive in six months' time?" I asked.

This was a stark case and my initial reaction was perhaps unhelpful. Faced with the same situation now, I would perhaps recommend that a second opinion might be useful – and not just a second opinion by another surgeon. It might in this circumstance be more valuable to find a doctor who was not dismissive of alternative approaches, who would know about other tests that might cast light on the situation. An advanced cancer stamps its signature on the body in many ways. We don't necessarily have to open up the rib cage for a visual inspection of the lungs to determine whether advanced lung cancer exists.

The Reporting of Tests

Finally, another problem with tests - one that is rarely mentioned - is the reporting of the results. Often this is done by a nurse to the patient over the phone. "The results are negative," my wife was told. She died, in part, because she accepted this information over the phone. If she had seen the test report she would have seen that there was a comment that indicated something was not 100 percent right. She would have had a retest. So do ask for a copy of the test results 'for your files'. A good doctor will welcome this as a sign that you are willing to take responsibility for your own health and well-being. A doctor who refuses needs to be removed from your environment.

A Closer Look at Some Specific Tests

The Pap Smear

This is the most common test for cervical cell analysis. Cells have to be removed through a surgical procedure that involves scraping and brushing the inside of the cervix to obtain cells for analysis. The removed cells are put on slides, stained with dyes and examined with a microscope. The cytologist will look for the characteristic appearance of malignant or pre-malignant cells. A pathologist should also examine the slides and either diagnose cancer or report a strong suspicion of cancer. According to conservative doctors, all women who are 18 or older or sexually active should have a Pap smear test every year or every 3 years after three normal yearly exams. Other doctors disagree vehemently with this suggestion, saying for instance that it is not "based on any acceptable clinical trial of the risks versus benefits of Pap smear" (Eugene D. Robin, 1984). The Pap smear is one of the most widely used of all cancer tests, and in Dr. Robin's view the dependency on the test is dangerous. The reason? It has a very high rate of false results.

How are these false results possible? Highly qualified specialists study the slides and the cancerous cells have a 'characteristic shape', so how is it possible for mistakes to happen?

First of all, Pap smears require interpretation. Different doctors examining the same specimen under the microscope will vary widely in their opinions. In one study, quoted by Dr. Robin, ten experts disagreed about the presence or absence of cancer cells in about 40 percent of the specimens.

One reason for the confusion is a non-cancerous state called dysplasia, which occurs in the cells of the cervix and may be difficult or impossible to distinguish from CIS - carcinoma in situ - a form of cancer or precancer where the cells remain localized; CIS does not necessarily become invasive cervical cancer (ICC). Abnormal cells can also appear in the Pap smear as a result of fungal infections, changes in the metabolic state of the subject, or for other reasons. As Dr. Robin remarks, "The possibility of finding in the Pap smear abnormal non-cancerous cells that can be mistaken for cancer is substantial." In the case of the Pap smear, the number of false positives and false negatives amount to over 30 percent of all test results.

A more recent test, known as liquid-based cytology (LBC), has demonstrated no meaningful improvement in reliability, according a report in *The Lancet*, January 2006.

The Mammogram

The mammogram test, in which breasts are X-rayed, has also been severely criticized for squeezing and bruising breast tissue - and in that way actually promotes the problem that it is supposed to be testing for. Physical trauma is considered to be one possible cause of cancer, and if there is cancer present it may also act to make the tumour more aggressive. Cancer incidence has been shown in some surveys to be higher among women who have annual check ups than among those who have never had a mammogram. The only group of women for whom regular mammograms have been shown to have any value is in the over 65, and then the degree of benefit is considered to be marginal.

Professor Michael Baum, a leading British cancer researcher, is horrified at the extent to which mammograms are promoted, without any evidence that they are beneficial, and despite a great deal of evidence that they pick up a great many non-invasive tumours which are then dealt with unnecessarily by radical surgery (reference: *Journal of the National Cancer Institute*, Vol. 96, No. 20, 1490-1491, October 20, 2004)

Cornelia J. Baines, M.D., deputy director of the Canadian National Breast Screening Study, writes: "an unacknowledged harm [of mammography] is that for up to 11 years after the initiation of breast cancer screening in women aged 40-49 years, screened women face a higher death rate from breast cancer than unscreened control women, although that is contrary to what one would expect... "Shouldn't women aged 40-49 years know that, three years after screening starts, their chance of death from breast cancer is more than double that for unscreened control women? Shouldn't they be informed that it will take 16 years after they start screening to reduce their chance of death from breast cancer by a mere 9 percent?"

For a fuller account of what should perhaps be referred to as 'the mammography scandal' go to www.rense.com/general64/mam.htm

Alternative Tests

There are a number of tests that are non-standard for a variety of reasons. I discuss these in greater detail on p. 103.

Tests for Prostate Cancer

The presence of prostate cancer is determined in the first place by a test known as the PSA (prostate-specific antigen) test. However, some men have been diagnosed with prostate cancer and yet have a normal low PSA reading, while others who have a high PSA reading have been found not to have the disease.

The simple fact is that most men, as they grow older, get prostate cancer. That's the bad news. The good news is that this form of cancer is usually very slow growing and not aggressively metastatic. You can live a long time with a cancer of this type and not even know it. So, the question is: who cares? There is no point in testing for something that is almost certainly present. Unfortunately, a very small number of cases of prostate cancer are aggressively metastatic.

The PSA is not the only way of testing for prostate cancer. Other tests include ultrasound and 'manual palpation' – this involves feeling the prostate to see if it is enlarged, asymmetrical, or nodular.

Summary

If you are asked to undergo any form of testing make sure you understand:

a)   The risks that the test may involve

b)   The reliability of the results

c)   The likely treatment you may require if the test shows you have cancer. If you do not wish to have the proposed treatment you may prefer not to undergo the test.

SURGERY

Historical Background

To put cancer surgery into some kind of perspective it is worth looking at its history. Surgery was known to the ancients but was expressly condemned in the case of cancer. Hippocrates' famous comment was: "It is better not to apply any treatment in cases of occult [i.e., hidden] cancer; for, if treated, the patients die quickly; but if not treated, they hold out for a long time." This is a conclusion supported by some contemporary medical statisticians. One researcher, Dr. Hardin Jones, professor of Medical Physics, calculated that cancer patients are on balance likely to live four times longer if they do nothing for their cancer than if they do something. This conclusion has never been decisively challenged in the four decades since he made this claim.

In Europe, medical practitioners between the twelfth and nineteenth centuries repudiated the use of any kind of surgery, leaving it to barbers to perform. Without asepsis or anaesthetics, it was cruel and generally unsuccessful. The great doctor Paracelsus (1493-1541) said, "It should be forbidden and severely punished to remove cancer by cutting, burning, cautery and other fiendish tortures. It is from nature that the disease arises and from nature comes the cure."

So doctors six hundred years ago were able to talk of curing cancer. It was also their combined experience of the disease that surgery was the wrong approach. Now it is considered the standard approach - and natural cures are considered beyond the pale. Clearly something has happened to medical thinking on the way.

It was only with the discovery of asepsis and anaesthetics that surgery, against much opposition, became accepted. It became accepted as a necessity during the Napoleonic wars - because men needed treatment for their battle wounds. Since then, surgical procedures and technology have improved by leaps and bounds. There is no doubt that for cases of severe physical trauma - resulting from war, traffic accident, or any other cause - surgery is essential if many victims are to survive. But cancer is not a severe physical trauma or a physical malformation that needs to be corrected. It matters not what great advances have been made in the area of surgery; the question of its appropriateness in the case of cancer remains contentious, and no amount of technological improvement can change that, because the problem relates almost entirely to the nature of cancer rather than to the nature of surgery.

The Dangers of Surgery

The simple fact is that surgery is dangerous and results in deaths. What is the combined death rate from all forms of surgery? Recent investigations in Britain suggest that the average surgeon has a patient mortality rate of between two and seven percent. This is measurably greater among those who have had the least experience. It is therefore better to go to a big hospital than a small local one. It is better not to be in hospital when medical students graduate and relieve their more experienced superiors. A specialist is always better than a general surgeon. Make sure any doctor doing surgery on you is a specialist. Insist on it.

Then there is the simple fact that surgery requires hospitalization – and hospitals are very unhealthy places to be. Apart from very real problems of dying directly from negligent treatment, drug overdoses, and so on, there is the increasing danger of hospital-acquired infection or, as doctors call it, nosocomial infection.

One of the most serious forms of infections that arises from a stay in hospital is MRSA (Methicillin-resistant staphylococcus aureus), which is a bacterial infection resistant to the antibiotic Methicillin. Staphylococcus aureus is a common bacterium found on the skin of healthy people. If 'staph' gets into the body, it can cause anything from a minor infection such as boils or pimples to more serious infections such as pneumonia or blood infections.

MRSA usually infects hospital patients who are elderly or very ill; specifically, you may be at more risk if you are a regular or long-term user of antiobiotics or you are immunosuppressed. Cancer patients fall right into the heart of this most vulnerable sector.

Symptoms of infection can range from red and inflamed areas around wound sites, fever, lethargy, and headache. MRSA can also cause urinary tract infections, pneumonia, toxic shock syndrome, and even death.

Within hours of admission to hospital, colonies of hospital strains of bacteria develop in the patient's skin, respiratory tract, and genitor-urinary tract. These are caused by such actions as intubation, urine catheterization and so on or by the administration of drugs that lower the immune response. Also there are the risks posed by neighbouring patients, poor ventilation systems, contaminated water systems, and above all inadequate sterilization procedures in the operating theatre and surrounding environment. Ironically, Intensive Care Units are the place you are most likely to be infected.

How frequent are Nosocomial infections? Official figures estimate occurrence at 5 percent of all acute care hospitalizations which in the USA alone, means more than 2 million cases per year, resulting, according to one calculation to added medical costs of over US$2 billion.

Mortality/Morbidity: Nosocomial infections are estimated to more than double the mortality and morbidity risks of any admitted patient. The official figures suggest that they cause about 20,000 deaths a year in the USA. It is also accepted that the real figure is very likely much higher. One estimate is close to 100,000. Deaths from nosocomial infections are always understated as this is rarely the reason given on death certificates, and only death certificate causes are counted for official purposes. If you have cancer but die of MRSA, the cause of death is still likely to appear as cancer.

Other common noscomial infections are vancomycin-resistant enterococcus (VRE), Pseudomonas, candidiasis, Legionella, respiratory syncytial virus, thrush, Clostridium difficile and necrotising fasciitis, the increasingly common flesh-eating, bacteria which is associated directly with surgical procedures. If you want to scare yourself, do a Google search for 'nosocomial infection' on the internet.

Since it is the most vulnerable who are most affected, it makes sense to take action to strengthen the immune system before going into hospital if that is unavoidable.

Some hospitals are recognizing the threat and are housing cancer patients in hotels where there is much less likelihood of infection.

Versus 'Radical' Surgery

Against this background we can now take a hard look at cancer surgery. Surgery can be categorized as localized surgery when it aims simply to remove the tumour and nothing else. It is called `radical surgery' when parts of the affected or neighbouring organs or lymph glands are also removed.

Localized Surgery

The argument for simple localized surgery to extract a tumour only - with only the minimum of surrounding tissue – (e.g., a lumpectomy, in the case of breast cancer) - appears to make a degree of sense. As long as metastasis has not occurred, the tumour is small enough to be removed, and the tumour is accessible, the chances, most surgeons say, are reasonably good that surgery will, on its own, be quite sufficient.

"Early stage tumours (e.g., carcinomas in situ) that have not yet invaded surrounding normal tissue can be completely removed and are virtually 100 percent curable" (Cooper, *The Cancer Book*, 1993).

This is comforting but unfortunately neglects an important point. Cancer tumours are highly individualistic. Just because a tumour is small does not mean it hasn't metastasized; just because it is big does not mean it is going to metastasize. And, in any case, most tumours are relatively far advanced by the time they are detected - even though they may appear small to the naked eye. So, it is not at all obvious before an operation which tumours are best treated by localized surgery and which are not.

Added to this is the question of surgical competence on the part of the surgeon. One American study suggests that even when a tumour appears to be singular and operable, in only 50 percent of cases is the entire tumour removed. In half the cases some cancerous cells are left to rebuild the tumour. In other cases the cancer tumour may be inadvertently cut, releasing cancerous cells into the bloodstream. The result? A cancer that spreads much more quickly. When this happens - and it undoubtedly does happen - the result is that surgery not only does not cure, it hastens death - just as Hippocrates observed.

As we have already noted, this caution applies even to diagnostic, incisional biopsies. The more aggressive the malignancy, the more dangerous the procedure is, and the more it must be avoided. In cases of testicular cancer, one of the most aggressive of all cancers, biopsies absolutely must not be performed.

It has also recently become apparent that a primary tumour in one site, in addition to seeding metastases to other sites, has the ability to control these metastases in such a way as to prevent them from growing. It does this by secreting two substances, angiostatin and endostatin, that inhibit the development of a blood supply. Once the primary tumour is removed, the means of control is also removed, and the result is that each metastasis quickly blossoms into a full-grown tumour of its own. A patient who has had one tumour successfully removed is therefore quickly inundated with numerous other tumours. This is another argument against proceeding automatically with surgery.

Radical Surgery

While some argument can be made in favour of localized surgery, the same cannot be said of radical surgery. Radical surgery is a desperate - and very likely vain - attempt to remove a cancer that has spread by cutting out all the tissue surrounding a tumour - or trying to locate and remove all the metastases of a tumour. With any major surgery of this kind the mortality risk must necessarily be greater. And for the patient the pain and suffering is greater – and for no good purpose. Patients may not only be seriously disfigured, lacking in basic bodily functions, and seriously weakened but, on top of that, they may have their remaining life-span reduced. The quality of that life will also be substantially impaired.

Dr. Hardin Jones, professor of Medical Physics at the University of California, studied the effectiveness of standard cancer therapies. It was his opinion - based on statistical analysis - that there was no relationship between the intensity of treatment and survival rates. Radical surgery, in short, does not improve one's statistical chances of full recovery. He is on record as saying: "radical surgery does more harm than good."

To conclude: For most cancer patients, the stated need for radical surgery will be for the reason that the tumour is known to have metastasized - or is strongly assumed to have done so. Once a tumour has metastasized, there is no knowing where the secondary tumours will appear. The tissue closest to the tumour will not necessarily be the tissue first affected by a new metastasis. The cancer cells will have been borne by the bloodstream to areas of the body far from the original site. Breast tumour cells may grow in lung tissue or in the bone - nevertheless it remains a breast cancer cell identifiable as such under the microscope. Once a tumour is suspected of metastasizing, surgery ceases to be an option that makes very much sense: what is the surgeon going to cut out? When will the surgeon finish cutting?

Modern Approaches to Surgery

As with any skill dependent on technology, there will continually be developments. In surgery, the use of lasers, computer-controlled radiation surgery and tissue-freezing techniques are areas where a lot of new work is being done. Some of these techniques, such as the cyber knife, are described later – and they certainly are a big step forward for the simple reason that they allow surgery to be done non-invasively and on an outpatient basis.

But, to repeat what I have said earlier, the problem is really not so much with the surgical procedures as with the nature of cancer. It therefore matters very little what the new developments are. These do not alter the basic question: is surgery the right thing to do?

The problem for the cancer patient is not just the problem of asking the right questions. There is the additional problem of who you ask – who you expect the answers to come from. A surgeon's job is to cut out cancer tumours. A cancer surgeon who believes that surgery is not an appropriate form of treatment would be arguing himself out of a job – and surgeons, like everyone else, have mortgages and children to put through school. Therefore, when we ask the surgeon: Is surgery the right thing to do? The surgeon, almost certainly, will say 'Yes, of course.' That's his job. What else can he say?

Mastectomy: A Special Case

The most common form of radical cancer surgery is mastectomy, the amputation of the breast. Any mastectomy could be termed 'radical surgery', as it involves removing tissue surrounding a tumour, but confusingly, there is a particular kind of procedure known as a 'radical mastectomy'.

Around the turn of the century, William Halsted of Johns Hopkins Hospital in Baltimore developed the radical mastectomy. His procedure involved removing the entire breast, removing the two underlying main chest wall muscles leading to the shoulder and removal of all the lymph nodes in the armpit. Ewan Cameron and Linus Pauling comment:

"This was an extensive and very mutilating procedure, leaving the woman not only without a breast but also with a deep depression where the underlying muscles had been removed, an ugly scar, and almost always a permanent brawny swelling of the arm because of the surgical interference with the lymphatic drainage."

What Cameron and Pauling don't say is that this swelling – oedema – is extremely painful and debilitating in its own right. In fact, it is a potentially permanent effect of any surgery that involves removal of lymph nodes. It needs to be repeated that this is a very painful condition that cannot be corrected.

After the Second World War, Scottish surgeons started to do a simplified mastectomy, removing the breast but not the underlying muscles or the lymphatic nodes. This was accompanied by radiation. The results appeared to be better than the Halsted procedure. In the 1950s, Finnish doctors developed the lumpectomy – and claimed even better results than with the mastectomy. This seems to have been supported by later studies.

Statisticians looking at the whole picture, comparing different cohorts of women with breast cancer choosing different treatments, have found that there is no difference at all in the death rate of women who have had mastectomies and women who have had no treatment at all. "There is no evidence that mastectomy affects survival. If women knew that they would probably refuse surgery" (Dr. L. Cunningham, *The Lancet*, 1980).

Despite this, until the 70s or 80s, American surgeons still tended to do radical mastectomies, while European surgeons tended to do 'simple' mastectomies or lumpectomies. The reason for American surgeons' preference for the radical mastectomy appears to be a combination of income - they earned more for doing more – and fear of litigation, you can't be sued for doing the maximum possible.

The current trend even in America is away from the Halsted procedure to lumpectomies or 'resections' – the cutting away of part of the breast. However, the Halsted procedure – or a modified, less-disfiguring version - may still be advised where there is significant spread. In such a case the patient might prefer not to undergo any surgery whatever, as there is no proof that extensive surgery in breast cancer has any impact on survival.

Amazingly, of those women who survive long-term after a mastectomy, 5-10 percent will later find a cancerous nodule on the mastectomy scar.

Despite this, in America, large numbers of mastectomies are performed as a preventative measure. Many women volunteer to have their breasts removed in order to avoid breast cancer. Figures from one New York hospital showed that such so-called `prophylactic mastectomies' accounted for 20 percent of the total! Ewan Cameron and Linus Pauling, who were by no means opposed to surgery as a first line of attack against cancer, had this to say: "The observations from Halsted on seem to be showing that the less that is done for breast cancer patients, the better their chances of survival. The damage done to the body by surgical or radiotherapeutic intervention may be greater than the benefit resulting from partial control of the disease. This trend has led many thoughtful surgeons to question seriously whether they should treat breast cancer patients at all – whether these patients might not better be left alone. The question is a serious one, demanding an answer" (Cameron & Pauling, *Cancer & Vitamin C*).

The conclusions we draw from the case of mastectomy will almost certainly be valid for any other surgery that may be proposed. While there may or may not be some argument for limited localized surgery, there is very little if any support at all for radical surgery.

Not All Doctors Approve of Surgery

Medicine is an arena of contending ideologies. One of these ideologies is the surgeon's creed that the best thing to do with a tumour is to cut it out. This belief has become so dominant that it is now almost unquestioned within the temples of modern medicine, but there have been many doctors along the way who have disagreed.

A hundred years ago, homoeopathic doctor Compton Burnett, a scathing critic of surgery for cancer, remarked: "Surgeons may think the cutting out and cutting off processes 'curing'; I think them a last refuge of helplessness."

He was not alone. Dr. Robert Bell, a senior staff member of the Glasgow Hospital for Women, agreed. In 1906, he wrote the following:

"I had been taught that this (surgery) was the only method by which malignant disease could be successfully treated, and, at the time, believed this to be true. But failure after failure following each other, without a single break, inclined me to alter my opinion. The disease invariably recurred with renewed virulence, suffering was intensified, and the life of the patient shortened." He went on to say: "That cancer is a curable disease… if rational dietetic and therapeutic measures are adopted and rigidly adhered to, there can be no doubt whatever."

It is not just doctors of a century ago who criticize surgery. Professor Michael Baum, a leading and very orthodox cancer specialist, published a report (*European Journal of Cancer*, March 2005) in which he argued that surgery – whether to to take out a lump or remove a breast -- could enable breast cancer to spread more quickly, especially in young patients whose cancer isn't advanced.

Baum's argument is that the body's response to surgery creates circumstances that help to stimulate the growth of tumours. For example, surgery creates a wound. The wound healing processs requires angiogenesis, the formation of new blood vessels, and these help to feed the tumours. Surgery also stimulates the production of growth factors as part of the postoperative wound healing process which in turn can promote tumour growth. "A likely trigger for 'kick-starting' the growth of micro-metastases could be the act of surgery itself," he wrote. Another way in which primary cancer tumours control metastasis is by releasing an antiogenesis inhibitor, angiostatin. When you remove the primary tumour – or irradiate it – the result is to stimulate the growth of metastases.

In short, surgery should not be an automatic knee-jerk response to cancer. Sadly, the desire to 'get rid of the damn thing' will in many cases propel patients unhesitatingly and unswervingly towards surgery. There is also the desire to eliminate this deadly 'poison' from the body. I would urge anyone contemplating surgery to re-read this section and meditate on the potential consequences of this act.

How Far Do You Want To Go? Putting Limits on Surgery

However, in a particular circumstance there may be very good reasons why cancer surgery is an attractive or at least the preferred option. Whether or not any major organ is removed is a matter for patients, not the doctors, to decide - although they will try to convince you otherwise. Every patient has the right to say that a procedure may or may not be done on his or her body. This decision should be made in writing, and if possible it should be witnessed.

Patients undergoing any form of surgery should therefore be very clear in their own minds as to how far they are willing to go. If a woman with suspected breast cancer, for example, is willing to have a lumpectomy but not a radical mastectomy, it is for that woman to write this down on the permission form before she signs it. Unfortunately, the legal protections for patients are not as strong as they should be. Doctors are allowed a great deal of leeway as to what they can do in the operating theatre, so it is best to get legal advice.

Surviving Surgery

The first step to ensure you survive an operation is to go into the operation with the most positive of thoughts. In your case, everything is going to work out fine. Positive thinking works. It helps to boost the immune system. Spend as much time as you can watching funny films and laughing your head off.

Another effective action is to take very large doses of vitamins C, and E starting a week or two before the operation and continuing for a month or so after. Similarly, acidophilus and other friendly bacteria should be taken in capsule form. Large doses of magnesium (1,000mg/day) are also highly recommended. Afterwards, you should also smear undiluted lavender essential oil on all the scars to aid healing. Lavender oil is a marvelous healing agent. The enzyme serrapeptase should also be taken after the operation, as it is a powerful anti-inflammatory and pain reliever.

Another precaution that you can take, especially if surgery is not scheduled for a number of weeks, is to build up a supply of your own blood to be used if necessary. This is to prevent the admittedly low possibility of catching hepatitis or HIV from infected blood. The estimated risk of HIV infection in the States is 1 in 225,000, while the risk of hepatitis is 1 in 6,000. Blood transfusion from other donors can also cause problems when there is a reaction to the foreign blood platelets and/or white blood cells - these may cause hives or fevers. The risk of one or other of these is apparently in the region of 1 in 15-20.

Finally, many testimonials relating to the Quantronic Resonance System testify to its value in helping people recover from surgery (see p. 294).

RADIATION

X-rays were discovered in 1895 by Wilhelm Konrad Roentgen and nowadays are largely restricted within the public domain to medical use - either diagnostic or therapeutic.

Diagnostic radiation uses very low doses - but even these low doses have been associated with a number of dangers, the two key ones being its potential for causing cancer and the possibility that it might cause genetic damage that may not reveal itself for generations. Since diagnostic radiation is used in mammograms, women who have regular check-ups for breast cancer may actually be exposing themselves to a higher risk than those who choose not to have a check-up.

Therapeutic radiation uses high-energy ionizing radiation to attack and kill cancer cells.

But even therapeutic X-rays have been implicated as a cause of cancer! Medical history contains many murky corners, and the following is a well-known case. In the 1940s and 50s it was common to irradiate the thyroid glands of children who were believed to have a particular thyroid condition. Many of these babies later developed cancer of the thyroid as adults. It was only when this connection was made that irradiation of children's thyroids was stopped. Subsequently it was discovered that the initial thyroid condition itself did not exist and had never existed - it had been a figment of the medical imagination. Bizarre but true!

Delivery of Therapeutic Radiation

Therapeutic Radiation is given in the form of ionizing radiation. This is radiation that has been 'accelerated' or increased in energy in such a way that it can ionize atoms or molecules (by removing electrons from their orbits). The process of ionization is very destructive to the DNA of all living tissue cells, but normal healthy cells are better able to repair the resulting DNA damage than are cancer cells. That is the theory. However, in practice many types of cancer cells are highly resistant to being destroyed by radiation. How they defend against the radiation is not yet known.

Radiation is normally given as external beam therapy in which a beam of high-energy rays is directed at the tumour. With the latest machines, the beam is rotated around the patient so that it irradiates the tumour from many different directions and so does not continuously pass through the same healthy tissues. Each patient undergoing radiation will have been individually assessed, and a total dose will be calculated. This total dose will then be divided into fractions, and each treatment will deliver one of these fractions until the total dose has been delivered. Once a tissue has been irradiated in this way it can never be radiated again.

In addition to external beam therapy, radiation can be delivered internally. Brachy-therapy uses sealed radioactive sources in the form of rods or small wires that are surgically inserted into a tumour to produce a highly localized dose. For cancers of the uterus and cervix, a machine called the Selectron will be placed in the vagina. Another way of delivering radiation internally is to give it in a form that will be selectively taken up by the target tissue. For example, radioactive iodine may be swallowed to treat cancer of the thyroid.

One of the problems faced by radiologists using older radiation machines is that of determining the exact spot where the tumour is. This has led to the development of a number of machines that combine a means of visualizing the exact location of the tumour. With three-dimensional conformal radiation therapy, the patient first undergoes a CT scan while lying in the treatment position. These scans are transferred to a computer, and the doctor can then plan a treatment that will allow the avoidance of organs that are more vulnerable to radiation damage – as the machine delivering the radiation rotates around the body. It is important to remember that these machines work with a virtual image of the tumour and surrounding tissues. If there is any change in real life this will not be taken into account. This issue has led to the development of a true image guided machine which have a CT scanner integrated with the treatment machine. This ability to correct for small movements means there are fewer set up errors–and consequently the likelihood of damage is decreased. Nevertheless, damage cannot be eliminated

This is admitted by the UK's Health Protection Agency whose website says this: "For a cure, sufficiently high doses must be delivered to kill all the living cells within the tumour and this will inevitably cause some damage to surrounding healthy tissues."

The Cyber knife or Gamma knife is a form of radiation technology that uses a beam of radiation to perform excisional surgery guided by a CT scanner.

Radiation Therapy for Cancer Patients: The Official Version

The U.S. National Cancer Institute publishes a booklet entitled "Radiation Therapy and You" where we are assured that radiation is an effective means of treating cancer.

"High doses of radiation can kill cells or keep them from growing and dividing...Although some normal cells are affected by radiation, most normal cells appear to recover more fully from the effects of radiation than do cancer cells. Doctors carefully limit the intensity of the treatments and the area being treated so that the cancer will be affected more than normal tissue.

"Radiation therapy is an effective way to treat many kinds of cancer in almost any part of the body. Half of all people with cancer are treated with radiation, and the number of cancer patients who have been cured is rising everyday. For many patients, radiation is the only kind of treatment needed. Thousands of people are free of cancer after having radiation treatments alone or in combination with surgery, chemotherapy or biological therapy."

On the question of risks, the brochure advises us that there are a number of side effects. But we are assured that "Your doctor will not advise you to have any treatment unless the benefits - control of the disease and relief from symptoms - are greater than the known risks. Although it will be many years before scientists know all the possible risks of radiation therapy, they now know it can control cancer."

The problem here is that the doctor assumes the terminal risk of malignant cancer is 100 percent. Therefore any amount of radiation risk, by this standard, would be acceptable. Also, we are informed that "it will be many years before scientists know all the possible risks of radiation therapy." Medical use of radiation therapy has been in existence for almost a century, yet the full extent of the risks is still not known. This is worrying. It suggests that no one has looked very carefully at the consequences of radiation. This does not sit well with orthodox medicine's claim to be 'scientific'.

What About the Side Effects?

Side effects, the National Cancer Institute brochure goes on to inform us, may be negligible, or they may be serious - but does not go on to elucidate how serious. The British Medical Association *Complete Family Health Encyclopaedia* is also reassuring: "...normal cells suffer little or no long-term damage (from radiation). [However,] Radiotherapy may produce unpleasant side-effects, including fatigue, nausea and vomiting (for which anti-emetic drugs may be prescribed) and loss of hair from irradiated areas. Rarely there may be reddening and blistering of the skin."

This is as much as the average cancer patient is told about radiation and its consequences. Certainly it is very reassuring - especially as the encyclopaedia goes on to say, "Radiotherapy cures most cancers of the larynx or skin. The cure rate for other types of cancer varies depending on how early the treatment is begun, but the cure rate can be 80 percent or higher."

So what's the problem? Eighty percent cure rate sounds good and a cure is worth a bit of pain. However, this contrasts with the 33 percent or the 40 percent or the 50 percent that various other experts say are being cured. The cancers where radiation is supposed to be particularly successful are cancers of the cervix, testicles, prostate, lymphosarcoma and Hodgkin's disease.

Other Views

Radiation is not without its detractors. Dr. Hardin Jones, a medical statistician, makes caustic comments on radiation: "Most of the time it makes not the slightest difference whether the machine is turned on or not." Another biostatistician, Dr. Irwin Bross, was quoted in 1979 as saying, "For the situations in which most radiotherapy is given, the chances of curing the patient by radiotherapy are probably about as good as the chances of curing him by laetrile...because the chances of curing any patient in advanced stages of cancer are very poor, regardless of the method employed."

Hang on! On the one side, we have a claim of a very-high success rate, and on the other side we have a claim that its success rate is close to zero. We need a third opinion.

Dr. Lucien Israel is a highly regarded French oncologist. In his opinion, radiation should be used in the early stages of Hodgkin's disease (he quotes a five year survival of 80 percent) but he is quite blunt in admitting that radiation is not a proven form of treatment: "... apart from Hodgkin's disease and lymphosarcoma, there is much disagreement as to its effectiveness - indeed there have been no conclusive trials - and many physicians prefer surgery, despite the mutilation it entails, because it has the advantage of making a clean sweep - total sterilization by radiation often remains problematical."

This is a less than ringing endorsement. Neither does research support the view that radiation is successful in extending people's lives. This question was studied by The National Surgical Adjuvant Breast Project, who, in 1970, summarized their findings in these words: "From the data available it would seem that the use of post-operative irradiation has provided no discernible advantage to patients so treated in terms of increasing the proportion who were free of disease for as long as five years" (Fisher, B. et. al., "Postoperative Radiotherapy in the Treatment of Breast Cancer; Results of the NSAPP Clinical Trial," *Annals of Surgery*, 172, No.4, Od. 1970). Although this study was conducted over 30 years ago, there has been no major change in standard radiation therapy since that time and no change in cancer's response to radiation. The findings then remain valid today. It is unknown whether new radiation technologies would make a difference.

Dr. Richard Evans of the Texas Cancer Center, a leading American cancer clinic – on his website at www.texascancercenter.com - says this of radiation in relation to breast cancer: "Radiation can reduce local recurrence with some patients, but it does not increase survival." And in the case of prostate cancer, he says: "Physicians at Stanford (University Medical Center) no longer recommend radiation for patients with curable prostate cancer." Clearly Dr. Evans is not convinced of the value of radiation.

Let us restate the situation. Radiation has been around for a very long time. It has been used medically against cancer for well over half a century and it is still not able to present a clear case that it is of curative value. In some cases, it is true, lung cancer being one, radiation does appear to extend life expectancy by a short time but generally, even here, it is used not to cure but to shrink the tumours and so hopefully extend the life of the patient. Radiation is good at shrinking many different kinds of tumour. The problem, unfortunately, is that when these tumours grow again, they grow more quickly and are more malignant. In exchange for the pain of radiation, some cancer patients may gain a limited period of life. This may seem to some to be worthwhile.

Non-Response to Radiation

Not all cancers respond well to radiation. Many cancers indeed are highly resistant to radiation. Also, any cancer that has already metastasized cannot be successfully treated with radiation – because radiation focuses a beam of ionizing radiation at a single spot or area in the body. It is most successful when used to slow down or reduce the size of aggressive tumours - and then its success may be, as we have seen, very short term. Some tumours - of skin, tongue and lips - respond very slowly to radiation treatment, but in these cases the radiation often appears to have comparatively good long-term results. In other cases, a tumour may appear to melt away only to return with greater force.

Radio resistance, as this effect is called, is a major problem and it has led some doctors to consider giving radiation in small daily doses rather than at intervals of days or even weeks. In this way the cells are given less time to repair themselves. Early evidence suggests that anyone deciding to take radiation should have many sessions with a small doses of radiation on a daily basis rather than fewer sessions of larger doses at longer intervals. However, pressure on radiotherapy services often makes this impossible. This is a case of health service administration procedures impeding possible beneficial medical practice.

It is possible to conclude the discussion so far by saying that radiation as a curative approach to cancer has not proven itself in any way, it has not even demonstrated much in the way of medium-term benefits for most cancers. As a short-term method for making tumours appear to go away it seems to be more successful.

Dangers

However, we need to note that there are a number of very serious dangers associated with radiation.

1) Radiation Can Itself Cause Cancer

Diagnostic radiation is known to be associated with cancer: First, it is known that radiologists as a profession have a higher than average likelihood of getting cancer. Frequency of radiation also increases vulnerability to cancer. A large scale study of 700,000 children compared children of mothers who had received pelvic X-rays during pregnancy with the children of mothers who had not been X-rayed. Cancer mortality was 40 percent higher among the children with X-rayed mothers (reference: figure quoted in *Death by Medicine*, Gary Null et al. 2003, www.garynull.com - MacMahon B., Prenatal X-ray Exposure and Childhood Cancer, *Journal of the National Cancer Institute* 28 [1962]: 1173).

Dr. John Gofman, in his book *Preventing Breast Cancer* (CNR Books, USA, 1996) argues that X-rays are very likely responsible for over 50 percent, and possibly even 75 percent, of all breast cancer cases. Dr. Gofman was Professor Emeritus of Molecular and Cell Biology at the University of California at Berkeley, so we should take his views seriously.

2. Radiation Makes Tumours More Aggressive

One problem is that many cancers treated by radiotherapy, with apparent success, return - some more quickly than others, and when they do so they are unstoppably aggressive.

American Senator Hubert Humphrey's bladder cancer returned three years after being irradiated. No further treatment was able to slow the progress of the disease. In my wife's case, her cervical tumour disappeared after radiation. However, within three months of stopping chemo-therapy, five months after completing the radiation treatment, a tumour five inches long was suddenly found to be wrapped around one of her ureters. She was given three months to live, and she in fact died almost exactly three months later. By that time the cancer had spread widely in the pelvic area.

This effect - of making a tumour more aggressive - should be kept firmly in mind by those patients for whom radiation therapy is advised.

3. Radiation Makes Tumours Impervious To New Treatment

Mice that have been irradiated do not respond at all to substances that have a beneficial effect on the cancers of non-irradiated mice. This is an important point to bear in mind for any patient interested in working with alternative approaches.

Most cancer patients go through variations of orthodox treatments before they think to tackle the alternative treatments.

4. Radiation Can Cause Severe Injury

One of the worst consequences of radiation is the injury it can cause. Injury, unfortunately, is not a random, rare and unforeseeable consequence of radiation treatment. It is an inevitable consequence. The fundamental fact is that radiation damage to normal tissues is a necessary and inevitable part of radiotherapy and this is clearly understood by all radiotherapists, but by very few patients. The reasons for this is as follows: One of the problems with radiation, according to Dr. Lucien Israel, is that each time a tumour is irradiated 37 percent of the tumour cells are not affected at all. The next time, 37 percent of this 37 percent is not affected - and so it goes on. Unless surrounding tissue is also attacked, it is impossible to eliminate all the malignant cells by radiation alone. From this we can see that radiotherapy can never succeed on its own if it is aimed only at the tumour.

If radiation is used to affect the surrounding tissue, then the likelihood of success increases dramatically. In fact, one can say that the success of radiation as a therapeutic tool rises in exact proportion to the amount of damage caused to surrounding tissues. Some damage will be discovered very quickly. Other damage may not appear for ten or twenty years - and may then not be attributed to the radiation treatment.

"Radiation can cause...loss of function of the irradiated tissues. The different organs vary in their vulnerability to this sort of complication. The liver, kidneys and lungs are particularly fragile; the muscles are also susceptible" (Israel, *Conquering Cancer*, 1976).

This damage may be very mild, or it may be permanently incapacitating or even life threatening. The fairly recent use of radiation and chemotherapy together has resulted in higher numbers of patients suffering from radiation-induced problems. Some doctors have established a grading for radiation damage:

Grade I: Minor symptoms that require no treatment.

Grade II: Minor symptoms that can be managed by simple outpatient methods.

Grade III: More severe symptoms. May have to be admitted for diagnostic procedures or minor surgery.

Grade IV: Prolonged hospitalization and major surgical intervention necessary.

Grade V: Fatal complications.

What this list tells us clearly is that some patients die from their radiation treatment and that for all patients suffering grade II, grade III and grade IV damage, pain - even extreme pain - and serious discomfort are the norm.

5. Radiation Can Cause Problems Five or Ten Years into the Future

Radiation damages healthy tissue–but this damage may not show up for months or even years. There are cases of radiation recipients suffering haemorrhages as blood vessels rupture. It is also well established that radiation to the chest area – particularly on the left side – creates a high likelihood of heart disease. Heart attacks are two and a half times more likely in irradiated groups compared with the general population. The problem is that when these effects occur it is not immediately clear that they have been caused by radiation. However, long-term comparisons of radiated and non-radiated groups of patients have established a clear picture that there are significant long-term risks – so great that they cancel out any presumed immediate benefit.

But What Exactly Is The Risk?

As we have seen this is a difficult question to answer because there is so much variation in therapeutic procedure from one hospital to another. But doctors have begun to state a figure of five percent. Five percent of patients undergoing radiation suffer some kind of serious complication. But this figure does not appear to have any basis in fact. One critic, Vicky Parker, believes that it actually represents a theoretical level of morbidity that would be professionally and ethically acceptable. Medical textbooks say that a morbidity rate of 10 percent is 'ethically unacceptable'.

One group which strongly suspects that the figure of 5 percent is a gross under-estimate is RAGE (Radiotherapy Action Group Exposure), a patients' rights group that, while it was active, advocated on behalf of people suffering from radiation damage and that organized mutual support groups in the UK for radiation-damaged patients (Sadly, the group is no longer active, as leading members have become too incapacitated to carry on their work). Their private estimate is that more than 10 percent of all people receiving radiotherapy are permanently damaged as a result. This figure will certainly be higher for women who have radiotherapy for cervical cancers, because of the number of organs so close together in the pelvic area that can also be irradiated. In their case, one would suspect a very high morbidity rate.

It is also becoming clear that some people are more sensitive to radiation than others. Different studies indicate that between 10 percent and 40 percent of women may be highly sensitive to radiation - and so will react more seriously to `normal' radiation doses. But the patient's own sensitivity to radiation is not taken into account when designing a course of radiotherapy treatment. The result of being overly sensitive to radiation is the increased likelihood of injury. Just how seriously debilitating some of these side effects and after effects are can be seen from the following examples. These are the words of one member of RAGE:

"I had my (internal radiation) in 1989. By 1992 I had lost my bladder, womb, ovaries and half my vagina. I had lost my career and my self-respect. I also almost lost my family, my mind and my sense of humour. "At least you don't have cancer," my urologist cheerfully informed me. No, I thought, I don't have a lot of things, like a sex life, or healthy kidneys. Is this the price for not having cancer? I wouldn't have minded so much but they insisted I didn't have cancer in the first place. Just a few suspicious cells which could turn cancerous if left untreated...." (Kath Ridgard. quoted in the Rage National Newsletter, Summer 1994)

A very common effect of radiation is that it damages or kills the body's glands. This is a very important consequence for patients receiving radiation in the area of the neck or head, as the salivary glands will be destroyed. In 1989, Ryan Werthwein, a ten-year-old American boy was diagnosed with a highly malignant brain tumour. He underwent radiation treatment, which proved to be ineffective. "The radiation burnt out most of Ryan's pituitary gland, stunted his growth, and hurt his mental functioning, We were never told about radiation's possible long term effects" (Ryan's mother, Sharon Werthwein, quoted in *Options*, Richard Walters, 1993).

Radiation of any of the hollow organs: intestine, bladder, ureters, uterus, fallopian tubes and so on will have the inevitable effect of damaging the mucous membrane which secretes the moisturising substance that protects the inside surfaces of these organs. Note that this damage becomes far more certain when radiation is combined with chemotherapy because chemotherapeutic agents are designed to attack cells that divide and multiply rapidly - such as the cells of the mucous membrane.

One form of damage is adhesion: where the sides of any tube stick together, another problem is that the cells lining the inside of the intestine can become fibrous, tough and rigid. When this happens in the intestine, blockage occurs, requiring urgent surgery to bypass the problem. The destruction of the organ linings is usually followed by erosion making perforations inevitable. This allows the contents of one organ to leak into another.

Damage to the lymph system is another common consequence of radiation. This results in extremely painful lymphatic swellings, called oedema - which vary in intensity and duration and which can be permanent.

Blood vessels are also vulnerable and haemorrhaging can also result - even as long as ten years or more later. Patients receiving radiation for brain tumours are therefore at risk of strokes.

Damage can also occur to the ureters, the tubes linking the kidneys and the bladder, so that they become blocked. Sometimes a straw like device called a stent is forced up to maintain the flow of urine. The problem is known as stenosis. Where stenting doesn't work, and where both ureters are affected, renal failure becomes a distinct possibility.

Radiation also can weaken tissues so that they fail at a later date. Intestines can rupture, for example: "Eighteen months after the radiotherapy, I started having violent abdominal pains followed by vomiting...Eventually...I was in absolute agony. The pain was indescribable. I began to vomit faecal matter and was rushed into hospital. On arrival the surgeon warned me that I needed life-saving surgery...when I came round from the anaesthetic the surgeon (informed) me that...the radiotherapy had burned my intestines resulting in the perforation, causing the bowel contents to leak into the peritoneal cavity resulting in peritonitis. The reason now, looking back, that I put up with the pain and vomiting...was because apart from being advised that there would be only some slight side effects during treatment, I was given no warning about long term side-effects...Had I been forewarned it would have saved me a great deal of both physical and emotional trauma" (`Mandy' quoted in the RAGE National newsletter, Summer 1994).

Mandy and Kath were victims of an iatrogenic episode resulting from experimental use of a new way of delivering radiation in a number of hospitals in Manchester, and elsewhere in England, using one or both of two new machines: the curiously named Hex 2 and the Selectron. Iatrogenesis is the term applied to diseases or harmful consequences that are directly caused by doctors or by standard medical practice.

The Selectron, which is still very much in use, is a way of giving radiation internally. In this particular case relatively high doses were given to the women. There was an economic basis for this decision. The bigger the dose, the fewer the number of sessions needed and so the greater the number of patients that can be treated within a given time span. Radiation machines are expensive. The budgets of radiotherapy units are huge. The problem with such high costs is that there will be continual pressures to find savings. The result was tragic: some 300 women were condemned to a life such as this: "My life is totally controlled by my condition. I'll never have sex, never marry and have kids, never work again. I'm luckier than some though - some of the women are housebound or bedridden. I can go out when I feel better, though I have to carry morphine syrup with me everywhere...The colostomy bag and my urostomy bag have burst when I've been out, so that's a constant worry and I have to use incontinence pads all the time. I can't start the day until about 2 pm and I tire very quickly. There's always something: vomiting, bleeding. I'm always back in hospital before my three-monthly appointment comes round...I've been in the operating theatre over 2 dozen times. Doctors say "but at least you're still alive." But this is no life. It's a nightmare." (Vicky Parker, one of the founders of RAGE).

No official figures have emerged from this disastrous episode - funds are rarely provided to investigate possible iatrogenic episodes - but one unofficial estimate is that nearly sixty percent of the women receiving this treatment up to 1982 subsequently suffered horrific damage to internal organs. Many are believed to have died. The hospitals in question have never offered apologies or explanations or in any other way accepted responsibility.

It is possible to argue that this is the sort of episode that one might expect from a monolithic state medical system, such as the NHS in Britain, and that it is most unlikely to occur in a freer, more competitive medical environment. However, even this episode would not have blipped on the radar if some very brave women had not organized themselves into an activist group. It is to honour the memory of these women that I dedicate this chapter. It may be that this was an exceptional episode, exceptional in the concentrated devastation that was caused. How common are such cases? Very likely they are not common at all. I certainly hope not. But I fear that they are more common than they should be. The truth is we shall never know.

Radiotherapy textbooks state very clearly that radiotherapy is an inexact science in which procedures are decided upon in an 'empirical manner' (i.e., if it works, it works, and if it doesn't, then tinker with it until it does work). There is very wide variance in practice between one centre and another. And it cannot be restated too often: fewer problems are associated with smaller fractions given frequently than larger fractions given at longer intervals.

Women undergoing radiation for breast cancers are also at risk. Radiation can damage the brachial plexus, a nerve tissue in a sensitive area which can be heavily irradiated in an attempt to kill a breast tumour. More than 1,000 women are known by RAGE to have suffered injuries in the brachial plexus. Some have lost the use of a hand or an arm, some suffer intractable pain, and a few have even had to have their arms amputated. This problem affects approximately one percent of all women irradiated for breast cancers - but this is only one of fifteen or more possible types of damage that can result from breast radiation.

Oedema of the lymph gland is another common result of radiation and the result is painful swollen limbs. This is an intractable problem that requires very careful management. Radiation of the neck, head or throat will almost certainly result in the destruction of all the salivary glands. The result is a very dry mouth and an inability to taste many foods. Very probably it will also result in the eventual loss of the teeth.

Finally, a number of less-well-known effects: If you have received radiation and you subsequently require surgery in that same area, complications are very likely to result as the body's healing powers will have been very negatively affected. Secondly, irradiation of the brain can lead to dementia or loss of the ability to maintain one's balance. The British politician, Mo Mowlam, died as a result of head injury caused by a fall. This happened eight years after receiving radiation treatment for a brain tumour which left her unable to control her balance.

If It's So Dangerous Why Is It Used?

One reason why such a dangerous form of treatment as radiotherapy is allowed to be used is that doctors assume that all cancers will inevitably lead to death. Professor Karol Sikora explains the general case thus: "For some forms (of cancer), such as cervical cancer, it is the only hope of cure and without it thousands of women would have died." But what this neglects to say is that cervical cancer is, generally speaking, a very slow growing cancer. Certainly women with this particular cancer in the early stages can afford to spend some time examining alternatives to radiation - such as the alternatives suggested in the second half of this book.

Another argument is economic. Large sums of money have been invested in some very expensive equipment, and in training people to use the equipment. How would the medical authorities justify a decision to stop using these machines? Unfortunately it is like a juggernaut. Once it has been set in motion, it becomes almost impossible to stop.

But perhaps I am wrong. Perhaps radiation makes sense as a key component in the war against cancer. That is for each reader to judge. I will leave the last word to John Cairns, a professor at Harvard University School of Public Health: "The majority of cancers cannot be cured by radiation because the dose of X-rays required to kill all the cancer cells would also kill the patient" (*Scientific American*, November 1985).

This contrasts markedly with the views of the U.S. National Cancer Institute quoted at the beginning of this chapter: "For many patients, radiation is the only kind of treatment needed."

New Developments

As with any other area of technology, there is a constant development of new machines that can do new procedures based on new assumptions. These are always tested empirically, that is to say they are tested out on patients—just as the Hex 2 and the Selectron were. It is a fair bet that almost every cancer patient that undergoes any form of treatment will, knowingly or otherwise, be part of an experimental study.

Having said all that, the move towards a reduced use of radiation has recently been reported: this is the use of a microbeam which fires a beam of helium ions just a thousandth of a millimetre wide, one at a time, at individual cancer cells. Apparently the cells that are killed send out 'suicide signals' which cause nearby cells to die as well. This is known as the 'bystander effect'. This is certainly a move in the right direction but there is, of course, no evidence as yet that it is effective, let alone safe. What will the side effects be? What damage might it cause? These are reasonable questions for each person discussing treatment options with an oncologist to ask.

Proton Therapy

Another development is Proton Therapy. The use of a proton accelerator to direct a stream of protons at hard-to-get-at tumours appears to have long lasting impact with minimal side effects. It is particularly used against prostate cancer tumours.

The key difference between proton therapy and standard radiation therapy is that X-rays affect everything in their path right through the body along the line they travel. Protons can be so focused that they do not affect anything in front of the target and come to a stop just beyond the target. There are testimonials to the effect that even many years later virtually no negative side effects have been experienced.

Most centres offering this therapy are in the USA but this may change with time. For more information, go to www.prostateproton.com.

CHEMOTHERAPY

According to the National Cancer Institute, chemotherapy drugs can produce cures in about 15 percent of cancer cases. According to less enthusiastic experts, the figure is really three percent. In fact, it is hard to see where the 15 percent figure can possibly come from, as only about five percent of the various types of cancer respond to chemotherapy to the extent that it can be called curative. But in none of these cases is it 100 percent effective. Against this, it has been estimated that 75 percent of cancer patients are given chemotherapy. This is not a very good success rate, especially as we know which five percent of cancer types respond well to chemo. Given the negative impacts of chemotherapy it is very possible to argue that chemotherapy kills more patients than it cures and injures very many more.

What Does Chemotherapy Involve?

Chemotherapy simply means that chemical substances are used to treat a medical problem. Taking aspirin for a headache is a relatively innocuous form of chemotherapy (though 750 people a year die in the U.S. from aspirin abuse!). But, as applied to cancer treatments, chemotherapy involves the use of very powerful chemical substances.

Over 100 different drugs can be used either alone or in combination. These drugs are used because they are poisonous. They kill cells. They kill normal cells in the same way that they do cancer cells because, to this date, it has not been possible to develop a totally cancer-specific chemotherapeutic agent.

Chemotherapy drugs act generally by killing DNA or the DNA synthesizing process. Those that focus on the synthesizing process will attack all fast-dividing cells, including the cells that line the intestinal tract, blood-forming cells and hair cells. The result is that anyone taking one of these agents will suffer some degree of nausea, infection and hair loss. The resulting infections are themselves potentially life threatening. It is not uncommon for people undergoing chemotherapy to develop pneumonia, for example - some dying as a result. Liver and kidney damage along with bone marrow suppression are the most widespread damage from chemotherapy.

Different agents have different effects. For example, Adriamycin (doxorubicin) is very damaging to the heart – serious cardiac damage occurs in over 20 percent of those taking it. This is one of a group of chemotherapy agents – the anthracyclines (epirubicin and idarubicin are others in this family of drugs) – that have been used almost as a default, against breast cancer in particular. Recent research shows that it has benefit (and benefit does not mean anything as wonderful as cure. It could mean something as little as a month or two increase in life expectancy) - for only a small percentage of breast cancer patients (8 percent is one quoted figure, 2 percent is another). Its nickname in some quarters is 'red death'.

Another example: A small percentage of those taking interferon will suffer psychotic breakdowns. In addition to these side effects, some, if not the majority, of chemotherapeutic agents are themselves carcinogenic (i.e., they will cause cancer themselves in a number of cases).

If anyone should doubt the reality of the seriousness of the side effects, let them consider this. According to Dr. Gerald Dermer, in some drug trials as many as 20 percent of cancer patients died not from the disease but from the chemotherapy - so-called 'toxic deaths'.

There appear to be a large number of deaths associated particularly with an intense form of therapy known as high-dose chemotherapy. Often the dose given is so lethal that it kills the bone marrow. This requires that patients undergo a further procedure known as autologous bone marrow transplantation in which some of their bone marrow is taken out before the chemotherapy treatments and cultivated. At the end of the chemotherapy treatments this marrow is then transplanted back into the patient. This is an expensive, high tech but grueling treatment which appears to have some short-term benefit in increasing disease free periods but long-term benefits in terms of substantially increased survival has not been clearly demonstrated for most cancers.

As with radiation, side effects are to be expected from chemotherapy, because damage to the body is inevitable. One study reported that between 1965 and 1969 the one-year survival rate for colon cancer was 68 percent but that this fell to 65 percent over the next two years, 1970-71, the reason being that it was now being treated more vigorously with chemotherapy.

The Successes of Chemotherapy

However, some cancers have shown a very positive response to chemotherapy. It has been shown to be very effective in the treatment of the following cancers: Burkitt's lymphoma, Hodgkin's disease, acute lymphocytic leukaemia, choriocarcinoma, embryonal testicular cancer, Ewing's sarcoma, lymphosarcoma, retinoblastoma, rhabdomyosarcoma, and Wilms' tumor. Unfortunately, together, these account for only about five percent of all cancer cases. There also appears to be a small sub-group of breast cancer cases who might benefit. In his January 2007 newsletter, Ralph Moss says "Current research indicates that the most commonly used breast cancer chemotherapy regimen almost certainly provides no benefit whatever to 92 percent of patients. A test is now being developed to identify the 8 percent of women who have the greatest chance of benefiting from chemotherapy." But even so the absolute benefit is not great (between 7-11 percent). Against this benefit has to be set the substantial risk of permanent damage caused by the chemotherapy drugs.

The cancers that respond best to chemo are penile and testicular cancer and the fast-growing lymphomas and the leukaemias. In the case of non-Hodgkin's lymphoma, low-grade (slow growing) tumours are incurable by any regime but medium- and high-grade tumours have a good response to chemotherapy, and cure rates are estimated at 50-80 percent. The form of leukaemia affecting most children is the form that responds best to chemotherapy. When leukaemia affects adults, it tends to be a form that is less responsive - though a 5-year survival rate of 50 percent is still claimed.

Unfortunately, chemotherapy will almost certainly cause serious side effects to children. Toxicity effects have been described as 'horrendous' - in one study 61 percent suffered seizures. Strokes and other 'acute mental status changes' are high-frequency effects. It also causes immune system collapse, and children often have to spend months at a time in germ free zones.

Its long-term effects are also serious. According to the largest study ever done on cancer survivors who have entered adulthood, only about one in three remain healthy. "Thirty years after their diagnosis, 40 percent of survivors have a serious health problem, and a third have multiple problems, including stroke, heart disease and kidney failure. It is now clear that damage to the organ systems of children caused by chemotherapy and radiation therapy may not become clinically evident for many years," said the research team, led by Kevin Oeffinger of the Memorial Sloan-Kettering Cancer Center in New York.

The survivors were 54 times more likely to have required a major joint replacement, 15 times more likely to have congestive heart failure or develop a second malignant tumor, 10 times more likely to have heart disease, and 9 times more likely to have suffered a stroke or kidney failure.

While it may appear that treating leukaemia with chemotherapy, horrible though it is, is the only way to deal with the problem, there are some who argue strongly that the fatal aspect of leukaemia is in fact a form of scurvy. This view is forcefully put by Dr. Irwin Stone, a long-time vitamin C advocate, as follows: "Leukemia is not a single disease but a combination of a neoplastic blood disease and severe biochemical scurvy. The scurvy can be relieved by massive daily dosing with ascorbic acid or sodium ascorbate. The secret is to employ 25 to 100 grams (25,000 to 100,000 milligrams) or more of ascorbate per day (spaced into four or five doses), given orally or intravenously or in a combination of both. Relief of the ascorbutic burden will give the patient a fighting chance for his body to battle with the neoplastic process. It may be found that without the severe biochemical scurvy, leukemia may be a relatively benign, non-fatal condition" (www.whale.to/cancer/stone.html).

Finally, it is worth quoting a Reuter's report: "Experts estimate that at least 25 percent of chemotherapy patients are affected by symptoms of confusion, so-called 'chemo brain', and a recent study by the University of Minnesota reported an 82 percent rate, the statement said. "People with 'chemo brain' often can't focus, remember things or multi-task the way they did before chemotherapy, " Prof. Silverman who led the study said. "Our study demonstrates for the first time that patients suffering from these cognitive symptoms have specific alterations in brain metabolism" (CNN, Reuters, October 5, 2006).

To put it simply, chemotherapy has a life-long impact on your ability to think straight.

The Failure of Chemotherapy

Even such a cancer research establishment figure as Harvard Medical School's Geoffrey Cooper has had to admit the poor prognosis for the chemotherapy treatment of most cancers. He says, "Unfortunately, curative chemotherapy for most common adult malignancies (eg breast, colon and lung carcinomas) remains elusive," he says in his book (*The Cancer Book*, 1993). "Chemotherapy of metastatic disease usually fails... Advances in chemotherapy have led to successes against a few malignancies, but not against the majority of common cancers."

One estimate is that 75 percent of cancer patients are prescribed chemotherapy (a figure that needs to be put against the recognized benefit to only five percent of all cancer patients – it is probably fair to say that more people are killed by chemotherapy than are cured by it). In many cases, doctors will point to its evident effects on chemical markers indicating the presence of cancer. But these effects are almost always too temporary. This must be a very frustrating experience for oncologists but it is certainly no reason for them to persevere in this futile exercise - yet persevere they do.

The Case of Breast Cancer

In the last decade, there has been an intensive focus on breast cancer and every week a new advance is announced in the press suggesting that some major improvement as been developed. It is very easy to find on the internet websites that say things like "Chemotherapy is effective against cancer cells because the drugs love to interfere with rapidly dividing cells" (www.breastcancer.org).

Uncritical statements of this sort are common on websites operated by cancer charities, cancer clinics and other sites wedded to the orthodox view. They give the patient who has been diagnosed with breast cancer an unrealistic view of the likelihood that chemotherapy will be effective in relation to their disease. However, this seductively rosy view is contradicted by other, less propagandistic sources: "In women with metastatic breast cancer, chemotherapy is usually given with palliative rather than curative intent. Cure (meaning that the cancer goes away completely and never comes back) is an unlikely outcome for women with metastatic breast cancer… Cure is possible, but uncommon in women with metastatic breast cancer…. Despite the disappointing cure rate, treatment most likely prolongs survival in women with metastatic breast cancer..." www.patients.uptodate.com.

This statement is very much at odds with other statements suggesting that, today, the woman diagnosed with breast cancer can expect to live another 20 years. Where does the truth lie? What does appear to be clear is that the form of chemotherapy known as high-dose chemotherapy is completely ineffective.

Two cancer researchers from Addenbrooke's Hospital, Cambridge, UK, Astrid Mayer and Helena Earl, published a paper in November 2000 (quoted in www.breast-cancer-research.com) in which they reported: "Four trials of high-dose chemotherapy with stem cell support in breast cancer in the adjuvant and metastatic settings have shown no long-term disease-free or overall survival gain."

Later in the same paper, these same researchers refer to: "the resounding failure of conventional high-dose chemotherapy approaches in breast cancer."

Certainly, the early approaches to chemotherapy in the case of breast cancer were not effective. As long ago as 1975, the British medical journal *The Lancet* reported on a study that compared the effect on cancer patients of chemotherapy versus no treatment at all. Those having no treatment at all had a better life expectancy and better quality of life.

So, has there been a chemotherapeutic revolution since then? The answer is no. As I write, a great deal of publicity has been given to a drug called Herceptin. Some cancer patients are reported as choosing to sell their houses to pay for this very expensive drug. The press is claiming that it improves survival by 50 percent. Yet the truth is rather different. First, Herceptin is potentially of use to only the 20-30 percent of breast cancer patients who have an aggressive form of the disease characterized by the overproduction of a protein called HER-2. In fact, Herceptin is an antibody to this protein and is used in addition to other chemotherapy regimes. According to the Genentech website, clinical trials demonstrated the following: With the addition of Herceptin to first-line chemotherapy, there was a significant improvement in median survival (the point at which half the group have died) to 25.1 months versus 20.3 months in the control group. The median time to disease progression was increased to 7.2 months in women treated with chemotherapy plus Herceptin, compared with 4.5 months in women treated with chemotherapy alone.

These results relate to women whose breast cancer has already metastasized and so does not apply to most breast cancer cases. But these figures clearly demonstrate the low expectations that anyone undergoing chemotherapy should have with regard to the effectiveness of the treatment.

The most recent analysis of the benefits of chemotherapy was conducted by three senior Australian oncologists: Associate Professor Graeme Morgan, Professor Robyn Ward and Dr. Michael Barton, was published in the journal *Clinical Oncology*. [Morgan G, Ward R, Barton M. "The contribution of cytotoxic chemotherapy to 5-year survival in adult malignancies." *Clin Oncol (R Coll Radiol)*. 2004;16(8):549-60. - This reference is for you to give to your doctor.]

They did a meta-analysis of *all* clinical trials of chemotherapy drugs for *all* the major cancers affecting adults that reported positive results for 5-year survival conducted in Australia and the USA 1990-2004. Their conclusion was that chemotherapy for the major cancers – breast, lung, colon, rectum, etc. – was responsible for increased survival in 2.1 percent of cases overall. For breast cancer, the figure was 1.5 percent. Of all the cancers studied, only testicular cancer and Hodgkin's disease showed significant benefit from chemotherapy.

But the general public is not told of any doubts about chemotherapy as a cancer treatment. On the contrary, they (we!) are fed an almost weekly diet of reports announcing the success of new treatments.

Ralph Moss has reported on this problem in his excellent newsletter, "Cancer Decisions" (www.cancerdecisions.com): "When physicians reporting the results of a major clinical trial announce a 23 percent improvement in survival for lung cancer patients taking a new drug, it would be hard to see this as anything less than a breakthrough. But examine this claim a little more closely and you will discover that the 23 percent improvement in survival actually translates into patients living for 12.5 months, rather than 10.2 months. Furthermore, a significant proportion - 4.5 percent—of patients receiving the new wonder drug can be expected to die as a direct result of the treatment itself, a mortality rate which, according to one of the lead researchers involved, is "well within accepted limits.""

So re-mortgaging your house to buy the latest wonder drug is not a very sensible decision.

So Why Is Chemotherapy Still So Commonly Prescribed?

The simple fact is: chemotherapy is big business. The chemotherapy business is worth literally billions of dollars to the pharmaceutical companies.

Then there is the cancer research industry. The major proportion of the money donated to cancer research goes to the search for chemotherapeutic drugs. It's a lucrative business for the institutes engaged in cancer research.

It's also a lucrative business for private oncologists. There have been accusations that patients have been put on ineffective low doses for long periods of time just to ensure the patient keeps coming back. No one wants to kill the goose that lays the golden egg.

This may seem like a cheap and unsupported accusation against respectable, hard-working doctors. Yet doctors have not been shy in stating publicly that it is better for a patient to be kept uselessly on a regime of chemotherapy rather than allow them to explore the unorthodox avenues.

Dr. Charles Moertel of the prestigious Mayo Clinic investigated the value of one of the most common of chemotherapy agents, 5-FU, in combination with other chemotherapy agents, and found that only about 15-20 percent of patients with gastro-intestinal cancers had any form of response and that for most of them these responses were only partial and transient. "There is no solid evidence that treatment with (5-FU and related compounds) contributes to the overall survival of patients with gastrointestinal cancer regardless of the stage of the disease at which they are applied" (Moertel, 1978, quoted by Pauling 1986). Moertel also, according to Pauling, came to the same conclusion with regard to the effect of 5-FU in combination with other chemotherapeutic agents for a variety of cancers from the throat to the rectum.

It would seem to follow that 5-FU and related chemotherapeutic agents were contraindicated for these cancers. But Moertel goes on to say: "By no means however should these conclusions imply that these efforts should be abandoned. Patients with advanced gastrointestinal cancer and their families have a compelling need for a basis of hope. If such hope is not offered, they will quickly seek it from the hands of quacks and charlatans" (Moertel, 1978, quoted by Pauling 1986).

In 1994, *Everyone's Guide to Cancer Therapy*, the official version of orthodox cancer medicine as seen fit for the un-medically-qualified member of the general public, mentions the use of 5-FU with the following cancers: anal, bile duct, bladder, breast, cervical, colorectal, esophical, gall bladder, gastrointestinal tract, head and neck, liver, ovarian, pancreatic, penile, small intestine, stomach, uterine, vaginal, and vulvar. To be fair, it doesn't always recommend its use. For example, in the case of bile-duct cancer it says, "Studies have not shown that chemotherapy can prolong survival, but the standard drugs used (mitomycin-C or 5-fluorouracil) may cause tumours to shrink and help about 25 percent of patients....however, patients may not be better off after chemotherapy. The treatment has side effects and the tumor ultimately re-grows" (Dollinger et al., 1994).

This means that, in the opinion of the best-informed doctors, a number of chemotherapy drugs, which are used sufficiently often so that they can be referred to as 'the standard drugs used', don't work. They certainly don't do what patients want them to do, which is to help them live significantly longer to justify the pain of undergoing the treatment.

The 2002 edition of the same book continues to refer to the use of 5-FU as an investigational drug in relation to colon cancer. The message seems to be: It hasn't worked so we must try harder to make it work.

It is extremely worrying that the medical profession seems so wedded to chemotherapy that they would rather use a useless chemotherapeutic than contemplate looking at alternative therapies.

How is it that this situation is allowed to continue? One reason is the baleful influence of the pharmaceutical companies who benefit from maintenance of the current situation. They are making huge profits, and it is reasonable to expect that they, like the tobacco industry, everything they can to defend themselves. They do this in a number of ways: combining political muscle with the power of the dollar. Politically, they have ensured that they are well represented on the executive committees of the National Cancer Institute (NCI) and the major cancer research centres in the USA—the Mayo Clinic and Sloan-Kettering, for example – as any analysis of membership of these committees will demonstrate. National cancer policy in the USA is largely in the hands of representatives of the drug industry. According to former NCI director, Samuel Broder, the NCI has become "what amounts to a governmental pharmaceutical company." Broder should know because, on leaving the National Cancer Institute in 1995, he went to work for IVAX Pharmaceuticals. In doing so he was following a well-worn track. This aspect of cancer, the politics and operations of the pharmaceutical industry and the major cancer charities, is further discussed in a later chapter.

But Why Doesn't Chemotherapy Work?

The main problem is resistance. Chemotherapy is often quite successful at first. After its use, the tumour shrinks and there is a decline in the chemical markers in the blood. These markers are indications of the cancers presence and degree of activity. But then, even though the drugs are still being given, there is a relapse and the cancer starts to grow again.

Resistance is not only very common; it is the normal result. This has led doctors to use two or more chemotherapy agents together in combination. The problem is that once resistance to one drug combination occurs, there is an increased likelihood that there will be resistance to other combinations.

The main problem is that most tumours contain a small percentage, approximately two percent, of cells that are resistant to multiple drugs. These are known, naturally enough, as multiple drug-resistant (MDR) cells. Since a tumour mass is composed of both normal and cancerous cells, most of which are vulnerable to chemotherapy, the first result of chemotherapy is a very much reduced tumour. Chemotherapy therefore can be said to have put the tumour into remission. The response will be good. Everyone will be happy. But the problem is that the MDR cells will now start to replicate themselves and the tumour will regrow. This time, however, the tumour is composed entirely of MDR cells. It is both more aggressive, because of the higher concentration of cancer cells in the tumour, and totally resistant to chemotherapy.

So, in the majority of cases, the end result of using chemotherapeutic drugs is to make cancer cells more cancerous. This is recognized by the experts. In 1985 a prominent cancer researcher named Robert T. Schimke publicly announced the problem in a lecture he gave at the National Institutes of Health. The problem, he explained, is that cancer cells resist chemotherapy and that resistance mimics the very processes of cancer itself. As a result, chemotherapy tends to make cancer worse.

yes

*Bill Henderson book names two alternative treatments for MDR cells.
Pg 151-155 But says it kills cells by reducing ATP = which is power-energy of all cells - need to talk to alternative Expert about these Graviola + Paw Paw*

Insulin Potentiation Therapy and Low-Dose Chemotherapy

It may be that, despite the discussion above, some cancer patients may still feel it is worth exploring the chemotherapy route. If so, they should perhaps consider Insulin Potentiation Therapy (IPT). In this therapy, a small dose of insulin is injected, causing a state of low-blood sugar, which leads to hypoglaecemic symptoms of light-headedness and weakness. At this stage, very-low doses of chemotherapy are administered. The cells, thinking they are going to get food, become more absorbent to the chemotherapy. In this way, low doses have an enhanced impact. In fact, they are capable of very substantially enhancing the effect of chemotherapy. This approach has been in use for over 75 years, and many patients claim to have been cured in this way, with no painful or harmful side effects whatsoever.

So, why isn't the IPT approach used all the time? Ask your oncologist. For more information on Insulin Potentiation Therapy, go to www.iptq.com and www.getipt.com/location.htm.

Conclusion

On examining this evidence, I can come to no other conclusion than that chemotherapy is a dangerous and desperate approach to the treatment of any cancer except for the treatment of a few cancers where its benefits have been well established.

Sadly, the oncologist, talking privately face to face with the patient, who recommends chemotherapy, as a wise precaution perhaps, will always carry a lot of weight. But do oncologists with cancer themselves opt for chemotherapy? No they don't.

In 1986, researchers at McGill University Medical Center in Montreal approached 118 doctors who routinely recommended patients for clinical trials involving chemotherapeutic agents and asked them to imagine that if they had cancer, which of six chemotherapy treatment plans they would choose for themselves. Only 79 replied and of these, 58 said they would choose none. The reasons they gave were the ineffectiveness of chemotherapy and the unacceptably high degree of toxicity.

Not All Doctors Have Been Silent.

Here are some statements that some very knowledgeable scientists and doctors have made about chemotherapy.

"If I contracted cancer I would never go to a standard treatment centre. Cancer victims who live far from such centres have a chance" - Professor George Mathé, French cancer specialist, 1989.

"Success of most chemotherapies is appalling...There is no scientific evidence or its ability to extend in any appreciable way the lives of patients suffering from the most common organic cancer..." - Dr. Uhlrich Abel, Stuttgart, 1990. Dr. Abel's conclusion was drawn at the end of the most comprehensive evaluation of chemotherapy ever undertaken by a single doctor.

"Aside from certain rare cancers, it is not possible to detect any sudden changes in the death rates for any of the major cancers that could be credited to chemotherapy. Whether any of the common cancers can be cured by chemotherapy has yet to be established." John Cairns, professor of Microbiology at Harvard University, *Scientific American*, Nov. 1985

"Most cancer patients in this country die of chemotherapy. Chemotherapy does not eliminate breast, colon, or lung cancers. This fact has been   documented for over a decade, yet doctors still use chemotherapy for these tumors," Allen Levin, M.D., - *The Healing of Cancer*, 1990

"We have a multi-billion dollar industry that is killing people, right and left, just for financial gain. Their idea of research is to see whether two doses of this poison is better than three doses of that poison." Glen Warner, M.D., oncologist

"As a chemist trained to interpret data, it is incomprehensible to me that physicians can ignore the clear evidence that chemotherapy does much, much more harm than good." - Alan Nixon, Ph.D., Past President, American Chemical Society.

"I wouldn't have chemotherapy and radiation because I'm not interested in therapies that cripple the immune system, and, in my opinion, virtually ensure failure for the majority of cancer patients." - - Julian Whitaker, M.D.

"Patients who underwent chemo were 14 times more likely to develop leukemia and 6 times more likely to develop cancers of the bones, joints, and soft tissues than those patients who did not undergo chemotherapy" (*NCI Journal* 87:10)." - - John Diamond M.D.

"My studies have proven conclusively that untreated cancer victims actually live up to four times longer than treated individuals. For a typical type of cancer, people who refused treatment lived for an average of twelve and a half years. Those who accepted surgery and other kinds of treatment lived an average of only three years" - Dr. Hardin Jones, Dept. of Medical Physics. University of California, 1969.

Final Comment

I was once asked by a woman who was preparing for chemotherapy to comment on whether vitamin supplements would interfere with the chemotherapy. I suggested to her that a better way of looking at the situation was to ask whether the chemotherapy would interfere with the vitamins.

OTHER TREATMENTS

a) Laser Therapy

This involves focusing a beam of high-intensity light at tumour cells. The use of laser is restricted at present to treating precancerous states and small tumours. It works by vaporizing tissue at very high temperatures. The result of laser treatment can be a hole or ulcer. The problem with laser treatment is that it can be used against only the portion of a tumour showing on the surface. But tumours are like icebergs. For cervical precancerous conditions it is claimed to be very effective – but the jury is still out as to whether or not it can be effective as more than palliative care.

In Germany, a technique called laser-induced interstitial thermo-therapy (LITT) has shown itself to be successful against liver metastases. In a study of 232 women with breast cancer who had a total of 578 liver metastases, 6 months after LITT treatment fewer than 5 percent of patients showed tumour progression, and no new tumours had developed.

b) Gamma-Knife Surgery

Developed in 1968 by Swedish professors Lars Leksell and Borge Larsson, the gamma knife is a highly advanced instrument used mainly to remove brain tumors. Without making any incision, it uses a concentrated radiation dose from Cobalt-60 sources. A total of 201 beams of radiation intersect to form a powerful tool focused on a targeted area of abnormal tissue within the brain. Clinics using this technology claim that the Gamma Knife is so precise that it damages and destroys the unhealthy tissue while sparing adjacent normal, healthy tissue. The success rate of the gamma knife, according to its advocates, is unprecedented. More that 41,000 patients have had gamma-knife radio-surgery with no mortality and minimal morbidity reported.

The risk of surgical complications is greatly reduced because the procedure is performed without having to make an incision. Therefore, gamma-knife radio-surgery is virtually painless. Patients routinely use only a local anesthetic along with a mild sedative to help them lie still during the procedure. Patients can undergo the procedure and go home in the evening.

A variation of this technology is called the cyber-knife. This system uses a miniature radiation machine and a robotic arm that moves around the patient's head while delivering small doses of radiation from hundreds of directions. During treatment a computer analyzes hundreds of brain images and adjusts for slight movements by the patient. This makes it possible to deliver the treatment without using a frame to hold the patient's head still. Only the tumor receives the high doses of radiation and healthy tissue is spared.

Given the apparently clear benefits of this approach, it is odd that it isn't used more widely for all tumours.

Another form of remote surgery is High Intensity Focused Ultrasound (HIFU). It has been used successfully in Japan for several years and is particularly used for the treatment of prostate cancer.

c) Photodynamic Therapy (PDT)

Can cancer be killed by a death ray? In his book *Light: Medicine of the Future*, Jacob Liberman reported that over 3,000 people with a variety of malignant tumours had been treated with a method known as photodynamic therapy and that the results had been very exciting: "Although they had been treated previously with surgery, chemotherapy, radiation, immunotherapy or a combination of these, their tumours responded positively to the light treatment 70 percent or 80 percent of the time, after only one treatment."

This therapy is based on two facts. The first is that there is a family of substances known as porphyrins which, when injected into the body, are selectively taken up by cancer cells -- but not by most normal cells. The interesting thing about porphyrins is that they are light sensitive to a high degree. They are not toxic in the dark but are highly toxic when exposed to light.

The second fact is that when the cancer cells have taken up the porphyrins they will fluoresce under ultraviolet light. This allows their position to be ascertained with a high degree of accuracy if they are not too deeply embedded in tissue.

Using these two facts, cancer patients are injected with porphyrins and then, once the sites of the cancer cells have been located, a red light, tuned to a wavelength of 630 nanometres, is delivered, using an argon pumped laser, directly to the treatment site using a fibre-optic tube no thicker than a hair.

"Within hours of the light treatment, the cancer cells begin to die, leaving most normal tissues unharmed. Even in tissues that are just partially cancerous, only the cancerous portion of the tissue will die. Since specific photosensitive dyes are combined with highly tuned laser light, the treatment is extremely precise"(Liberman, 1991).

One problem with this therapy is the fact that the liver, kidneys and spleen also retain porphyrins. For this reason a gap of 24-72 hours between injecting the porphyrins and turning on the red light. This time lapse allows the normal tissues to clear out the porphyrins. The second problem is that patients undergoing this treatment suffer from increased skin sensitivity to sunlight, which may result in intense skin irritation for 4-6 weeks after.

A combination of photodynamic therapy and hypothermia is offered under the name LIESH therapy (The acronym standing for Light Induced Enhanced Selective Hyperthermia) by Lase Medical Institute. Using a non-drug method - they use nano-particles instead - they claim to be able to attack large tumours with "100 percent effectiveness". However, this therapy is most suitable for cancers on or near the surface of the skin. The treatment requires daily sessions for 5-10 days and is pain-free. To obtain a free phone consultation, call 1-702-953-0267. This therapy is available only in Jacksonville, Arkansas. For further details go to www.lasemedinc.com.

d) Hyperthermia

This refers to the raising of the temperature of the body to about 108 F (42 C) - and sometimes higher - by various means. The whole body may be heated or localized heating can be achieved using microwaves. There is some disagreement as to its usefulness. At present, heating treatments are generally limited to one hour sessions, but it appears that longer sessions have achieved some exciting results - the longer the better. This is, in fact, a therapy that has crossed the orthodox-alternative divide and is recommended by both. Since the high heat interferes with the cell's ability to repair itself after radiation treatments, it is now being used along with radiation, and it appears that immediate response rates nearly double as a result.

One study showed that radiation on its own had a 31-37 percent response rate, while radiation with heat treatment had a response rate of 63-71percent. Response rates, however, as we have seen, mean little on their own. Nevertheless, some studies claim long-term benefits. This suggests that, if radiation is to be chosen as the form of treatment, the best way of conducting it would be to have very small fractions of radiation everyday with long-term hyperthermia treatment in between.

Hyperthermia may be used regionally, in a part of the body only, using microwaves, or may involve the whole body. In the case of liver cancer, this method is being used, apparently, with some success in those cases, the majority, where surgery cannot be undertaken because of the cancer's spread. The side effects of hyperthermia are minimal.

Radio-Frequency Ablation (Rfa)

This technique involves the use of a high-frequency electric current to heat tumors and kill them. It was at first used to provide palliative relief to terminal patients, particularly those with liver cancer. However, its effects were so positive that it is now being considered as a replacement of both surgery and radiation.

The Life Extension Foundation website (www.lef.org) describes the advantages of the therapy: "Because of its therapeutic value and cost effectiveness, along with its noninvasive, low-risk profile, RFA has the attention of both physicians and patients. The National Institutes of Health consider RFA the most predictable, safest, and simplest method for thermal ablation in bone, liver, kidney, prostate, breast, and brain cancers."

In this therapy an MRI scanner is used to pinpoint the location of the tumour and a titanium electrode is then inserted into it. The radio-frequencies transmitted through the electrode to the tumour can in a matter of 10-12 minutes kill a sphere of 1-2 inches. In the case of a large tumour the electrode is moved to a number of sites in the tumour until the whole tumour is killed. Radio Frequency Thermal Ablation is another way of inducing highly localized increases in temperature. For more information about Radio Frequency Thermal Ablation, visit www.cancerablation.com.

e) Hormones

Hormone treatment is often recommended with breast and prostate cancers.

Hormones for Breast Cancer

Hormone therapy is designed to inhibit oestrogen and progesterone which, in some cases of breast cancer, are having the effect of promoting cancer cell growth. In some cases doctors will prescribe drugs to turn off the production of hormones from the ovaries—alternatively they will recommend the surgical removal of the ovaries to achieve the same result. If diagnosis shows that the cancer cells have oestrogen or progesterone receptors, it means that growth of the cancer tumour will be stimulated by these hormones. If a cancer is found to have these receptors, hormone therapy is recommended as part of the treatment plan.

Unfortunately, although the theory may be sound, the practice is less than perfect. Tamoxifen is the best known hormone treatment for breast cancer. Sherrill Sellman, a health writer, has investigated the subject intensively, and I recommend that you read her article in full. It can be read at www.all-natural.com/tamox.html . She concludes that Tamoxifen has shown a very marginal benefit—but only for post-menopausal women - but that it comes with such serious side effects (risk of blood clots, endometrial cancer, uterine sarcoma and fibroids) that it should almost certainly be avoided. More recently two similar drugs appear to have better results with reduced negative impacts: Raloxifene and Anastrozole (Arimidex). However, the list of side effects for these two drugs still makes for sober reading:

Side Effects of Raloxifene:

More common: Bloody or cloudy urine; chest pain; difficult, burning, or painful urination; fever; frequent urge to urinate; infection, including body aches or pain, congestion in throat, cough, dryness or soreness of throat, and loss of voice; runny nose ; leg cramping; skin rash ; swelling of hands, ankles, or feet; vaginal itching. **Less common:** Abdominal pain (severe); aching body pains; congestion in lungs; decreased vision or other changes in vision; diarrhea; difficulty in breathing; hoarseness; loss of appetite; nausea; trouble in swallowing; weakness. **Rare:** Coughing blood; headache or migraine headache; loss of or change in speech, coordination, or vision; pain or numbness in chest, arm, or leg; shortness of breath (unexplained).

Side Effects of Arimidex

More common: Abdominal pain, accidental injury, anxiety, arthritis, back pain, bone pain, breast pain, cataracts, chest pain, constipation, cough, depression, diarrhea, dizziness, dry mouth, flu-like symptoms, fractures, headache, heart disease, high blood pressure or cholesterol, hot flashes, infection, insomnia, joint disease or pain, loss of appetite, nausea, osteoporosis, pain, pelvic pain and stiffness, "pins and needles," rash, shortness of breath, sore throat, stomach and intestinal upset, sweating, swelling of arms and legs, urinary tract infection, vaginal discharge or inflammation, vomiting, weakness, weight gain. **Less common or rare**: Blood clots, bronchitis, confusion, drowsiness, feeling of illness, fever, hair thinning, heart attack, increased appetite, itching, muscle pain, nasal or sinus inflammation, neck pain, nervousness, severe blisters in the mouth or other mucous membranes, sluggishness, stroke, temporary tumor growth, tense muscles, vaginal bleeding, vaginal dryness, weight loss.

Hormones for Prostate Cancer

Hormones cannot cure prostate cancer but they can slow the growth. The idea behind the treatment is that the male hormone, testosterone, helps prostate cancer cells to thrive. Removing this hormone slows the rate of growth. One way in which this can be done is through surgical castration. Another way is through oral hormone pills that feminize the patient.

The side effects of this therapy are severe: besides breast development there is deep-vein thrombosis (blood clotting). In fact the side effects of all such drugs should be read with care. Those for hydrocortisone, one of the hormone drugs used includes raised blood pressure, heart trouble, mood changes, blood clots, thinning of the bone leading to increases in fractures, bruising, changes in vision and acne. Loss of sexual interest too will almost certainly happen

The problem is that these hormones have to be taken for life. The fact is, taking hormones for prostate cancer is a tough option - very severe side effects have to be borne for a less than satisfactory objective.

f) Biological Therapies

The idea behind biological therapies is that the immune system can be activated to target cancer cells - and if these defences can be activated the cancer tumour would be destroyed by the body's own immune system. Sometimes this happens spontaneously.

In 1986 Molly O'Connor, a five-month-old baby, was diagnosed with a neural blastoma which had already spread to the liver. The cancer tumour swelled up and distended the stomach. The specialists, however, detected certain signs that were positive and decided not to proceed with chemotherapy. Instead they observed her. At a certain point the cancer stopped growing and retreated of its own accord. She is still alive to this day. This was a case of spontaneous remission. Somehow the immune system kicked in and once it had done so the cancer tumour retreated and finally disappeared.

In order to replicate this process, a large number of biological substances, extracted from tumour and immune cells, have been investigated: interleukins, interferons, tumour necrosis factor, prostaglandin and others. All of these substances have been trialed on cancer patients. Some have very minor side effects, some cause flu-like symptoms and some, such as interleukin-2, has severe and life-threatening effects. To date, this approach has not been particularly successful

Vaccination

Vaccination is another form of biological therapy. Cancer vaccines are different from other prophylactic vaccines in that they are not preventive. Rather, cancer vaccines are therapeutic - they are used to treat the disease rather than prevent it.

One pioneer in this field is Dr. Donald Morton, Director of the John Wayne Cancer Institute. He has used the standard BCG vaccination with some success against malignant melanoma - four of the first seven patients to receive the BCG survived. Analysis of the results showed that those patients whose melanoma was confined to the skin recovered but those whose melanoma had struck deep into the body - particularly the brain - did not.

However, while orthodox cancer clinics have been prevented by lack of FDA approval from offering vaccine therapies, this is not the case with scientific pioneers who are forced to practice outside the USA. Vaccination plays a key part in the therapies offered by the ITL Cancer Clinic in the Bahamas, which is carrying on the work of Lawrence Burton (see p. 271). For more information go to www.immunemedicine.com.

g) Bone Marrow Transplantation

There are two reasons why a patient may be advised to undergo bone marrow transplantation. One is allogenic transplantation, in which new bone marrow - usually from a close relative without cancer - is transplanted into the patient to help the body to fight the cancer. Identical twins are fortunate in having a walking supply of perfect bone marrow to draw on.

The more common autologous transplantation is used when the doctors want to use massive doses of chemotherapy - dose levels that would normally kill the bone marrow cells. In this case the bone marrow is taken out before the chemotherapy course and replaced afterwards.

h) Anti-Angiogenesis Agents

This is a new but promising area of attack. It is known that solid tumours need to develop their own blood supply—a process known as angiogenesis - in order to fuel their growth. By attacking this development of blood vessels, using an anti-angiogenesis agent, the tumour can, in theory, be prevented from growing. However, it still remains to be seen whether or not attacking the blood supply will be effective in eliminating tumours.

However, this approach opens up another interesting avenue. It is known that inflammation induces angiogenesis, which in turn increases the risk that a cancer will spread - and this may explain why physical trauma is associated with cancer. This has led some researchers to hypothesize that anti-inflammatory agents may help prevent increasing angiogenesis of pre-existing tumors. It should be mentioned that there are many natural anti-inflammatory agents (e.g., lavender essential oil, ginger, curcumin, fish oils, the Ayurvedic herb boswellia serrata, and bindweed, among others).

Interestingly, among drugs being tested for anti-angiogenesis effects is the notorious Thalidomide.

i) Smart Drugs

The latest scientific research buzz-word is 'smart drug'. The idea is that so much is now known about cancer that to talk of lung cancer, for example, no longer makes sense to a cancer researcher. He will want to know whether you are talking about lung cancer type A2 or Type B3. These different types are distinguished by molecular peculiarities. It is these peculiarities that are now becoming the focus of intense research activity. Drugs will target the specific molecular vulnerabilities of each different type of cancer. Great things, according to research spokesmen, are expected.

One new smart drug is a breast cancer treatment called Herceptin. It targets cancer cells that make too much of a protein called HER-2 which is found on the surface of cancer cells. This effect occurs in about 25 percent of breast cancer cases. Herceptin is designed to slow or stop the growth of these cells. And has it been successful? Sadly, it is not a cure. It has demonstrated some short-term benefits in relation to tumour shrinkage but these benefits are not earth shaking. On its own, only 14 percent of women taking it demonstrated a significant response. For patients taking it in addition to chemotherapy there was a slight improvement in life expectancy after one year (76 percent as against 68 percent of women taking chemotherapy alone).

Unfortunately, there is a big fly in the ointment. It is no longer possible to talk even of a lung cancer type A2, for example. Every tumour contains cells that are genetically heterogenous. Put simply, there are many different types of cancer cell within each tumour. And your tumour is different from mine. In addition the cells that leave the primary tumour – the ones that will eventually create the metastases that will, possibly, kill the patient - are different again. And not all cells that go on the journey away from the primary tumour will create metastases. Given this complex genetic cellular reality no one smart drug can possibly work. This is a case of researchers knowing more and more about less and less until they are close to knowing almost everything about virtually nothing. The level of focus is too precise. Scientists need to lift their eyes from these tantalising details to look at cancer once again within the framework of its context.

What Orthodox Treatments Are Recommended for Your Particular Cancer?

As cancers at various sites differ from each other in many ways, so too do the treatment protocols for these cancers differ. Chemotherapy may be very effective in treating some (i.e., testicular cancer), but totally ineffective in treating others, even though they may initially provoke a response. Remember, response rates are a meaningless measure of therapeutic effectiveness and have little if any correlation with long-term survival of the patient, or even with extending life. A tumour may respond initially but then return with renewed force.

The problem is that doctors are part of a system – and that system is wedded to the use of surgery, radiation, and chemotherapy. The availability of other therapies may only be open to patients who persist in looking for options, or for those who are considered 'terminal' and for whom the other therapies have been tried and have failed.

The medical establishment requires obedience by individual doctors to generally agreed treatment protocols. Doctors cannot, therefore, be trusted to be open and truthful about the impact of these therapies and the damage they can cause. Their careers – their ability to pay mortgages school fees, etc. - depend on going with the institutional flow.

The patient undergoing treatment should take note of the words of one of the founders of modern medicine, Sir William Osler: "In today's system of medicine a patient has to recover twice: Once from the disease and once from the treatment."

However, many readers will nevertheless want to know more about the latest treatments for their own cancers. Rather than attempt to provide inadequate summaries of these standard treatment protocols for the various cancers, I will here direct you to sources of information of the latest approaches.

1. The U.S. National Cancer Institute at www.cancer.gov. provides detailed descriptions of the standard treatments and prognoses for each cancer. It is updated monthly, so you can be sure this is the very latest information.

2. Two books that are aggressively in favour of the orthodox protocols and which give an impressive amount of information are:

a) *Everyone's Guide to Cancer Therapy*, by M. Dollinger M.D. et al., and

b) *What You Really Need to Know about Cancer*, by Dr. Robert Buckman

When reading these books, you should be alert to the fact that where there are no figures of success for a treatment, there is very likely little chance that this treatment will be effective. Where there is no standard treatment, that means none has proven itself to be effective. That when it says clinical studies are ongoing, that means patients are being directed to treatments so that they can be studied. Also, it has been brought to my notice by a doctor that these books tend to recommend the most aggressive approaches and there are private clinics where less aggressive approaches are preferred.

3. A book you really should read before undergoing chemotherapy is

Questioning Chemotherapy, by Ralph Moss.

4. Another book, one that is stridently in favour of orthodox treatments but which, blow by blow, describes how painful undergoing such cancer treatment can be, is:

C, by John Diamond.

REDUCING THE SIDE EFFECTS

Although I have been very critical of standard cancer treatments - and have argued that surgery, radiation and chemotherapy are forms of treatment to be regarded with great caution, many patients have undergone these therapies, their tumours have disappeared (for the time being) and they appear, for now, to be living comfortable lives. In America it has been estimated that there are 8 million people who have apparently recovered having gone through some form of orthodox treatment. The therapeutic conveyor belt will continue to channel patients to these therapies in large numbers, and many patients will feel happy that their cancer is in the hands of experts who know what they are doing. For these and other reasons, radiation and chemotherapy will continue to be performed in large numbers for the foreseeable future. However, since these forms of treatment are hazardous, anyone deciding to undergo radiation therapy or chemotherapy should consider the advice of a number of complementary therapists and take the following precautions before, during and after treatment.

For Serious Damage

plus cancer hates oxygen

In the event that serious damage is caused by radiation, you should know that oxygen is considered to have enormous healing properties. One way to make use of this knowledge is to get a referral to a hyperbaric oxygen unit. These units use the oxygen chambers familiar to divers who rise to the surface too quickly and are in danger of 'the bends'. These chambers increase oxygen levels throughout the body and could be very beneficial for anyone suffering serious damage from radiation treatment. Similarly, drinking water containing a few drops of 35 percent pharmaceutical grade hydrogen peroxide may be a simple way of achieving the same end. Some private clinics offer ozone treatments that are also said to be beneficial.

Damage Prevention

Grapes: Doctors at The Institute of Cancer Research in London believe the antioxidants in grapes may protect against radiation fibrosis, a condition that causes tissue around the breast to become hard and stiff. It can be very painful. The problem can appear many years after the treatment. Eating grapes or taking grape seed extract appears to be highly effective as a preventative – but doctors are not entirely sure why.

Glutamine: This is a common amino acid. Supplementing 25-30 grams a day 35 (or 0.3 grams per kilo of body weight) is highly recommended for anyone undergoing radiation or chemotherapy. Very important for healing. It is recommended to combine this with isoleucine, another amino acid.

Co-enzyme Q10 (CoQ10): CoQ10 provides important protection for the heart. For anyone taking Adriamycin/doxorubicin or any other cardiotoxic drug, this is a must. 200-400mg a day.

Lactobacillus acidophilus: These are the friendly bacteria. L. acidophilus and L bulgaricus have a noted effect in cleaning out the toxic wastes that result from these therapies. As a result, the toxic impact of the treatments is reduced. Start taking before any treatment is started.

Potassium: Radiation causes problems for the sodium-potassium balance of the body. Potassium is a very important mineral, which is essential for nerves, muscles, regulation of osmotic pressure, maintenance of the acid-base balance of the body and also for the proper levels of blood sugar. Ocean fish, seaweed (kelp, dulce, etc.), beans, whole grains and dried figs and bananas are good sources. For a protective effect, 3-6,000 mg a day is required. Overdosing can be a problem above this level, so it is best to monitor your intake carefully. A normal dietary intake (from fruits, vegetables, nuts and whole grains) should provide around 2-3,000 mgs.

Magnesium: Magnesium deficiency can be caused by drinking too much milk, coffee, alcohol, and fluoridated water. Many chemotherapy drugs cause loss of this mineral. Deficiency can cause a loss of calcium and potassium, kidney disease, muscle cramps, irritability, depression and even heart disease. It is an important mineral and needs to be taken as a supplement unless your diet also includes a lot of sea vegetables, soybean products or nuts. The truth is most people are deficient in this vital mineral. For more information on the importance of magnesium go to www.mgwater.com.

Selenium: This has a protective effect against mercury - as in dental fillings. It also helps protect against radioactivity. 100-200 mg a day. Indeed it is one of the most significant anti-cancer minerals (and depletion of selenium has been associated with higher incidence of AIDS and many other diseases). Do not take at the same time as vitamin C, as vitamin C interferes with the absorption of selenium.

Iodine: Iodine deficiency can also occur as a result of radiotherapy, and some form of supplementation should be considered. Iodine in particular affects a large number of the body's metabolic processes. For this reason, it is recommended that seaweed products such as kelp or dulce, available at any adequate health store, should become a regular part of the diet - also green vegetables, and egg yolks. A tincture of iodine called Lugol's solution is recommended by some. If the local chemist shop won't supply it, try the internet. Iodoral tablets are another useful way of taking iodine and potassium. These are easily available from internet suppliers. Finally, many people advocate the benefits of Atomic Iodine, or Nascent Iodine as it is sometimes referred to. This comes in 1 percent and 7 percent solutions. Cancer patients will want the 7 percent solution. As it is a liquid it can be administered to the skin as well as taken internally. Dr. Albert Szent Györgi, the Nobel Prize-winning biochemist who isolated vitamin C, wrote, "When I was a medical student, iodine in the form of KI (Potassium Iodide) was the universal medicine. Nobody knew what it did, but it did something and did something good." In those days the standard dose was 1 gram – which contained 770 mg of iodine. For more information on the health benefits of iodine go to www.health.groups.yahoo.com/group/iodine.

Sodium alginate: Sodium alginate is another highly recommended substance, as it helps reduce the impact of radiotherapy on the bones and, in small doses, is known to act as a cancer preventative. Brown sea vegetables such as kelp are a good source of sodium alginate. There are a number of concentrated brown seaweed extracts—which incidentally have strong anti-cancer activitities: Modifilan and U-Fn Fucoidan are two such products.

Aloe Vera: Some people recommend drinking aloe vera juice regularly for its healing properties. We have already noted the terrible impact of radiation on the intestines. It is also recommended that aloe vera gel should be rubbed into skin areas affected by radiation half an hour before exposure. In addition to its anti-cancer activity it also protects people with weakened immune systems against infection. It is a powerful protector against free radicals and is an excellent source of glyconutrients.

Slippery Elm: Since damage to the mucous membranes lining all the hollow tubes in the body is inevitable, some complementary therapists recommend that radiation patients should constantly drink slippery elm, a herbal compound that should also be available at your local health shop, and olive oil. These are obviously intended to replace the natural mucous material lining the insides of hollow organs and so avoid the worst consequences of radiation treatment. Black currant juice is also recommended for this purpose.

Transfer Factors: There are stories of people sailing through chemotherapy and radiation with very few side effects because they were taking transfer factor supplements (see page 199)

Vitamin A: The main problem of both radiation and chemotherapy is that it attacks the epithelial cells that line the inside of the intestines and which produce the mucous membrane. Vitamin A is necessary for the growth and maintenance of epithelial tissue, and it is therefore necessary to take this vitamin, either as vitamin A or as beta carotene, in large quantities while undergoing either treatment; several glasses of fresh carrot juice a day throughout the treatment would be sufficient. For cancer patients, real Vitamin A is better than beta carotene, because conversion of beta carotene into vitamin A may be, and often is, problematic.

Vitamin C: Chemotherapy patients are often urged not to take any anti-oxidant vitamins, particularly vitamin C, during their chemotherapy, as it is believed these will reduce the effect of the drug. Critics, meanwhile, suggested that it was the chemotherapy that was interfering with the benefits of vitamin C! However, a recent study shows that vitamin C not only supports the body but aids any chemotherapy regime by making cancer cells more sensitive to the toxic impact of the drug. If you need to, direct your doctor to the following reference: Abdellatif et al. "Vitamin C enhances chemosensitization of esophageal cancer cells in vitro." *J Chemother*, 2005; 17 (5):539-549.

Vitamin E: This vitamin helps the body to recover from post-irradiation anaemia and helps to protect red and white blood cells. It has been found to protect the heart against damage and lower skin toxicity from the doxorubicin agents, and protects against lung fibrosis from use of bleomycin.

Taking 1,600 IU or more, starting one week before chemotherapy treatment, has a significant impact on hair retention. However, a number of alternative cancer therapists believe vitamin E protects cancer tumours and even promotes their growth. On the other hand, there is evidence that vitamin E in the form of Vitamin E Succinate does inhibit tumour growth. This demonstrates very clearly that all forms of any vitamin are very far from being equal.

See Blaylock book pg 12 about types of vitamin E.

Herbs: A number of herbs are useful as protective agents: Siberian ginseng, panax ginseng and chaparral. In the case of panax ginseng, a Korean study found that a normally fatal dose of radiation would leave 5 percent of mice alive in the control group compared with 82.5 percent in the group given the herb. Chinese herbs - especially blood strengtheners and kidney tonics - have shown great ability to support the body.

Maharishi amrit kalash (MAK): This is an Ayurvedic food supplement made up of a variety of herbs and minerals. According to its manufacturers it has 1,000 times the antioxidant power of vitamins C and E.

The All India Institute of Medical Sciences in New Delhi did a study comparing breast cancer patients, some of whom received only chemo while others had chemo plus MAK. The MAK was found to cut the number of people who suffered vomiting by almost half. It also helped reduce appetite loss and increase overall quality of life. It had no effect on hair loss, diarrhoea, mouth ulcers, and low blood counts. It is available at www.mapi.com.

Triphala: This is another ayurvedic preparation that helps to maintain good health and which has demonstrated strong anti-cancer effects of its own.

Nutritional Yeast: Nutritional yeasts bond with pollutants and heavy metals. Mixed with brown rice, this has protective value for the liver. Bio-Strath is a Swiss herbal product that contains a good yeast (saccharomyces cerivisiae) and 15 herbs. The production of Bio-Strath requires two months of fermentation. In one study, a group of radiation patients who took Bio-Strath suffered no weight loss, or depression of the haemoglobin. It also helped to enhance the assimilation of nutrients. It also has been shown to retard tumour growth in mice - and mice on a diet of Bio-Strath - did not develop as many cancers as a control group.

Reishi Mushrooms: In Japan, drinking tea made with Reishi mushrooms (aka Ling zhi) is also often recommended for radiation patients as it protects the white blood cells.

Green Drinks: Green drinks based on chlorella, spirulina and barley sprouts and which also contain vegetables rich in chlorophyll such as green cabbage, broccoli and alfalfa have been shown to reduce radiation damage by 50 percent in studies on guinea pigs. Chlorophyll is very similar in its molecular composition to haemoglobin. This should be near the top of the list. There are a number of different brands. I am familiar with Barlean's Greens and Green Defense, both of which are good.

Olive Oil: When this comprises 15 percent of total calories of a daily diet it provides optimal protection against radiation. In one study with mice which received from 0 to 30 percent of their diet in the form of olive oil, those mice that had no olive oil all suffered radiation damage to liver, kidneys, lungs, skin and hair. Olive oil demonstrated strong protective properties.

On a side note, the incidence of skin cancer among Mediterranean populations is low, and it is speculated that this is because of the high olive oil consumption. Olive oil contains significantly higher amounts of squalene than seed oils. Virgin olive oil (cold pressed) applied to the skin after sunbathing may protect against skin cancer.

Olive oil may also protect against bowel cancer by regulating the enzyme diamine oxidase, which in turn may be linked to cell division in the bowel.

When buying olive oil make sure it states on the container that the oil was extracted by mechanical means and not by heat. Cold pressed extra virgin olive oil is best. Extra virgin olive oil is the only vegetable oil that does not go through chemical processing - peanut, safflower, and canola oil all go through chemical processing to remove toxic substances. Many cheap commercial olive oils may also have green dyes added to them to make them look more authentic.

Garlic: Garlic promotes healing and protects against radiation damage. It is a very powerful food medicine, and you should eat as much as you can tolerate. It contains two powerful substances: allicin oil and organic germanium. It also contains a substance that Russian scientists have called vitamin X, because its functions are not yet fully understood. Kyolic brand deodorized garlic capsules are highly rated and aged garlic extracts are reputed to be highly effective as protection against DNA damage that the radiation causes. However, there is nothing wrong (and a lot that is right) with eating fresh, preferably organic, raw garlic. Another product that claims to be very much more effective in crossing the stomach barrier is alkaline buffered garlic powder. This is available under the name, Real Garlic, from Purity Products www.purityproducts.com.

DMSO: DMSO, dimethyl sulphoxide, an organic sulphur compound of great therapeutic value, has shown itself to be valuable both in alleviating the side effects of radiation and being an anti-cancer therapy in its own right. There is evidence that, when combined with low doses of chemo-therapeutic agents, it is also highly effective against cancer.

Immune-system Boosting Drugs: Isoprinosine®: This is marketed under the trade names Methisoprinol and Inosiplex. It is used for anyone with a compromised immune system - AIDS and cancer patients - as it has demonstrated a strong anti-viral activity and is valuable for restoring and strengthening the immune system. It is even used to treat some cancers – particularly melanomas. It is often used postoperatively and with radiation and chemotherapy. Discuss the availability of these drugs with your doctor. It has few side effects – or as doctors like to put it, it is 'well tolerated'. The few side effects reported included: itchiness, dizziness, and problems with digestion (slight stomach pain, feeling full after eating only a small amount of food).

Seaweed: Lots of sea vegetables (seaweed) are recommended. Anecdotal evidence strongly suggests that side effects are much reduced if the patient takes large quantities of seaweed during treatment. Modifilan and U-fn Fucoidan brown seaweed extracts are highly recommended.

Ice-pack: Some people have suggested that keeping an ice-pack on the head during the chemotherapy sessions and for an hour or so after may prevent hair loss (as does vitamin E).

Lifewave Patch & Ice-Wave Patch: One of the problems patients face with these grueling treatments is that they feel completely depleted of energy. Lifewave patches, developed to enhance athletic performance, will give much needed energy. These are not transdermal patches in that nothing in the patch is physically absorbed through the skin. Instead, they use a proprietory technology involving minute quantities of certain organic compounds that are programmed to send frequencies into the body. These in turn stimulate the body to produce ATP, which is the fuel needed for cellular energy. The result is increased energy, stamina and strength. These patches are used mainly by athletes to promote performance–and they have testimonials from quite a few well known athletes such as veteran tennis player, Fred Stolle - but they will be particularly beneficial to those who are energy depleted as a result of medical treatment. Go to www.lifewave.com for more information. The Ice-wave patch is based on the same technology and has been developed for pain relief.

Kinotakara Foot Patches: Two Japanese researchers Dr. Takao Matsushita and Dr. Kawase Itsuko have developed a patch that they claim gives a major boost to the wearer's energy levels while at the same time helping detoxification. The patches are placed overnight on the foot (usually) or anywhere else where there are swellings. In the morning, the white patch is generally found to be stained with toxins it has drawn from the body. The patches, which combine 'wood vinegar essence' – from oak, beech and sakura trees – with a number of other ingredients including pearl powder, tourmaline stones and negative ions. It may seem bizarre and exotic but they have become big business in Japan. For more information go to www.kinotakarafootpatch.com.

Traditional Chinese Medicine/Ayurvedic Medicine: Both these forms of traditional medicine - which use diet, herbs, breathing, exercise and other modalities such as acupuncture – are extremely helpful in counteracting the negative effects of chemotherapy and radiation. Look in the Yellow Pages for a local practitioner.

Visualisation: Finally, anyone opting for radiation and chemotherapy should develop a positive attitude to these treatments and visualize how they are working against the cancer.

RESEARCH & POLITICS

Cancer Research

Underlying all orthodox cancer treatment is the belief that it is scientific in some way. Both patients and doctors base their faith in modern medicine on this credo. It is presumed that behind everything that doctors do there is a vast machinery of scientific expertise that is creating, testing and evaluating products and processes. And which, in the case of cancer, is going all out to find a cure with no other consideration being allowed to hinder this effort. Certainly this is the picture that is created by news reports and advertisements for cancer research charities.

But inevitably the truth is a little baser than this idealistic image. Even a casual look at modern medicine will find very little that is based on such scientific procedures. Dr. Luisa Dillner, an assistant editor of the *British Medical Journal*, explains: "Less than half of what doctors do now is based on solid scientific evidence...This is not to say that doctors are lazy or incompetent. It is partly that medicine moves so fast it is hard to keep up with the latest evidence of what works and what does not" (*Guardian*, October 1995).

The simple fact, as we have seen, is that there is no proof that surgery and radiation are effective methods of treatment of cancer. Chemotherapy, on the other hand, has been very heavily tested by scientific methods of extreme rigor – and the results effectively amount to a disproof of the value of chemotherapy as a curative treatment for the vast majority of the cancers for which it is used.

The American analyst of medical statistics, Hardin Jones presented a paper nearly 30 years ago arguing that his statistical analysis overall suggested that no treatment was better than any treatment - indeed it was four times better! People who received no treatment were likely to live four times longer than people who did receive treatment. There has been no marked change since then. That is the closest thing to a scientific analysis of the benefits of modern medicine as we are likely to get.

Yet doctors continue to insist on the necessity of treating cancer with the weapons of surgery, radiation and chemotherapy. Now, it may be that doctors and statisticians are looking at different things. Since doctors are focused on the tumour, not the patient, they may be able to claim successful treatment (talking of remission and regression) even though a patient's total life span may not be affected at all. The treatment was a success even though the patient died.

The question of the interplay of medicine and science is a complex one. Should medicine be seen as an art or as a science? When doctors treat patients are they serving the cause of the patient's health alone or a higher god of scientific truth? Should a doctor, when all else fails, give a sugar pill under the guise that it is an effective medication?

Deepak Chopra tells the story that having cut open a patient he found that she was so riddled with cancer that there was no point in continuing with the surgery. He agonized over what to tell her and in the end he lied to her saying that he had removed the cause of her problems. He fully expected her to die within a matter of months. A long time later he found her once again a patient. He did some tests and found her cancer had completely disappeared. She confessed that she had previously feared that she had had cancer but that his reassurance had so cheered her up she had felt a new person altogether. So his lie had cured her. Is this science? Clearly then there is more to being a doctor than simply being a technician of health procedures. This is an extreme example of the placebo effect. Many doctors actually feel that it is somehow wrong to make use of the placebo effect. It is unscientific therefore it is fraudulent. The patient of course doesn't care if the cancer has gone away as a result of a placebo effect. He is just damned pleased to be free of the cancer.

But science is of course central to what doctors do. We want them to be armed with the facts, with an understanding of the truth. Without that how could we trust them? But how can we discover the truth of any matter? I suppose we can say that what is true is what has been demonstrated to be true—demonstrated absolutely so that we can say it has been proved. Let us now look at this question of proof in a medical context.

The Concept of 'Proof' and the Clinical Trial

Proof, in the context of medicine, has a very specific meaning. It means that something has been demonstrated to be true in a double-blind clinical trial. This is a specialized experimental procedure that is the end result of a series of other clinical trials. It will help if we have an idea of the whole process. The double-blind clinical trial can, in theory, be applied to any practice or treatment. However, since most of these trials relate to the development of drugs, we will see how it is applied in this area.

Usually the initial idea is developed in the laboratory. A scientist has found a chemical agent that appears to be toxic to cancer cells in Petri dishes. This is tried out on rats or mice to see if the effect persists and also to see what dose levels might be appropriate for humans. This is the preliminary stage. Once a drug has passed this process, it is given a phase I clinical trial. About 20 humans are given the drug. They are terminal patients who have volunteered. The sole purpose of this trial is to determine dose levels. It is not expected that any of the phase I patients will actually survive.

The next step is to see which cancer tumours are likely to be the most responsive to this new drug. Different groups of about 20 patients each, all having the same type of cancer, are tested to determine what the response rate is. Does the drug work better for breast cancer or colon cancer or what? This is the objective of the phase II trials, which again are conducted on patients who have no further orthodox treatment options. They have been treated, the treatments have been ineffective and they are now considered terminal. If the results are acceptable then the process moves to the last phase.

The phase III clinical trial focuses on one particular drug regime and applies it to thousands of patients - all with the same cancer - over a period of time. These patients are in two groups: the experimental group - which receives the new drug - and the control group, which doesn't. Instead this second group gets a placebo which appears identical to the drug but which contains nothing of any known medical benefit. It is best if the patients don't know who is receiving the drug and who the placebo. This is known as a blind trial. The trial becomes double-blind when even the doctors dispensing the drug don't know who is getting the new drug and who isn't.

In very simplified terms this is the process that all new drugs go through in order to get approval for their general use. It is also the procedure used to assess the value of the drug. However, once a drug has been approved in this way, doctors will start using it in different unapproved ways. This is admitted by the authors of *Everyone's Guide to Cancer Therapy*, who write: "...many drug programs in standard use are not listed as 'approved'. They are used because experience with patients has shown they are effective."

This applies to about half of all current uses of anti-cancer drugs in North America. Where is the science there? The critic may ask. The treatment is based solely on 'experience' - and this experience must first have been obtained by applying the drug randomly in an empirical - let's see what happens if we do this - manner. Clearly at this stage, what they are doing may be rigorous, it may be analytical, rational and scientific but it is not based on proof or even evidence. (Furthermore, while this may very well be a valid way of proceeding, doctors are a little dishonest because they attack other people's use of 'experience' on the grounds that it is merely anecdotal evidence.)

For patients recommended to join a clinical trial, the key implications of all this has to be taken on board. First, they should understand that apart from the clinical trial, their doctors have run out of ideas about what to do with them. Their cancer is 'terminal' (I have put the word in inverted commas because some patients undoubtedly owe their lives to being classified as terminal. They have therefore been saved from grueling radiation and pointless chemotherapy and they have been free to look at the unorthodox treatments). Secondly, patients should remember that no standard chemotherapy regimes have established themselves for the vast majority of cancers over the last twenty to thirty years. They have not established themselves because they have not been adequately successful. Since the clinical trials of the past two to three decades have not been successful, the chances of a new drug being successful are also remote. But why not? If the general theory makes sense why haven't they been able to convert that into a practical cure? In short, how is it that rigorous scientific procedures are not producing the goods?

It is hard to imagine that there should be any problem with modern scientific research and the means it uses to advance knowledge and thereby, hopefully, help the development of cancer treatments. Unfortunately, a closer examination reveals fundamental flaws.

Flaw 1

Dr. Gerald Dermer, who published his views in his book, *The Immortal Cell*, pointed out one major flaw, a flaw so great it invalidates all laboratory-based cancer research. When most people talk about cancer they are, correctly, thinking about the tumours in people's bodies. These tumours consist of rapidly reproducing cells, which have specific characteristics depending on what kind of cancer they are. If a breast tumour spreads to the lung, the resulting tumour is still composed of cells that have the characteristics of the original breast cancer cell. However, when cancer researchers think of cancer cells, they are thinking of the cells they observe in Petri dishes in their laboratories, cells that derive from cell lines.

What Are Cell Lines?

In 1951, a woman by the name of Henrietta Lacks became a patient at Johns Hopkins Hospital in Baltimore, Maryland. She had cervical cancer and she eventually died of this disease. But her cells live on. Cells from her tumour were removed and placed in a Petri dish with a culture to feed them. All previous attempts at trying to establish living colonies of live cancer cells in a test tube environment had failed. Mrs. Lacks' cells successfully made the leap from existence in vivo (i.e., in the living body) to existence in vitro (i.e., in a Petri dish). 45 years on, these cells – known as the HeLa cell line - continue to reproduce and continue to be used in research.

It is not easy to create a cell line. Tumour cells will generally live a short time in a Petri dish before dying off. But very occasionally, something else happens. One or more cells display different behaviour. They keep on dividing and do not die off. The result is a cellular culture that has evolved to living in a Petri dish. It is effectively immortal. It just keeps on dividing. This is the birth of an ancestral line of cells all of which derive from this individual parent. This is known as a cell line.

It is the fact that these cells grow quickly and are standardized that makes them attractive. Scientists can then conduct daily experiments on them and publish monthly papers. (The rule of the research game is `publish or perish'.) Cell lines then provide an efficient source of cancer cells to work on. The alternative of using fresh tumour cells is less appealing. Malignant cells living in a tumour, just removed from a patient, are more difficult to work with. Real tumours do not just consist of malignant cancer cells. Various types of normal cells are also present. Another problem is that the tumour itself remains alive for only a short period of time, so it is difficult, if not impossible, to measure the effects of experimental procedures on these living cancer cells while they are alive. These difficulties slow the work and limit the kinds of experiments that can be performed. As a result, fewer papers are published by the even fewer scientists who study tumours than are published by the vast majority of researchers who study cell lines.

So using cell lines seems to make a lot of sense. However, in order for a cell to adapt to life in a Petri dish it has to change. It has to change at a very fundamental level. That change makes the cell very different from a normal tumour cell. It displays very different characteristics. Those changes completely invalidate the results gained from research on cell lines. The information gained applies to cell lines - but does not apply to real living cancer cells in real living tumours in real living people. This is a fundamental flaw.

How Different Are Cells In Vitro From Cells In Vivo?

Dermer points out a number of differences. First, cancer cells in the body are genetically stable. Their characteristics remain fixed. A breast cancer cell that metastasizes in the lung five years later will be identical to the original breast tumour cells. In contrast, cells in cell lines are notably unstable at the chromosomal level. The number and structure of the chromosomes in the cells change in a random way over time. Scientists working with such cells assume the genetic instability derives from the original breast cancer cell. Pathologists know that's not true.

Another important difference is that cancer tumour cells taken from the body have clear sex chromosomes; cells in cell lines commonly lose these sex chromosomes altogether.

A third difference is that when fresh from a living human, a breast cancer cell is very different from a lung cancer cell and is different from a rectal cancer cell. In cell lines they are indistinguishable. This fact led to an amusing, but costly, result. For a decade or more many scientists who believed they were studying prostate cancer cells or liver cancer cells or bladder tumour cells were actually studying the HeLa line of cells. What had happened was that contamination had occurred and the HeLa line is a particularly dominating cell line. If a cell from HeLa gets into a Petri dish containing cells from another line, it quickly colonises the dish and annihilates the other cells. This is what had happened at a number of institutes - and they never noticed. They didn't notice because there was nothing to distinguish one cell line from another. It was only when the weight of anomalous results became apparent over a period of a decade or more that the problem was discovered.

But it may be that this contamination continues. Who knows? Who cares? As long as papers are accepted for publication, nothing matters. Except that the possibility of a cure remains forever a mirage and people will continue to die of cancer in large numbers. Dermer's comment: "The cancer research community is almost devoid of people who understand human cancer."

Flaw 2

If we then turn to animal studies, there would appear to be a great deal we can learn from these. They are based on a simple premise that all mammals share a great many physical similarities and that what is true for one species has an increased chance of being true for another. The problem is that there are substances that are seriously toxic for rats that have no affect on mice. There are viruses that will devastate man, which are quite innocuous for other primates - AIDS being one. Malaria is another. Almost every ape and monkey has its own susceptibilities to a different type of parasite - but very few species share susceptibilities with each other. In short, what is true for rats and mice has no necessary predictive value for man.

This is a serious issue. Unfortunately, most of the attacks on animal experimentation have focused on the emotive issue of cruelty. While this an important issue it has rather left the public thinking that animal experiments are deeply unpleasant but nevertheless necessary if we are to properly test drugs to make sure they are safe for humans. The truth of the matter is that animal testing serves only two functions. It allows experimenters to produce research studies that can be published at a great rate — hough everyone knows that these studies are useless as far as the development of drugs for humans is concerned. Secondly, animal experiments allow pharmaceutical companies to claim that they have done due diligence. Useful insurance for when things don't turn out as expected.

Testing drugs on rats, rabbits, guinea pigs and even chimpanzees provides absolutely no valid data in relation to the effect and effectiveness of any drug on a human being. Thalidomide, for example, was widely tested on animals before being approved. It simply does not have the effect on any other of the normal experimental species that it has in humans. Because of this, Thalidomide remained on the market even when everyone knew it was to blame for the damage it caused. The animal data, unfortunately, refused to validate this conclusion.

The reverse situation is also a danger. If penicillin, for example, had been tested on animals before being made available to humans, its devastating effect on guinea pigs would very likely have stopped research on this drug in its tracks. In fact the development of penicillin was delayed because it was tested on rabbits and found to have no effect whatsoever. It is odd to think that if Fleming had not taken a chance and tested it on a human being, the development of antibiotics might never have occurred.

Cancer research focuses an enormous amount of attention on cancer tumours in rats and mice. But, to take one example, a breast cancer in a rat or mouse is a very different thing to a human breast cancer. The biochemical context of the mouse provides lessons that are only applicable to mice. We are spending vast sums of money looking into cancers of mice and rats; very little into understanding the real cancers of human beings.

Animal testing is an enormous scientific cul de sac. But the name of the game for most scientists is to knock out papers. That is the currency of their careers. As long as this fact remains unchallenged the pressure to persevere with animal experiments will continue.

Scientists and medical researchers need to get their houses in order. If they don't, we will all suffer.

Flaw 3

And then we come to the human phase of the double-blind clinical trial. Medical science has built a cult around this specific test. Nothing else can replace this experimental procedure and hope to achieve acceptance. The reason for its status is that it is assumed to provide results that are irrefutable. But is this true? Can we rely on the results gained from double-blind clinical trials?

To answer this question I am going to compare two trials that were conducted to see if vitamin C was an effective agent in the fight against cancer. One of these trials was not double blind, though it was a controlled study–that is an experimental group was compared with another group. This trial was conducted by the famous vitamin C protagonist, Linus Pauling. The other was a double-blind clinical trial conducted by Dr. Charles Moertel, a noted opponent of vitamin C - and of anything else that smacked of the unorthodox. These two trials came up with very different results. The former showed that vitamin C had the power in some cases to cure terminal cancer patients and for many others to extend their lives. The latter appeared to show that it didn't have this effect at all.

The Pauling trial was conducted in cooperation with Dr. Cameron at a Scottish hospital. Cameron, like Pauling believed in the efficacy of vitamin C. He could not therefore ethically refuse to give it to any of his patients for the purposes of a double or even a single blind clinical trial. However, he reasoned that the other doctors at the hospital did not share his views and since cancer patients were distributed to doctors on a random basis, he could simply compare his vitamin C taking patients with the patients being seen by other doctors. In addition, he also asked another doctor to compare his patients against 1,000 past patients who had already received treatment and who were matched by age and disease with his patients.

Because the trial was not double-blind, the normal demeanour of the presiding doctor ceased to be a factor. Both Cameron and Pauling made a point of encouraging and exhorting their patients to feel hopeful about the potential for a cure. The result was very positive. A small number of these patients were still alive ten years later compared with none from any of the other groups.

The Mayo Clinic trial was, however, a true double blind trial conducted by doctors sceptical of the value of the substance they were testing - and dealing with patients who had no idea what they were taking. So, in the Cameron-Pauling trial the patients became involved. They bought into it. Doctors and patients were partners fighting for the same cause. In the Mayo Clinic trial, on the other hand, the doctors remained aloof, patients remained passive. We can therefore assume that the patients in Cameron-Pauling's test felt better about their situation. This 'feeling good' response may have had a critical importance as we can see from the following.

It has been argued by Hans Selye in a book called *The Stress of Life* that the body goes through three stages in responding to stress:

1. Alarm Reaction
2. Stage of Resistance
3. Stage of Exhaustion.

Most terminal cancer patients are in the final stage. Stages one and three are typified by overproduction of corticoid hormones. Corticoids are stress hormones and they depress the immune system. This explains the link between stress and illness. They make the body feel bad to tell the mind that it is time to take a rest. In the Stage of Resistance, however, corticoid hormone levels are normal. Now, vitamin C has among its many functions the regulation of the production of corticoid hormones.

So, in Stages 1 and 3, the vitamin C intake may be used to produce corticoid hormones rather than going to the aid of the immune system. It may therefore have no protective value to the patient. Indeed it may hasten death. The only way to make it valuable is to force the patient back from the stage of exhaustion into the stage of resistance. This can be done only by psychological means: the emotions reflect the physiological status of the body and, similarly, the physiology reflects the emotional status of the body. Happy, involved people are resisting. Tired, frustrated, depersonalized people are exhausted. Hopeful patients live, hopeless patients die.

And so double-blind studies, that deliberately keep patients in a state of uncertainty and helplessness, that see patients as mechanical objects not as active biological beings, cannot detect the value of chemicals that to be effective depend on the patient's own psychological attitude. People are not things but clinical trials assume they are. That is the flaw.

Flaw 4

There are flaws of omission as well as of commission. The key flaw of omission is that the whole focus of attention is on the cancer cell - not on the person who has cancer. The biochemical terrain in which the cancer cell develops and lives is hardly considered. If we believe that the cancer cell arrives in the body as an act of God - and has no biochemical origin - this might make sense. This of course is one of the dividing lines between orthodox and unorthodox medicine. Orthodox researchers focus on the problem in its most reduced state - the chemicals in the cancer cell. Unorthodox researchers look at the whole body of the person who has cancer and seek to determine what is different about that body. As a result they have found that trace minerals and omega 3 oils, for example, are deficient in people with cancer. By restoring the balance of these chemicals they claim to obtain good results. But this is not mainstream research and so gets little funding.

To put this in another way, let us take an analogy. The modern scientific cancer researcher is in the position of a Martian who, seeking to understand the game of tennis, approaches the task by minutely analyzing a tennis ball. He may come up with fascinating information on the performance potential of the ball and the industrial processes required to produce it - but none of this will lead to any real understanding of tennis as a game.

Flaw 5

Clinical trials are a cumbersome method of progressing from one truth to another. Ultimately, they require vast resources of time, effort, people and money. If we were to depend entirely on clinical trials, scientific progress would slow to a snail's pace. Problems are subjected to a reductive analysis in order to ensure that all possible variations are controlled and that any result that emerges can have only one cause - and the means of action of that cause are clear. Requirements such as these enable science to take leave of common sense.

This point is well made by Harry Clayton, Director of Patient Experience and Public Involvement at the UK's National Health Service. He says: "The randomized control trial can only ever answer one question at a time. To get a good answer to that question it eliminates all the variables. The problem is that in real life our health care is surrounded by variables. Although (it) remains the gold standard for pure scientific research, it is not necessarily better at answering the questions of what works in the real world" (*Sunday Telegraph*, Oct 19, 2003).

There are also other requirements that have to be satisfied before and during the human phase clinical trials. One of these requirements is that the exact means by which the drug achieves its effect has to be described.

Some years ago, a report appeared in the newspaper to the effect that some scientists at the University of Texas had successful results using certain un-named Chinese herbs against cancer. The project director was quoted as saying, "We have something that works, or at least seems to. Our problem, however, is that we do not know why or how it works, and until we do, we cannot develop this as a modern medicine." So, these Chinese herbs are kept away from patients even though there is scientific evidence - based on scientifically controlled tests - that they work. Is this a sane way to go about the management of our health profession? As consumers of the work of doctors we are entitled to ask this question. Clearly the risk-benefit question is not being applied to the problem: what is the risk involved? What is the potential benefit? The search for truth has deposed the original goal (i.e., the search for cures).

If 'proof' is the only acceptable standard then there is no reason for assuming that smoking causes cancer. The association of tobacco with cancer is statistical. No proof of a classical nature exists - yet 99.99 percent of scientists believe that tobacco causes cancer. Thalidomide was withdrawn from the market - but there was never any proof that it caused birth defects - yet there is no doubt that thalidomide caused those defects. So when doctors and scientists insist on the necessity of proof, they are being seriously dishonest. Perhaps we need proof that the concept of 'proof ' is a useful concept.

Flaw 6

Even the results of clinical trials cannot be accepted uncritically. As Dr. Steven Rosenberg, Chief of Surgery at the U.S. National Cancer Institute says in his book *The Transformed Cell*: "I think as many as 30 percent of scientific articles contain results or conclusions that are wrong and are not reproducible. A good many more stretch their conclusions far beyond what their evidence will support."

Flaw 7

This is perhaps the biggest flaw of all. A method is successful only to the extent that it leads to a good result. The final flaw of the whole edifice of medical research as it applies to cancer is that it has not developed anything that remotely looks like a cure for cancer. I see it as a highway that is perfect in its proportions, made from the very best materials, precisely engineered in every way but which, in the end, leads nowhere - certainly nowhere very useful to you or me if we have cancer. Is a highway to nowhere a good highway?

But how is it possible that billions have been poured into research with no results? This frustration with the current state of research methods and objectives is shared by many others who have read widely around the subject. For decades now, the general public has been told that cancer research is getting closer and closer to finding a cure. But the sad fact is, despite the billions poured into cancer research, it is unlikely that there will be any sudden breakthrough in the near future. That is the simple truth but how is this possible?

A Question of Ethics

In addition to these flaws, there is growing concern about the ethical questions relating to clinical trials. Because of their size, large numbers of people need to be drawn into these trials. Many of these people are desperate. The existing protocols for most cancers are not curative so there is a constant search for new treatments. The result, as one leading British hospital, Addenbrooke's, explains on their website: "Many patients who have cancer will be asked by their doctors whether they wish to enter a clinical trial or clinical study." That is to say, the carrot of possibly benefiting from a new successful treatment is dangled in front of patients who are offered no other choice apart from the existing protocol of which the same hospital says: "...for many cancers, the commonly used treatments offer a smaller chance of cure than we would like."

As we shall see in the second half of this book, there are many very promising approaches to the treatment of cancer – but patients are not properly informed of these options (in fact, to the extent that doctors do discuss them it is simply to deride them). Instead patients are encouraged to take part in large scale trials in which they don't know which group they would prefer to be in: the experimental group which gets the new treatment (but which may be more dangerous, or less effective) or the control group which gets the 'standard treatment' which is admitted to be inadequate.

Given the size of trials and the expense of running them, many are now being subcontracted to specialist agencies who conduct their trials off-shore in third-world countries – especially India. Issues of whether patients are really given 'informed consent' have recently come to the fore. Many patients do not even know that they are taking part in a clinical trial. As one Indian patient explained: "We just sign because I believe the doctor takes the signature to help us. That's why I sign it...I don't know a lot about all these things. I am poor and I live in a small hut and I don't understand many things. The doctors are intelligent. They write the drugs for me so I have to take them accordingly" (quoted in a BBC report 22nd April 2006).

Control of Research by Drug Companies

How is it possible that after decades of research and billions of dollars spent, a cure for cancer still remains a mirage shimmering on the horizon? One answer that has been put forward is that pharmaceutical companies have no desire to find a cancer cure - unless it is a cure that they can profit from. It doesn't take too much cynicism to see the validity of this argument. If it became possible to turn the clock back 200 years when cancer incidence was in the region of 1-2 percent of the population - compared with 40-50 percent today - the pharmaceutical industry would suffer grievously. No industry will support the means by which its own profits will be threatened. On the contrary, it is very much in the pharmaceutical industry's interests to impede any such work. The most benign way in which this work can be impeded is simply to starve it of funds. In this way, interesting but unprofitable possibilities are sidelined in favour of research into patentable drugs.

Most cancer research is conducted under the umbrella of one or other of the pharmaceutical companies. They provide much of the financing and the means by which a drug can be developed. If their search for a pharmaceutical cure is fundamentally flawed then all the money put into this kind of research will be wasted. The pharmaceutical companies are very happy with the current situation as the profit margins on the anticancer drugs they are currently marketing are very fat. Cancer is good for profits.

Many people will consider such a conclusion to be overly cynical, even paranoid. And it may be that the truth is slightly more prosaic. One writer who knows the drug companies very well, who writes for *Fortune* and *The New York Times*, who according to the blurb on the back of the book in front of me 'has connections deep within the business and financial communities' and who has written in-depth studies on both drug companies and the FDA, is Fran Hawthorne. In her 2005 book, *Inside the FDA*, she discusses a cancer drug, Erbitox. In passing, she makes this comment: "Erbitox does not "cure" colon or rectal cancer. It did not even extend patients' lives significantly in clinical trials. Oncology drugs rarely do. But measured by the yardstick generally used for cancer treatments – how they shrink tumours – Erbotix seemed promising."

Read that statement again, very slowly. "Oncology drugs rarely do [extend patients' lives significantly.]"

It seems that the pharmaceutical companies have slightly but significantly changed the rules of the game. Success is measured in tumour shrinkage not cures. That's the word from as close to the horse's mouth as any of us will get.

If anyone should doubt the controlling influence of the drug companies on cancer research they should look at who is on the controlling boards of the largest cancer research institutions. Certainly, it is common for senior officers retiring from American regulatory bodies such as the FDA to be given directorships on the boards of the drug companies. So commercial interests and their influence in the halls of power must be accepted as one of the problems a new idea seeking acceptance must overcome.

The Question of Status

But money and commercial interests are not the only obstacles. Another obstacle relates to the status of the person demonstrating the proof or the institution where the work is undertaken.

We can see this clearly if we consider the following argument. It seems sensible to say that results emerge from effort and that therefore the greater the effort, the greater the results must be. If we follow this logic then we can also argue that the greater the amount of money we spend on a project, the greater the amount of effort that will result. So it follows that the places attracting the largest amounts of research money must be the places where the greatest scientific advances will take place. And since those institutes will also be where the scientists with the highest reputations will be employed, because their presence will attract research funding, we have a very tidy and comfortable picture of scientific eminence and scientific breakthrough walking hand-in-hand.

Conversely, of course, a poorly funded individual of little eminence cannot be expected to achieve much. Certainly, such a person cannot be expected to solve problems that elude the great minds supported by access to large resources.

As a result of this and related, possibly unconscious, prejudices, established bodies will not accept any 'proof' simply because it has been demonstrated. They will, instead, be highly suspicious of any evidence that does not come from certain accepted sources. This is quite explicitly stated by Dr. Robert Harris of the then Imperial Cancer Research Fund (now part of Cancer Research UK) who rejected the value of the work of Dr. Joseph Issels. "But you must remember that millions of pounds are spent on cancer research every year, and you can't expect anybody in this field to seriously believe that somewhere in Bavaria there is a man who's got hold of something which has escaped the rest of us."

Curiously, however, there does appear to be a consistent pattern where the poorly funded individual of little eminence, either through rigorously logical reasoning, great genius, bold experimentation, rare opportunity, simple accident or plain dumb luck, does indeed find the answer - often only to be ridiculed or ignored by the great.

The most famous case in medical history concerns a Dr. Ignaz Semmelweiss. It was in a Viennese hospital that Semmelweiss's attention was drawn to a curious fact. There were two maternity wards in the hospital. One was attended to by the doctors, and the other was attended by midwives. No doubt the wealthier ladies were favoured by the doctors while the poor had to make do with the midwives. Semmelweiss discovered that women patients who should have been clamouring for the attentions of the doctors were actually seeking to get admitted to the other ward. There were two possible reasons for this. Either it was a matter of modesty or ill-informed nonsense - as the Professors insisted - or the women's excuse that fewer women died in the midwives' ward had some merit.

To determine the matter Semmelweiss studied the records and observed the matter in person. The results were clear. The women patients were right. A great many of the women in the doctor's ward died of puerperal fever, relatively few from the midwives' ward did so. What could account for this strange fact? Semmelweiss saw that the main difference was that the midwives washed their hands while the doctors did not. Worse, the doctors when not attending to their patients were in the next room doing postmortems on patients who had died of puerperal fever to discover the cause of death.

Semmelweiss started to wash his hands and the result was that few of his patients subsequently got puerperal fever. He therefore theorised that some form of invisible contagion was the cause of the disease - at that time, 1848 - Pasteur had not yet convinced the world of the germ theory of disease. Puerperal fever was common. 40 percent of women giving birth in hospital got it and more than a third of those died.

Semmelweiss, sought to persuade the other doctors of his findings - but he was a young provincial Hungarian in the best hospital in Vienna. His views were derided. When he published the results of ten years of observation in 1861, he suffered vicious attacks on his integrity and was forced to flee Vienna. He eventually suffered a complete psychological breakdown and committed suicide.

Semmelweis couldn't prove he was right. He didn't understand why he was right. But he was right. The sad truth is that experts resist change.

And as a postscript to this story it should be noted that it was the women patients who saw the truth first. They saw the simple truth that medical experts refused to see for several decades longer.

Dr. Eugene Robin calls events of this type `iatro-epidemics' - large scale attacks on public health caused by doctors or the medical system itself. He lists radical mastectomy and tonsilectomy as two other common, unnecessary procedures which resulted and continue to result in unnecessary deaths. His calculation for 1984 was that 1 child in 10-15,000 died as a result of a tonsillectomy, and, as 400,000 such operations were conducted annually, the result would have been around 30 children dying needlessly each year in the USA.

Other doctors think radiotherapy will one day in the future also be seen as an iatrogenic episode. Biostatistician, Dr. Irwin Bross, who tried to investigate this question of whether radiation therapy was iatrogenic, had his research funding cut off by the National Cancer Institute. Bross wrote: "It is almost impossible to get `peer review' that will accept a study of iatrogenic disease...For

30 years radiotherapists in this country have been engaged in massive malpractice - which is something a doctor will not say about another doctor" (quoted in Moss, 1982).

The Problem of Conformity

So, why is it that simple evident truths - or interesting possibilities - are so hard for the medical profession to accept?

One answer is conformity. Medical researchers conform to the same goal - to seek chemotherapeutic agents that will kill cancer (they test out 50,000 substances each year); they conform to the same method - the use of cancer cells that reproduce themselves in Petri dishes; they conform in their funding sources - in America these must be approved by the National Cancer Institute and in Britain by the Medical Research Council. These deciding bodies are run by groups of respected scientists who have a shared vision of how the goal of cancer cure will be achieved. Anyone who does not share that goal will not get funding. Indeed, as Gerald Dermer discovered, they will be cold-shouldered. In this way an entire industry quickly develops a single perception.

Most cancer researchers wish to advance in their chosen careers. They wish to go from working as part of a team, to leading a team to heading an institute. To do this they need to publish results. In order to publish results they must persuade their mentors to add their names to their research - only the previously published get subsequently published. Their articles must also receive the go ahead from colleagues under the 'peer-review' system. So, they need to know the right people, they need to say the right things. If there are any fundamental flaws in fundamental assumptions, perceptions or methods of research then these flaws will invalidate the work of the entire industry. The laws of conformity will ensure that everyone is wrong.

If this is true, then the individual working far from these centres and uncluttered by a ruling theoretical orthodoxy is the one most likely to come up with something interesting, something that works, something true. However, this scientist would not find it easy to inform the world about his discovery because the same people who fund science are those that also validate and publish its results. New discoveries that are foreign to normal practice tend to be ignored or sidelined. Peer-review journals will not publish papers that go against the prevailing ethos. Conferences will not accept such papers. Research-funding bodies will not provide the necessary funds to continue the work. So the new discovery has to wait in the wings for unconscionable periods of time before it gets accepted - if it ever does. If the researcher attempts to go public by announcing the discovery to the world at large, he or she is vilified.

Another force working against the development of new interesting ideas is that institutions are highly competitive. If the idea has emerged from a rival institution there will be a natural attempt to discredit it. If that doesn't work then it must somehow be taken over. Current research work is a highly prized secret that must not be revealed to the outside world. Failures are buried. Successes applauded unduly.

The Authoritarian Personality

The structure of the scientific and medical professions is very hierarchical giving great power and authority to those at the top and requiring submissiveness from those below. At the bottom is the patient. Since doctors and scientists live and thrive in professions that are highly hierarchical and authoritarian we must assume that they feel comfortable in such a structure. Science writer Richard Milton thinks this is the case. He believes that scientists with authoritarian personalities will tend to do better in the scientific world than scientists with democratic personalities.

He quotes the case of a postgraduate student in the 1980s seeking to get support from his professor for permission to study hypnosis. The professor refused to allow it on the grounds that it was not a respectable field for research. It was not respectable because there was no serious literature, and there was no serious literature because no one had done any research, and no one had done any research because it was not a respectable field of research. Joseph Heller coined the term Catch-22 to define this form of circular argument. In this case, a potentially serious study of a subject about which little is known is starved of funds and professional support because it contravenes conventional attitudes.

Compare this with the following words from Professor John Huizenga: "It is seldom, if ever, true that it is advantageous in science to move into a new discipline without a thorough foundation in the basics of that field."

Huizenga appears to be saying that we should study only what we already understand, and we should ignore what we don't understand. This is troubling because, at the time he made this statement, Professor Huizenga was co-chairman of a committee set up to investigate whether funds should be directed into new areas of research. Clearly, no new area of research can ever satisfy the requirements required to obtain funding.

Doctors, and even entire medical establishments, have a history of allying themselves with the most authoritarian political structures within any given society. This tendency is also clear in the practice of their profession. The doctor and the surgeon like to be in charge. They don't like patients who do not cooperate immediately. As Dr. Steven Rosenberg says: "Too many doctors are comfortable dealing with patients only when they can assume an air of unquestioned authority. Surgeons tend to be particularly authoritative." Knowing this, we can see how a profession can persevere for 25-30 years with a treatment like chemotherapy that they know doesn't work for the majority of cancers, and that they also know will kill a significant number of their patients.

Some research has been done on medical students and their attitude to authority. This research has found that first and second year medical students have a strong sense of ethical sensitivity but that this deteriorates as they progress through the next three years of their medical studies. Obviously, the doctors that most patients first see, their GPs, have to a certain extent opted out of this hierarchical world but only at the cost of being permanently last in the medical pecking order. The views of a GP carry no weight whatsoever in the medical field.

So...?

I will end this section with the following observation: "A solution to cancer would mean the termination of research programs, the obsolescence of skills, the end of dreams of personal glory. Triumph over cancer would dry up contributions to self-perpetuating charities....It would mortally threaten the present clinical establishments by rendering obsolete the expensive surgical, radiological and chemotherapeutic treatments in which so much money, training and equipment is invested.... The new therapy must be disbelieved, denied, discouraged and disallowed at all costs, regardless of actual testing results, and preferably without any testing at all." - Robert Houston and Gary Null

And lastly, those who still believe that 'scientific research' is an honest enterprise should look at the blog of Dr. Aubrey Blumsohn at www.scientific-misconduct.blogspot.com.

The Politics of Cancer

The medical profession is socially and politically powerful. The scientific community is entrenched, competitive and defensive. The drug companies wield a great deal of financial clout. Together they are a formidable social force.

A war has waged in America for several decades between this orthodox establishment, on the one side, and proponents of alternative or complementary medicines on the other. The details of the war are far too long and complex to go into in this book. Anyone seeking a good account of its impact in the U.S. should read *The Cancer Industry* by Ralph Moss, very much an insider's account, and for the way the war is being waged (with the full backing of the national 'quality' press).

One of the most extreme – even rabid – organizations hostile to alternative medicine is the Campaign Against Health Fraud, who consider themselves to be 'quackbusters'. They seek every opportunity to attack alternative treatments seeking always to pin the label 'unproven' on them.

For the non-aligned spectator, this is unedifying – and indeed worrying. If the general public, through charitable donations and taxes, are supporting the major cancer research charities, then surely they have a right to expect these charities to engage in testing all the unpatentable ideas that might show anti-cancer activity. Yet these charities appear to be locked into a dance with the pharmaceutical companies. If big pharmaceutical companies can make profits from anti-cancer drugs, surely cancer research charities, at the very least, can benefit from royalties on any patentable drug they find effective and at the same time plough these surplus sums into looking at vitamin C, colloidal silver, herbs and indeed anything else that comes along. It seems to me that the onus for doing basic research belongs to that very medical/scientific establishment that is rejecting alternative therapies until they are proven.

Whether or not the Campaign for Health Fraud is itself responsible, the war against alternative thought has intensified in recent years. The means used are the smear campaign and outright harassment. Harassment of alternative practitioners or of anyone associated with unorthodox ideas has also occurred. In the US, doctors who mention vitamins in a positive way are in danger of losing their license to practice.

In the USA, the FDA frequently raids alternative clinics. This is why most alternative therapy clinics have had to move to the relative freedom of Mexico. There they cluster in Tijuana, just across the border. For a list of these clinics see www.cancure.org, www.CancerControlSociety.com, and www.ThirdOpinionGuide.com.

Then there is the manipulation by the medical authorities of our legal freedoms. Over the last decade or more, there have been several attempts in the USA and Europe to limit access to high-dose vitamin supplements by changing the law. Constant vigilance is required to ensure some sneaky piece of legislation is not passed through on the nod (most senators and congressmen are far too busy to read and analyze all the legislation they are required to vote on). The politics of medicine are as vicious as politics in any other arena of endeavour.

'Unproven Therapies'

One of the key concepts in the dispute between orthodox medicine and alternative medicine is the concept of 'proof'. The idea is generally put forward that orthodox methods of treating cancer are `proven' methods and that all other methods are 'unproven'. We have already seen that most orthodox methods are unproven by any standard. There is a widespread medical myth — that, in contrast to complementary therapies, conventional therapies are all evidence-based, founded on a bed rock of sound science. But even the *British Medical Journal's* website Clinical Evidence (www.clinicalevidence.com) has reported that, of the 2,404 treatments they have surveyed, only 15 percent are rated as beneficial, while 47 percent are of unknown effectiveness.

However, the term `unproven therapies' is used by the American Cancer Society (ACS) to label methods of treatment which it has decided to oppose. This term is used in much the same way that the word `Communist' was used by Senator McCarthy in the 1950s. It is used as a slur.

'Unproven' of course means simply that no proof has been obtained. It does not mean that a therapy's effectiveness has been disproved. Yet many writers who put forward the establishment view appear to think it does. They also confuse the words `evidence' and `proof'. We may accept that there are very hard standards that have to be satisfied before proof is established - but on the way to proof we collect evidence. We collect this evidence through tests. These tests must follow accepted scientific procedures. It is common therefore to have scientific evidence without necessarily having scientific proof.

There is something curious and indeed unacceptable about the speed with which therapies are rejected. Why are they being rejected? What is the agenda of the people rejecting them? These are valid questions which need to be answered. Yet there appears to be very little desire among the hundreds of thousands of scientists working in the field of cancer research and medical doctors working in the leading hospitals of North America and Europe, to demand an answer or to challenge these rejections. One former official of the American Cancer Society, Pat McGrady, Sr. has written: "[The American cancer establishment] has turned the terror of [cancer] to its own ends in seeking more and more contributions from a frightened public and appropriations from a concerned Congress. Still, undismayed by the futility of funds dumped into the bottomless pit of its 'proven' methods, it remains adamant in refusing to investigate 'unproven' methods."

Every book written from a staunchly orthodox stance contains warnings to patients that they should not entertain any thoughts of going down the route of 'unproven' therapies.

"Keep in mind that accepted medical treatment for your cancer is the best scientifically tested treatment....The best way to determine whether a treatment is proven or unproven is to ask your family doctor. Doctors rely on scientific proof before they use a treatment. Unproven methods lack such proof." So says an American Cancer Society pamphlet. Other warnings suggest that 'unproven' methods can cause harm either directly or indirectly, by seducing patients from proper treatments. Dr. Friedberg is so concerned to dissuade the potentially errant patient that he produces the ultimate argument.

"[E]ven if the "treatments" are not in themselves harmful, a serious consequence of their use, and one that is insufficiently recognized by cancer patients and their families, is that those who use them are wasting valuable time" (Friedberg, 1992).

They are, he goes on to say, wasting time that should be better used in continuing 'accepted' forms of cancer treatment but also, more importantly, time that should be spent getting used to dying. Clearly Dr. Friedberg assumes that unproven remedies are necessarily ineffective. This is, as we have seen, an unscientific position to take.

The problem is that by having a list of unproven therapies, and by using this list as a blacklist to stop further funding, we have a self-fulfilling prophecy. They are unproven because there is   no institutional will to seek proof. There is, instead, an institutional will to prevent such proof being established. Disproof is assumed. That is one of the rules of the game. Another rule is that anyone who proposes or uses an unorthodox approach has to be slandered as a 'quack' and/or a 'charlatan'.

Underlying this game of name calling is a profoundly false assumption. It is one thing to say that a doctor needs scientific proof that a drug is effective - a point that is itself debatable - It is quite another thing to demand this of patients. Patients don't need proof - not when the price of proof is so high. Anecdotal evidence is quite sufficient for most aspects of life. If Mr. Brown took substance X and was cured and Mrs. Smith took substance X and was cured of the same thing,   you can bet your bottom dollar I also will try substance X the next time the need arises. I wouldn't think of waiting thirty or a hundred years for science to get its act together to prove that it worked. To repeat a point I made earlier, patients perhaps need proof that 'proof' itself is a valid validating concept.

Are We Missing Opportunities?

One of the first examples of a well conducted controlled test was conducted, in 1747, on twelve patients suffering from scurvy. Dr. James Lind placed all of them on the same diet except for one item - the supposed remedies that he was testing: citrus fruits, cider, vinegar, sea water, a mixture of drugs. He gave each of these remedies to two patients. At the end of six days the two who had been given citrus fruits were well, while the others were still ill. Lind published these results in 1753. This was not of course a double blind trial. Both Lind and the sailors knew exactly what they were receiving but as a trial it was rational, rigorously carried out and easily repeatable. It therefore has all the hallmarks of classical scientific testing. It is now hailed as the moment the cause of, and cure for, scurvy was established beyond doubt.

Yet, as we have just seen, such a test today would carry little weight with the elders of the accrediting committees that govern the practice of medical science. First the elders would note that it was a lowly and insignificant naval doctor who had done the experiment and simply ignore it on that ground alone. If however, they were feeling generous, they might admit the result was interesting but certainly not conclusive. It does not establish proof, once and for all, that lemons cure scurvy. Under current protocols, many more years of testing would be required to establish such proof. Scientists would need to know why lemons cured scurvy. The active ingredient would have to be isolated and then tested on cells in laboratories, in animal studies and then experimentally in human trials using double blind procedures. This is where science and common sense start to follow different roads. All this time, the doctors would be warning patients not to take any form of unproven treatment - like lemons - for their scurvy.

As it happened, Dr. Lind's demonstration that the answer to scurvy lay in the lemon was not accepted despite its elegance. On the contrary, since fresh fruits - and fresh fruit juices – were expensive there were pressures on ship owners and the established authorities not to accept the results. However, eventually, in 1795, over 40 years after Lind published his results, the British Admiralty ordered that a daily ration of fresh lime juice be given to all hands. As a result, scurvy disappeared from the Royal Navy. The merchant navy, however, was under the control of the Board of Trade. It wasn't until 1865, a full 120 years after the original experiment, that the Board of Trade also passed its own lime-juice regulations.

Putting It All Together

We can now appreciate what Linus Pauling meant when he suggested that there is a fundamental, organizational blindness that prevents science and medicine developing except along narrow, well-trodden, safe pathways through the confusing forests of reality. "The National Cancer Institute is not operated in a way as to favor the discovery of new methods of controlling cancer...In my opinion the NCI does not know how to carry on research nor how to recognize a new idea."

This, then, is the scientific research that is eating most of the money donated to cancer research. This is the research that despite an expenditure of thousands of millions of pounds has not resulted in any fundamental advance in cancer treatment for the last 20 years.

"It is gradually dawning on the donors that for the past 20 years practical benefits have not followed (from medical research). During that time there have been no substantial improvements in morbidity or mortality from major disease that can be attributed to public funding of medical research" (Dr. David Horrobin, 1982, quoted by Milton, 1994).

But one can also see the problem from the orthodox side. If surgery, radiation and chemotherapy are to be set aside, what can the doctor do to help the cancer patient? The answer appears to be nothing - especially if that doctor rejects all unorthodox approaches. How could the medical establishment possibly address the world and say: we have nothing in our techno-pharmaceutical armoury that is truly effective against cancer? The uproar would be deafening. The courts would overflow with lawsuits. We can see that such a situation is impossible. No establishment in its right mind would voluntarily bring such a response down on its own head. In brief, no matter how damaging and ineffective conventional treatments may be, the orthodox medical practitioner must persevere in directing patients down this path. He must do this, or change his specialty or leave the profession.

All of this is simple logic. From this it follows that the fact that a treatment is offered by a consultant in a leading cancer institute does not in any way indicate that it is necessarily effective. The patient must always ask for proof or evidence of effectiveness. Usually, as with chemotherapy trials, the result may or may not indicate increased survival - by a week or a month, by 2 percent or 4 percent. This is not worth fighting for if the previous six months are full of suffering.

If doctors are not going to change standard medical practice, then patients must. Every single one of us has the right to choose the therapy we wish for ourselves based on our own understanding of the facts and awareness of our needs, fears, desires and even prejudices.

But if patients are to reject one form of treatment they must have some idea of the options. And there are options: in fact there is a dizzying array of options. Many promise exciting results. For the patient with courage the picture is not bleak. I describe these possibilities in the second half of this book.

Summing Up

It is clear from the preceding discussion of orthodox approaches to cancer that on the whole, with about a dozen notable exceptions, chemotherapy is useless and extremely damaging. Surgery and radiation can claim to be more successful, perhaps, but they too can be very damaging, and they too may have results that are seriously negative.

Last year, more than one million Americans were diagnosed with cancer and probably the same number of Europeans. With or without treatment, these people will not die immediately. Many will undergo orthodox treatments and feel saved when the cancer appears to have gone. For some of these people the cancer will never return but for most it will come back. They will undergo further treatment and again, for some, this treatment may be successful in the long term. There are therefore going to be many millions of people who will swear that their cancer has been cured by orthodox means—and that therefore this is the only sensible way to proceed. That is of course for each person to decide but, as we shall see in the remainder of this book, there are many 'alternative' or 'complementary' approaches that also claim to be curative without any of the damaging side effects.

These approaches have almost all been attacked as 'unproven' - but almost never as being disproved — but survey after survey has shown that patients are moving very strongly in that direction. The rest of this book looks at all the many different approaches that go under the heading of alternative or complementary therapy.

MEDICINE AND MONEY

Our image of the doctor is an amalgam of *ER*'s frenetic interns desperately dealing with casualty victims and the calm competence of their family doctor or a senior consultant. Whatever the personal flaws of the individual, it's generally a picture of solid professionalism. But this image has in recent years come under strong attack – and the fiercest critics are themselves distinguished doctors, like Jerome Kassirer M.D. whose credits are hard to fault. He is Distinguished Professor at Tufts University School of Medicine, Adjunct Professor at Yale University School of Medicine and was for eight years Editor-in-Chief of the *New England Journal of Medicine*. His 2005 book, *On The Take*, has the following subtitle: "How Medicine's Complicity with Big Business Can Endanger Your Health." Another critic is Marcia Angell, M.D., who is on the faculty of Harvard University School of Medicine and who is another former editor of the *New England Journal of Medicine*. Her 2004 book, *The Truth About the Drug Companies*, has the subtitle: "How They Deceive Us and What To Do About It".

These books are blunt and trenchant in their attack on the tight embrace of medicine and the pharmaceutical companies. These and other critics make the following points:

1. Doctors make a lot of money from complex incentive schemes designed to reward them for prescribing particular drugs. This is so endemic it constitutes a serious conflict of interest that negatively affects their relationship with their patients. This conflict need not be at the level of the individual doctor but at the level of the medical institution as a whole. Patients are directed to protocols that benefit pharmaceutical companies. (For cancer patients going to specialist cancer clinics, this spectre is particularly frightening.)

2. Pharmaceutical companies provide agreeable doctors with all-expenses-paid 'conferences' in exotic locations and pay large consulting fees . Often the drug companies write up the research findings on their own drugs and then go looking for doctors to put their names to the research. There is no shortage of doctors willing to engage in this practice. (*The Lancet* recently expressed concerns at this practice, suggesting that as many as half the articles they published were not in fact written by the person whose name appeared on them.) This means that the higher up the medical ladder a doctor goes, the more likely he or she is to be compromised.

3. Most continuing medical education is funded by the drug companies and is effectively a covert marketing strategy to promote their drugs. Studies show that doctors' prescription behaviour is influenced.

4. Most medical charities and patient activist groups receive a great deal if not most of their funding from pharmaceutical companies or companies with a potential interest, and this undoubtedly influences their behaviour.

To take one obvious example: The American Council of Science and Health, which bills itself as "a consumer education organization concerned with issues related to food, nutrition, chemicals, pharmaceuticals, lifestyle, the environment and health" is financed mainly by, as one critic puts it, 'corporations with specific and direct interest in ACSH's chosen battles'. Since its creation in 1978, it has stated:

a) That there is no proven link between heart disease and a diet high in fat and cholesterol.

b) That there is no truth that saccharin is potentially carcinogenic. This research was financed by Coca-Cola, Pepsi, NutraSweet and the National Soft Drink Association

c) That Bovine Growth Hormone is perfectly safe, despite clear evidence that it substantially increases the IGF-1 (Insulin Growth Factor) content. IGF-1 is known to be a risk factor in breast and prostate cancer.

5. Almost all research on any drug is done by doctors and scientists who are paid by the Pharmaceutical companies who tie those researchers to contracts that prevent them from making public any negative findings – even where patients' lives are placed at risk. Negative findings are routinely hidden. Pharmaceutical companies also routinely request changes to results or changes of wording.

6. Universities have been known to fire faculty who raise issues about drugs or research that conflict with the views of pharmaceutical companies. University research funding is highly dependent on maintaining good relations with the pharmaceutical companies. When truth is the victim, who can we trust?

7. Many supposedly objective research studies published in major peer-reviewed medical journals are reviewed by peers who themselves have financial interests in the drug companies whose drug is being reviewed. As we have already noted, often the drug companies write the research on their own drugs and then go looking for doctors to put their names to the research. There is no shortage of doctors willing to engage in this practice.

Section 3: Complementary & Alternative Approaches

Introduction

The term 'complementary/alternative therapies' (CAM) covers a wide range of approaches and ideas. Most, but not all, of these therapies take as a central concept the idea that cancer is a disease of the whole body and that the tumour is simply a symptom. After all, we don't treat measles by cutting off every itchy red spot on the body. Why do we think cutting out tumours is going to work any better? The cause of measles is recognized to be a virus – when the virus has run its course the symptoms disappear. Unfortunately, cancer is usually not self-limiting in the way measles is. Nevertheless the same logic applies. If we can find the cause of cancer and can eliminate it in some way, the symptom (ie the tumour) will disappear of its own accord. To the extent that these approaches concentrate on the whole body, they are referred to as 'holistic' (or sometimes 'wholistic'). However, as we shall see, not all 'alternative' approaches are holistic.

These treatments may be used either as a truly alternative treatment that completely replaces orthodox treatment or in addition to orthodox treatment - in which case they will tend to be referred to as 'complementary therapies'. It is now also common to refer to this area of medicine as CAM (Complementary/Alternative Medicine).

Nutrition is central to the alternative approach. Many people find it difficult to comprehend that food can be more powerful than chemotherapy drugs. We have already seen in the previous section the almost total failure of chemotherapy to adequately control the vast majority of cancers. If chemotherapy is so unsuccessful, how can a simple diet be successful? For me, the following children's story provides a useful metaphor. Winter and Summer were arguing as to which was most powerful. Finally, they decide on a test. Which of them can force a man to take off his coat? Winter goes first and lashes the man with searing winds and driving rain – all to no avail. The man hugs his coat tightly too him. The stronger the wind the more he clutches to his coat. In the end Winter fails and it is Summer's opportunity. Summer brings out the warm sun and soon the man is so hot he gladly takes off his coat. Summer wins this contest – not by attacking the man with any weapons but simply by creating an environment that is conducive to the result it wants.

The story of beri beri, the disease that is now known to be caused by vitamin B1 (thiamine) deficiency, is instructive. It was a serious life-threatening disease with multiple manifestations: wasting away, paralysis, heart disease and so on. For decades it existed in epidemic proportions, causing vast numbers – millions - of people to die horribly and painfully. It was thought to be bacterial in nature, and many different drugs were tried out. Eventually the true cause was discovered – the lack of a single food nutrient. Given the increasing impoverishment of our own food supplies, it would be no surprise if cancer was also found to be caused by specific nutrient deficiencies.

Sadly, over 95 percent of cancer patients do not even think of taking the alternative route until they have been told they are terminal by their mainstream oncologist – and he hangs on to them for as long as he can, trying out two or even three courses of chemotherapy before he allows them to go. Having neglected to research this area, largely because they have taken on their doctor's prejudices against the alternative approaches, they will often try the wrong things, or do too little – and of course it is very, very late.

Before continuing we need to confront one of the false assumptions that many cancer patients have – that the world of cancer therapy is divided into two areas. One is science based and is the preserve of doctors and organized medicine. The other is a lot of airy-fairy, New Age nonsense that sounds fine but is really just pie in the sky.

This is a very false image. The truth is that the alternative approaches almost certainly have more good science on their side than organized medicine. Many of the supplements, chemicals, therapies and approaches described in the following pages are based on hard research by a wide array of scientific researchers. The truth is that we are in the midst of a scientific revolution - but the old guard and the old institutions need to die out before the new ideas can be more widely accepted. Until that time they remain beyond the pale. The story of how science progresses is well told in a classic text, Thomas Kuhn's *The Structure of Scientific Revolutions*. It would be nice if science progressed in a simple rational way but it doesn't. Instead, as Kuhn demonstrates, old concepts ('paradigms' is the word he uses) do not go gently. Egos, inertia, institutional reputations and the pursuit of profits all impede the progress of knowledge. That is very much the situation we find ourselves in today with regard to alternative approaches. It is not a stable state of affairs and the dynamic is very much powering the development of alternative therapies, formulas and technologies. And there is a continual state of seepage across the line from alternative into mainstream medicine.

The problem is that there are few organized channels that lead from these researchers to you through the systems of organized medicine. As a patient you will meet surgeons (who believe in surgery), oncologists (who generally speaking are confined to the use of chemotherapeutic drugs unless the hospital is equipped to provide other forms of treatment) or radiologists (who use machines that deliver ionizing radiation). There is no general cancer doctor who has knowledge of diets, vitamins or any other of the following suggestions. So, valid though they may be, you will not hear of them through the normal channels.

And for those of you who have a powerful respect for doctors, you might wish to consider the following. In 1973, doctors in Israel went on strike for a month – and the number of funerals dropped by 50 percent over the same period. Coincidence? No. In 1976, in Columbia, a doctor's strike led to a 38 percent drop in the death rate. Again, in 1978 British doctors went on strike – and funerals dropped by 40 percent. Think about it. These statistics are well known to the medical profession.

And here is the comment of a retired doctor, Alan Greenberg:

"In almost every area except for treatment of acute trauma, mainstream medicine is a gigantic fraud. Why do I believe this? I practiced medicine for about 40 years in the areas of neurology and psychiatry. I also studied biochemistry for several years under a National Science Foundation fellowship. I saw people improve with better nutrition and healthier lifestyles, but not with the use of drugs. Treatments sanctioned by mainstream medicine - such as drugs, surgery and radiation - target symptoms, not the underlying causes. In fact, not a single cure for a major degenerative disease has been accomplished in the past 100 years. Recent research on mitochondrial function shows that almost without exception, synthetic drugs are toxic to mitochondria and lead to impaired ATP synthesis, free radical formation, cytokine release with resultant chronic inflammation, tissue damage, chronic fatigue and degenerative disease.

If you look carefully, you will see that Allopathic Medicine has systematically suppressed every cure for degenerative disease and particularly for cancer since the early part of the 20th century. Check out www.williamfkoch.com and Barry Lynes' book, "The Cancer Cure That Worked". In the case of cervical cancer, it has been known since about 1938 that abnormal Pap smears are associated with folic acid deficiency and that treatment with folic acid causes reversion of the Pap smear to normal. Withholding folic acid is known to cause progression to outright malignancy. Yet women with abnormal Pap smears are almost never prescribed folic acid. It has been known for many years that Vitamin D significantly reduces the risk and incidence of cancer as well as many other problems such as autoimmune disorders, heart disease and hypertension. Yet doctors in prestigious medical institutions regularly write articles advocating sun avoidance and the use of sunblockers, which are actually carcinogenic. Prozac and other antidepressant drugs are regularly prescribed for depression although there is clear evidence that they increase the risk of suicide because long-term use causes the depletion of serotonin in the CNS and blood platelets. Mercury is known to be highly toxic to the body and a vast body of scientific research confirms the toxicity of amalgam fillings (50 percent mercury), yet the American Dental Association persists in claiming that amalgams are safe and the AMA and related organizations support this position. It is known that toxic metals are responsible for 82 percent of degenerative diseases (WHO Report on Toxic Metals, Florence, Italy 1974) yet chelation is not taught in medical schools and state medical boards have systematically attempted to suppress its use.

Most people in this country still have the expectation that their physician will have the ability to cure whatever ails them, but they are sadly mistaken. Although the vast majority of physicians are dedicated and conscientious, they lack the knowledge and training to cure any disease and because of the enormous pressures on their time, are unable to do the independent library research needed to find real solutions. Many are either brain-washed to believe they already have the answers or are intimidated by the medical establishment, which strongly discourages independent thinking. The use of nutrients, herbs and a host of alternative treatments is much safer and generally more effective than mainstream treatments, but their use is strongly condemned by the medical establishment. In short, our mainstream medical system is hopelessly inept and/or corrupt. The treatment of cancer and degenerative diseases is a national scandal. The sooner you learn this, the better off you will be." (Personal communication)

This is a strong statement of an opinion that is rarely given room in the mass media. It demonstrates that there is a case for being cautious with mainstream medicine and that looking at diet, vitamins, herbs and so on makes a lot of sense.

But now, let's return to the question of alternative approaches to cancer. The good news is that there can be little doubt that people have been cured, or had their life extended, or had the quality of their lives improved using many, if not all, of these methods either on their own or in combination with each other. What is hotly debated is whether or not any of these methods can claim to consistently cure cancer. Certainly, many of these approaches do claim not only consistency but an extraordinary level of effectiveness. Some claim to be able to cure over 70 percent of patients who have been dismissed by mainstream medicine as incurable – and have evidence of a sort to support these claims. However, it should also be said that since this consistency is absent from mainstream methods, a lack of proof of consistency is not a fatal criticism.

Few of these therapies have been clinically tested to any great extent, so none of them can claim to have 'proof', but the anecdotal evidence that supports them is often very persuasive.

And although many of them have been put forward by orthodox medical practitioners or biochemists, people who espouse these therapies are often labeled 'quacks' or 'charlatans' by ultra-orthodox critics. These are emotive terms and largely meaningless. The war of medical philosophies deserves a more honest debate than it tends to get.

Choosing the alternative path to recovery and wellness is an act of faith. But then again so is the decision to have radiation, chemotherapy and surgery. There are no studies that directly compare surgery to the grape diet and there never will be. The question nevertheless remains: How can one choose these alternative therapies (if one wishes to) over orthodox approaches?

Obviously it is for each person to weigh up the pros and cons for him-or-herself. On the one hand, you have therapies that are supported by the doctors who are self-assured and insistent that their way is best and supported, they say, by science. On the negative side, we can see that all is not well in the halls of medicine and the influence of the pharmaceutical companies has meant that more and more people are choosing to question the degree of trust they wish to place in their doctor. Then too there is the question of the damage to the body that these orthodox treatments inflict–despite which, in the case of many, indeed most, cancers, there is often a less than fifty percent chance of success.

So the decision to at least consider the alternative approaches is a sensible one. And as you will see, the promise they hold out is a cure that is lasting, a cure that looks at causes of cancer, a cure that doesn't cost an arm and a leg (or a lung or a breast) and most importantly a cure that isn't horrendously toxic.

In my view, it is valid to approach these therapies on the basis of a risk-benefit analysis. If the risk appears to be low and the potential benefit high then there is nothing to lose from following a particular course of treatment. Belief is certainly not a requirement. Doctors who insist that proof of value must precede the use of any mode of treatment utterly miss the point. As long as there is no proof that a particular therapy is of absolutely no value - and negative proofs are harder to arrive at than positive proofs - and as long as there is little or no danger, then any course of action that makes sense (to you) should be followed - as long as you accept responsibility for yourself. That is all that is required.

For the cancer patient, alternative therapies offer the prospect of cure without the fearful damage that often accompanies mainstream methods; while complementary use of these therapies offers the promise of some lessening of the damaging effects of orthodox treatments.

A Warning

However, a word of warning is necessary. Since the first edition of this book was published, the internet has exploded. This has the benefit of allowing us easy access to many valuable and useful sources of information and products. But there is a downside. The freedom of the internet has allowed many unscrupulous people to make claims for products that are wholly spurious and to sell these products through websites and multi-level marketing schemes that are in my opinion bordering on the unethical. Sometimes, products are marketed as containing X, Y and Z when they do not. Testimonials can be invented. Copying of information from one site to another is another vice of the medium. You may find ten sites all claiming that something works – and then you see that they all use exactly the same wording! It is not wise to accept information at face value. It is also important, when buying herbs or supplements, to deal with companies that are reputable. Time spent on reading around a subject is never wasted. There are many good internet suppliers of herbs. Also, it should be noted that some common supplements (e.g., calcium) for which big claims are made by some, are not supported by other evidence. Do not assume that anything alternative must be OK.

The profit motive is not confined to the pharmaceutical companies whose profit margins are renowned for being outrageous. There are also self-proclaimed healers who prey on the vulnerabilities of the desperate. One example that came to my attention related to a young British woman whose therapist was asking £1,000 (US$1,800) to obtain injectable ginseng from China.

When dealing with alternative remedies, it is sensible to do as much research as possible. You should also consider the following advice:

1. Do not inject anything herbal into the bloodstream unless your own independent researches suggest this will be all right. There can be – and have been – fatal consequences.

2. Do not be suckered into paying out large sums of money for specific treatments unless you feel that you are going to get value for money and something of well attested benefit. Many people, I believe, have been cured of their cancer for no more than the cost of their groceries. One man calculates that his cure for cancer costs him less than US$1 a day.

The Herxheimer Response: The Healing Crisis

Negative symptoms don't necessarily indicate toxicity. An effective healing program may nevertheless result in negative symptoms: headaches, stomach gas, skin rashes, nausea, etc. This should not be taken as necessarily indicating toxicity of the food or herbs being taken. Nor is it necessarily an allergic reaction. Almost every effective healing program will induce some symptoms of this sort. This is known as a healing crisis. The symptoms are the body's reaction to the elimination of toxins. This crisis should not last longer than a week or so. However, if the symptoms are severe, it might be wise to reduce or stop the program for a period of time.

How do supplements and herbs compare with mainstream medicine on the question of safety? Certainly, most vitamin supplements are entirely safe. Mineral supplements need to be taken with a bit more caution but herbs cannot be presumed to be safe – let's face it, some herbs are poisonous. Socrates killed himself by drinking a herbal potion. Between 1994 and 1998, the FDA recorded 184 deaths from the use of dietary supplements (i.e., an average of 46 a year). In 1998, the American Association of Poison Control Centers received nearly 7,000 reports of adverse reactions with 1,369 cases involving hospitalization. Most of the problems relate to Chinese herbal combinations and to weight management supplements.

However, let's put this in context. Compare those figures with the following: In 2004, Dr. Lucien Leape, a Harvard University professor, who is considered to be the world's leading expert on medical errors, announced the following figures: American doctors write about 3.5 billion prescriptions every year. Nearly one percent of those prescriptions is wrong, either the wrong drug, the wrong dose or the wrong patient. Of the 28 million wrong prescriptions about 21 percent - nearly 6 million--contain "serious errors." One calculation of annual deaths in America caused by medical failings is that roughly 100,000 deaths occur as a result of adverse drug reactions in hospital and a further 200,000 from adverse drug reactions among outpatients. In addition another 100,000 die as a result of hospital acquired infection and another 100,000 from malnutrition while in hospital. In fact, according to these figures, medical error was the leading cause of death in America.

As more than one person has commented: if we say that we've got an AIDS epidemic, shouldn't we also say we've got an epidemic of medical error? So it seems reasonable to say that the alternative approach is a great deal safer than the standard medical route.

Large numbers of people are taking both herbs and drugs and there is the danger that particular combinations may have serious side effects. The truth is that no one knows what interactions there might be – not the herbalist, the pharmacist or the doctor. Close monitoring of the situation by yourself is necessary – and it would be wise to take advice from doctor, pharmacist and herbalist.

Let us now turn our attention to the alternative approaches to cancer. In this section of the book we will be looking at diets, herbs, supplements, formulas, specially designed anti-cancer programs, mind-body approaches and electromagnetic interventions. There are a lot of ideas out there. They may be clinically untested in large-scale randomized double blind trials but, despite all that, the sheer weight of evidence that they work requires that we take them very seriously. They hold out the great promise of long-term health and freedom from cancer. Indeed, in America, for over 15 years more money has been spent on alternative health than on mainstream health – and doctors are taking note.

ALTERNATIVE TESTING PROCEDURES

I first thought of calling this section Alternative Diagnostics, but the word 'diagnosis' tends to be reserved for the identification of specific diseases or illnesses. Most alternative tests do not diagnose disease conditions but rather they analyze aspects of the body's biochemistry to determine if everything is as it should be. We diagnose herpes, for example, but test to evaluate the pH of the body's tissues.

Just as the orthodox doctor relies on information derived from blood and urine tests, X-rays and CAT scans, so too do practitioners of alternative medicine rely on information gained from an array of testing procedures and equipment. We will look at some of these procedures that are useful for the person who has cancer.

Bloodwork

'Bloodwork' is the American slang word for blood tests. Regular blood tests have a strong role to play in an overall anti-cancer strategy.

If we go back to the very definition of cancer, you will remember that there are two opposing views. The first is the view that the tumour represents the disease. Once you have rid the body of that object, then the cancer can be considered cured. Opposed to this is the view that the tumour is only a symptom of the disease. The cause of the cancer is an unhealthy body. Eliminating the symptom will do nothing in the long run. It may delay the inevitable for a while but the ill-health of the body will eventually provoke new cancer tumours. In this view only by returning the whole body to a state of health can cancer be truly cured.

The relevance of this to blood tests is that instead of doing tests simply to detect the chemical markers for various cancers, we need to do tests that will measure the overall health of the body's ecology – the terrain in which the disease arises. This is the area where it is good to have the cooperation of a friendly doctor who will agree to carry out these tests while you experiment with the diets, supplements, herbs and other alternative strategies listed in the following chapters.

There are a number of tests that should be done regularly (i.e., once a month or possibly even more frequently) to keep track of the body's basic health. In this way you can see clearly if what you are doing is working. However, remember that all tests suffer from the problems of false negative and false positive results so, if there are anomalous results, get re-tested. It is also a good idea to use two tests that may test the same thing in different ways so that you build in a degree of redundancy. This will help you see more clearly where the problems may lie – in the body or in specific test results. So what blood tests will measure the basic health of the body?

Blood Sedimentation Rate Test

The Erythrocyte Sedimentation Rate (ESR) test, which in medical jargon is known as the 'sed rate', measures the speed at which red blood cells settle at the bottom of a glass tube. The speed of sedimentation reflects the concentration of certain proteins in the blood.

This is a screening test for overall health. It is not specific to any one illness. A slow rate of sedimentation is good. Speedy sedimentation may be caused by infection, inflammation and the presence of cancer.

Complete Blood Count

This test will determine the quantity of red and white blood cells – which in turn will provide useful information on the general health of the body.

AMAS

AMAS (Anti-malignin antibody screen) test is able to detect cancers well in advance of other signs and symptoms, and months before other conventional medical tests can detect it. However, it remains the preserve of a single laboratory, Oncolab, which developed the test, and has not gained wide acceptance. You may therefore have to bring this test to the attention of your doctor. See www.oncolabinc.com for more details. You should also note that it appears to produce a relatively high number of false negatives – so don't assume a 'no cancer' result means what it says 100 percent of the time. Get a re-test in three months time just to be sure.

DR-70

The DR-70 is a simple blood test that screens for 13 different cancers all at the same time. Clinical studies have been conducted all over the world and the results showed that it detected cancers of the lung, colon, stomach, liver, pancreas, rectum, ovaries, oesophagus, cervix, uterus, thyroid, breast and even malignant lymphoma. The test is simple, noninvasive, and costs around $100. It is highly 'sensitive' in that it will detect most cancers (so the risk of false negatives is low) and 'selective' in that it will not say cancer is present when it isn't (so the risk of false positives is low).

C-Reactive Protein Test

The liver produces C-reactive protein in response to acute inflammation. The presence of this protein is therefore a good sign that there is acute inflammation. Since inflammation is strongly associated with cancer it is a good to be able to detect the extent of inflammation in any part of the body

CEA (carcinoembryonic antigen) Test

This is a back up test that measures inflammation. Although low scores cannot be taken as evidence that there is no cancer in the system, and high scores cannot definitively point to which cancer is present, if you already know where the tumour is, a high score will generally indicate that inflammation is present. Note that pregnancy will also cause high levels of CEA.

Liver Tests

The liver is a key organ. If the liver is unhealthy, the whole physical system suffers. It is therefore vital that the liver be returned to good health as quickly as possible. This is something that most detoxification regimes do not fully recognize. It is no good attempting to flush toxins out if the liver, whose job is to deal with these toxins, is unable to deal with them. There are a number of tests that look at various liver functions. The following tests are usually undertaken in tandem and are known by the initials of the enzyme markers they relate to: GGT, AST, ALT, ALP and LD. The levels of bilirubin are also tested for. Taken together these provide a detailed picture of liver health. GGT, in particular, is an extremely sensitive test. When cancer develops, the liver finds itself forced to work harder and harder to try and maintain normal functioning. GGT is the test that reveals overactive liver action.

Other Tests

i. Interleukin 6.

This is a measure of angiogenesis activity. Angiogenesis is the process by which a cancer tumour creates a blood supply to support its growth. The IL6 tests for activity in this area. By itself, it should not be taken as an indicator of cancerous activity simply because it can give false readings. However, when used in conjunction with other tests, it is a very good indicator that something is going wrong. If cancer is present and active, it will inevitably be growing its own life support and IL6 levels will become elevated. It is important to get this marker into the normal range. If you can do this, you will win the fight against cancer. If you can't, your cancer wins.

ii. Biological Terrain Assessment (BTA)

There has long been a dispute between the supporters of Louis Pasteur - who argue that diseases are caused by viruses, bacteria and so on – and the supporters of Pasteur's rival, Claude Bernard, who argued that the terrain in which the viruses are found is the real cause of disease. According to this view, the viruses could not flourish in a cellular terrain that was healthy. The diseased terrain allows the agents of disease to operate. Pasteur is often quoted on his death bed as having admitted that his rival was correct: "The germ is nothing, the terrain is everything."

Taking the logic of this one step further, it follows that a sick terrain will lead inevitably to ill health and that a plant is only as healthy as the soil it grows in. And so, we can conclude, to cure the unhealthy plant it is more effective to fix the soil than to treat the plant itself.

This idea that disease may first be detected in the cellular terrain has led to the development of BTA. BTA does a computerized analysis of blood, urine and saliva looking at three specific features: the pH of the cellular environment; the degree of oxidative stress and mineral concentration levels.

Obviously, results of this test will not diagnose any specific disease but they will reveal areas of the body's ecology that can be improved by means of diet, supplementation or other intervention. Generally speaking this is not a test that your doctor will carry out. An internet search will be needed to find a therapist near you who offers this type of analysis.

Digital Infrared Thermal Imaging (DITI)

This is a non-invasive scanning technique that measures changes in the surface temperature of skin. It converts the infrared radiation that is emitted from the skin into visual images that look like a Technicolor weather map. This visual image is called a thermogram. The body is usually symmetrical in its functioning so any asymmetrical patterns that appear on the thermogram demonstrate areas of concern.

The value of this to a person scanning for cancer is that a hot spot can be detected long before a cancer tumour has grown to the size where it can be picked up by standard scanning equipment. The precancerous activity shows up hot because it is developing its own blood supply – a process referred to as neo-vascularisation.

A DITI thermogram provides a visual picture of what's going on in the body rather than being a precise diagnostic technique—but for the purpose of acting as an early warning system for cancers close to the skin surface it is an excellent tool. For deeply rooted cancers it is less useful.

This is a technology that is developing fast both in complexity and in popularity. It is entirely non-invasive and does not traumatize tissue - unlike the standard mammogram.

At present, it is still viewed with suspicion by mainstream diagnostic centres – though this is likely to change rapidly in the coming years. One reason for this suspicion is simply that the technology detects precancerous changes far earlier than they can be dealt with surgically. You can't take out a lump before a lump has formed.

It is also a testing procedure with an excellent record of accuracy. Only 9 percent of test results are false (either false positive or false negative) according to research at the Pasteur Institute in France. It can clearly distinguish between cancer (which is hot) and fiberadenoma cysts (which are cold). In this way it eliminates 80 percent of the false positives which result from mammography.

For more detailed information and to view some example thermograms go to www.healthybreasts.info.

That is the positive spin on thermograms. However, some critics have pointed out that it does not pick up more deep seated tumours – so an all clear is not in any way conclusive. Also, an asymmetrical heat pattern can have a number of causes and do not necessarily indicate a precancerous situation. Finally some slow-growing cancers do not show up on thermograms. The DITI should therefore be viewed as only one test among several.

Bio-Resonance Testing

Bio-resonance testing (also known as Autonomic Response Testing) is one umbrella name for a number of different practices which measure bio-feedback, usually using some form of equipment: Applied Kinesiology, EAV (Electro-acupuncture According to Voll), Electrodermal Screening, Contact Reflex Analysis, Omura O-Ring Test, QXCI, VEGA and others. Here I will look at the first two.

i. Applied Kinesiology

Most cancer patients see their problem in the following way: I have cancer. I want to get rid of it. I wish I knew of some way of just eliminating the cancer – I just want it to go away so I can get on with the life I was leading before it came along.

The problem with this way of thinking is that, almost certainly, it was precisely the way of life you were leading that gave rise to the cancer in the first place. Something, possibly major, maybe very minor, happened that eventually led to the cancer forming in your body. If that is the case then just getting rid of the cancer isn't going to work. If the conditions remain unchanged the cancer is almost certain to return. This is one of the problems that orthodox medicine signally fails to recognize. They – the oncologists – are focusing all their attention on making the tumour go away so that you can get on with your life. Sadly, they are unable in the majority of cases to do even that - but that's another issue.

This may be very annoying but it is a fact that those cancer patients who survive generally come to terms with. They need to know what it is that's going wrong in their body. Once they know that, they can correct it. Now, the exciting possibility is that once they have got rid of the causes of the cancer, the cancer itself might go away.

Dr. Max Gerson explained his own realization of this truth in these words: "I gradually came to the basic conclusion that, in a body with normal metabolism, cancer cannot develop. The normalization of the damaged metabolism is therefore the essential aim of any therapy."

This is one of two basic assumptions underlying Applied Kinesiology. The second assumption is that the body knows what is wrong with it and will tell you if you ask the right questions in the right way.

Kinesiology, therefore, is a system of evaluating the body's weaknesses and strengths using the body itself as a sounding board. The basic idea is that the body is wise. It responds to contact with any item in one of three ways. If the body needs a substance, it will show this by strengthening the muscles. If it finds the substance detrimental in some way, it will weaken the muscles and if it is neutral to it there is no response. The kinesiologist therefore approaches the diagnostic problems posed by a patient by taking a muscle group (i.e., an arm or a leg) and exerting a little pressure against it while the patient resists the pressure. Then substances that will reveal the inner workings of the body are placed in contact with the body and the effect on the muscle is tested – does the muscle remain strong or does it weaken?

The kinesiologist doesn't, however, use a lump of lead, if he's testing for lead toxicity. Instead he will use a small glass vial containing a homoeopathic concentration of lead. The skin as an organ is known to be a crude photosensitive receptor (people have, for example, been taught to read shapes using the palms of their hands) and the idea is that the skin records the light waves that pass through the homoeopathic substance and sends a signal to the brain. The brain evaluates it and then responds according to whether it likes the signal or doesn't.

Having personally undergone a kinesiological evaluation, I can tell you that the muscle responses appear to be consistent and repeatable. Indeed, if it didn't work, it is unlikely that it would become widely accepted as a health promoting approach – but it has. A large number of otherwise orthodox doctors have also trained in kinesiology. The founder of the approach, George Goodheart Jr, is still alive today and was the first chiropractor to serve on the US Olympic medical committee. Nevertheless, it is fair to say that it has not conclusively proven its claims and that a number of clinical trials have been done and the results have tended to be negative.

But what makes applied kinesiology potentially such a powerful and important weapon is that it may be able to reveal very subtle biochemical problems immediately – there's no waiting for days or weeks to get lab results - and without the necessity for invasive procedures. Indeed, if it is not a sham, the analysis is at levels of precision way beyond what most orthodox doctors will do, or indeed can do using orthodox means. Perhaps it is this potential that seduces us to ignore or question the negative results of clinical trials. It is not my desire to undermine the idea of kinesiology – but I do wish to point out that it is one of the most contentious areas of alternative medical practice.

To help you understand kinesiology a little better, I will give an example. The body is a system in which every cell is both manufacturing and breaking down numerous hormones, neurotransmitters and other biochemical molecules necessary for the body to function. To take a specific example, the amino acid tyrosine that is extracted from food is transformed in the body first into L-dopa, which in turn is transformed into dopamine, which is transformed into noradrenalin, and that is then transformed into adrenalin. Once each of the chemicals in this chain is no longer needed there is a three stage process by which the chemical is changed to make it capable of being eliminated in the urine. That is just one of thousands of cycles that the body does seemingly effortlessly all the time. However, each of these transformations requires other substances to be present – vitamins, minerals and so on. If these other chemicals are not present then the result is that one of the intermediate products can not be broken down for elimination and so it remains in the body – usually in the fatty tissue – such as the breasts for example. The problem is that these intermediate products are toxic and have the potential to cause precancerous changes, among other things. So, the lack of a vitamin or a mineral can have very serious consequences. The point needs to be made here that a serious result may have an apparently minor cause. One boy losing his balance on a trampoline may simply bounce on the sprung surface and think it's funny while another boy, falling on the same trampoline, might crack his neck against the steel rim and be paralysed for life. Same cause different results.

Unfortunately, the orthodox doctor ignores this level of biochemistry completely. One way, potentially, of finding out what is needed is to undergo a kinesiological evaluation.

The kinesiologist also understands that each body is unique. For him it is not sufficient to say, for example, that magnesium is required. In my own case, further testing showed that the common supplement magnesium citrate would be of no value to me. For me, magnesium chloride and magnesium oxide were the preferred salts. For you, the answer would be different.

Depending on what the kinesiologist discovers you might be directed to nutritional supplements or osteopathic manipulation or other forms of therapy. A list of trained Applied Kinesiologists can be found at www.icak.com

ii. EAV (Electro-Acupuncture according to Voll)

Hans Larson, editor of *International Health News*, puts the matter succinctly: "Imagine if you could go to your doctor, sit for an hour in a comfortable chair where you are hooked up to some highly sophisticated electronic equipment, and then receive a detailed assessment of your health status. Sounds far fetched? Perhaps, but thousands of progressive practitioners around the world are already providing this service."

The machine Larson describes is an EAV machine which measures the electrical impulses found in acupuncture points and other locations. It is able, very quickly, to tell the therapist about the patient's toxic metal loads, the health of the organs (particularly liver function), the presence of any inflammation, fungi, food intolerances, and mineral deficiencies.

It was developed initially in the 1950s by a German doctor Dr. Reinhold Voll while studying the electrical properties of acupuncture points.

With this machine, the patient holds a brass bar and a probe is then placed on a suitable acupuncture point. A wide range of subtle frequencies are then fed into the patient's body and the body's responses to these are noted by the computer that is hooked up to the machine. The result is a global health analysis in well under an hour.

What this means is that the complex of energy patterns in the body reveals the health or otherwise of every component and process in the body. The EAV machine measures these energy patterns.

But EAV is not just an assessment tool for diagnosis. Actually diagnosis is not the right word for what it does. EAV cannot tell you that you have cancer or diabetes or TB. What it can tell you is the specific problems facing specific parts of the body. Together all the information might add up to a probability of a particular disease but the EAV practitioner cannot definitively draw that conclusion.

EAV is also a means of providing treatment. If a disharmony is detected, the practitioner can reverse the procedure, using the EAV machine to create homoeopathic-strength vibrational remedies which will help to reverse the energetic imbalance and so correct the original health problem. This is, in fact, a form of energy medicine and not a form of chemical medicine. The results are at levels of sensitivity far exceeding what is possible in any other way. Because of this the results cannot be checked to assess whether the results are true or false. Using the modality therefore becomes an act of faith. Both Kinesiology and EAV are challenging modalities – challenging to our sense of the world. However, the proof of the pudding is whether or not they work – and, in the absence of clear proof or disproof, each person needs to decide that for him- or herself.

Live Blood and Dried Blood Analysis

These are two techniques for looking at the blood using different types of high-resolution microscope. Dried blood analysis uses a light field microscope while live blood analysis uses what is called a darkfield microscope. In both cases, using only a small amount of blood – a single drop of live blood from the patient's finger – the therapist can see the vital components of the cell clearly. These can be viewed on a video monitor. The blood analysis provides information about the condition of the red cell membranes, the activity levels of white blood cells and the quantity and quality of various blood plasma elements.

Both tests allow even very early signs of ill health to be picked up. It is possible to see free radical damage, vitamin deficiencies, hormonal imbalances, digestive problems, the degree of toxicity, pH and mineral imbalances, as well as the extent of parasite, fungus and yeast infestation. These provide information relevant to immune system function and nutritional status.

These blood tests are good basic screening tools that provide information that can help the therapist target more specific tests. When abnormalities or deficiencies are detected in the blood the therapist will seek to provide treatments the aim of which will be to bring the blood quality back to that associated with normal good health. While a live blood test cannot make a definitive diagnosis of cancer it provides important information about the basic biological terrain of the patient's body and is therefore a useful and relatively cheap clinical tool.

Hair Analysis

Hair is a highly metabolically active tissue and an analysis of hair will normally reveal significant details concerning the nutritional and endocrine status of a patient well before these abnormalities will be found using standard blood tests. It will often also disclose information that cannot be easily determined from more conventional diagnostic tests.

Hair analysis simply involves cutting off some hair–a small clump is required - from the scalp, sending it to a laboratory where it will be tested for mineral and toxic metal content.

This is an analytical tool that tends to be frowned on by doctors but is used by forensic scientists as a matter of course. American law enforcement agencies have used hair analyses for decades considering them conclusive as evidence in crime investigations and for drug testing. Death by poisoning can be determined conclusively only by means of a hair analysis. A three-inch strand of hair will contain a record of chemical exposure over the previous six months (hair grows at an average rate of half an inch a month).

The purpose of a hair analysis is to determine whether metal and mineral contents indicate an overload which may impact on our health. Once identified, detoxification can be done through herb and vitamin supplementation or dietary changes.

Saliva & Urine Hormone Analysis

For many health investigations, it is necessary to determine the levels of a range of hormones in the body, and their ratios. Normally, in mainstream clinical settings, this is done using blood tests but in fact the hormone fractions (unbound fractions) present in saliva and urine provide a better picture of what is happening hormonally in the body than those found in blood (bound fractions). Saliva and urine tests can therefore provide useful information about the biochemical functioning of the body.

DETOXIFICATION

The food and drink we consume and the air we breathe are all contaminated with chemicals that we would normally not choose to take into our bodies. The more toxic our bodies, the less able they are to be brought back to a state of health. If we want a cancer-free body, we need to help the body to become cleansed internally. That means detox. Here are some of the procedures people with cancer should be thinking about.

Colon Cleansing

Purification of the liver is the key step to a cancer-free existence. But before we look at liver detoxification, it is reasonable to ask what causes the liver to become toxic and so dysfunctional in the first place. The answer is poor elimination of waste in the colon. Poisonous materials are trapped in the large intestine and reabsorbed back into the bloodstream where they again go through an increasingly weakened liver. As it becomes less and less able to keep up the work of cleaning the blood, the whole body becomes more toxic. According to Professor Serge Jurasunas, writing in the Townsend Letter for Doctors and Patients "There is a definite correlation between breast cancer and chronic constipation. My own observation leaves no doubt about this. There is hardly a case of breast cancer with good bowel function."

If you attempt to clean your liver, blood, or lymph system without first addressing a waste filled bowel, the excreted toxins will only get recycled back into your body. So, before attempting to detoxify the liver, you need first to cleanse the colon.

There are a number of different approaches to resolving this problem. Enemas help clean out the end of the colon, colonic irrigation helps clean the whole of the large intestine using warm water pumped in under pressure and there is colonic cleansing which uses herbs or clay to achieve the same object.

The most famous exponent of colon health was Norman W. Walker. On the first page of his book *Colon Health: the Key to a Vibrant Life*, he says: "Few of us realize that failure to effectively eliminate waste products from the body causes so much fermentation and putrefaction in the large intestine, or colon, that the neglected accumulation of such waste can, and frequently does, result in a lingering demise."

Norman Walker's prescription for a healthy life included half-yearly colonics, vitamin C and raw vegetable juices, particularly carrot juice. Since he lived actively to the age of 109, it is hard to argue with him. Clearly he was doing something right.

An efficient colon will eliminate food 16-24 hours after it has been ingested. Very few British intestines work at this rate. According to the Dunn Nutritional Institute at Cambridge, they average, 60 hours, and 5 days is not unusual. In France, studies indicate that over 35 percent of the population suffers from constipation regularly. According to the 1991 National Health Interview Survey, about 4.5 million people in the United States say they are constipated most or all of the time.

Colonic therapist Pauline Noakes, likens the situation to having the dustmen permanently on strike so that the rubbish piles up in the street.

"Many people don't realize they are carrying around impacted faecal matter in their colons and that their lack of energy, their irritability, their aches and pains...and various ailments are due to the toxic waste in the bowel." (P.Noakes, *Positive Health* magazine, April/May 1995)

There is evidence to support this view. Two doctors from University of California, Nicholas Petrakis and Eileen King, writing in *The Lancet* in 1982, reported that they had studied the breast fluids of 5,000 women. They had found that women who had two or fewer bowel movements per week had four times the risk of breast disease (benign or malignant) as those who had one or more bowel movements per day. They also found that the bowels of people who ate meat contained greater amounts of mutagenic (potentially harmful) substances than did those of people who abstained from eating meat.

Enemas can be undertaken at home with an enema kit bought at a pharmacy. Easier and more effective is to go to a colonic cleansing clinic, but make sure the person giving the therapy is a registered colonic therapist. And how do you feel after a colonic? Carol Signorella, writing in *Cosmopolitan* October 1979 wrote: "After a year of colonics, my appearance and energy levels were both radically improved. No more draggy mornings or late afternoon slumps. I seem to think more clearly now and I need less sleep. In a word my body and mind feel marvellously clean."

Wouldn't laxatives work just as well? The answer is a definite no. Colonics clean out the large intestine but laxatives also interfere with the small intestine which is where digestion and absorption of nutrients occur. Also laxatives are, in a sense, addictive - for them to continue to be effective, you need to take larger and larger doses.

A word of caution: colon hydrotherapy is not suitable for people with the following conditions: severe cardiac disease, aneurysm, severe anaemia, severe haemorrhoids, cirrhosis, carcinoma of the colon, fistulas, advanced pregnancy, kidney problems and hernia.

There are perfectly good alternatives to a full colonic. One is to drink a colon cleansing treatment. A suspension of Bentonite mud and dried psyllium husks does a good job of taking waste material out of the digestive system. For those who like a ready-mixed product will find any number on the internet. One that boasts a lot of testimonials can be found at www.drnatura.com.

However, when doing colonic cleansing it is important to replace electrolytes, perhaps by drinking raw fruit and vegetable juices.

Magnesium Oxide

Magnesium oxide is one of the best and easiest ways to flush out the intestines. When mixed with water it produces large amounts of oxygen. In the intestine, the effect of this is to promote healthy aerobic bacteria and at the same time inhibit the growth of unhealthy anaerobic bacteria and fungi (especially Candida Albicans).

The freed oxygen in magnesium oxide reacts with hydrogen to form water in the intestinal tract. This helps to soften and cleanse the intestine's contents and walls. Unlike other laxatives, Magnesium oxide is both safe and gentle.

Magnesium oxide is a white powder. Dissolve half a teaspoon in a glass of water. Add lemon juice or cider vinegar as desired and drink on an empty stomach. This can be repeated several times a day. The aim is to achieve two or three bowel movements a day.

It is safe to use on a regular basis but anyone doing so should ensure their potassium and electrolyte levels don't fall too low. Drinking fresh fruit juices will help achieve this.

Charcoal

Charcoal is a traditional remedy for many gastric and other ailments. It is used for resolving dysentery and eliminating stomach upsets. Less well known is the fact that has a wide ranging action that is both healing and detoxifying. For all types of skin ailments including cancer, it can be used externally in a poultice (mix olive oil and charcoal powder and soak a cloth in the mix. Add a heating pad to help absorption through the skin). Charcoal, taken both internally and externally, has been successfully used against a variety of cancers and can help reduce swellings of the lymphatic system. A good source of charcoal powder is www.buyactivatedcharcoal.com

Castor Oil

For a stronger purging of the contents of the intestines, castor oil is highly recommended. A few tablespoons mixed with juice or water should be sufficient. It has memorably been described as WD40 (a brand of household lubcriating oil) for the gastro-intestinal system.

Naturally, for obvious reasons, no laxative or purgative should be taken during pregnancy.

Once the colon has been flushed out it is important to maintain a regular and frequent pattern of elimination. Twice a day is considered healthy. Unfortunately, constipation is a problem that seems to go hand in hand with the Western diet. Green drinks filled with enzymes (see p. 161) are one answer to regular bowel movements. A couple of apples a day should also do the trick.

Caster Oil as a Healing Oil

On the subject of castor oil, you should note that it is a healing oil in its own right – and can be applied continuously – particularly to any tumour on the surface but also for cancers lying below the surface. Famously, castor oil was promoted by the mystic Edgar Cayce, whose instructions on how to make a castor oil pack was as follows: "Heat the Oil; dipping two, three to four layers of flannel in same, wring out and apply directly to the body."

Castor oil is also a solvent so it is possible to add other ingredients to the oil and these will also soak into the tissues through the skin. Some use raw crushed ginger and I personally have used tea tree oil, propolis and the grapefruit seed extract, Citricidal, to very good effect against a fungal infection. Herbalist Dr. Richard Schulze promotes the use of cayenne pepper tincture. There are stories on the internet claiming that castor oil has cured even deep seated cancers such as carcinoma of the kidneys.

Cellular Drainage Therapy

Once we have flushed the colon out we can now start to address the problems of the liver. Can you mop up a pool of water with a soggy sponge? Obviously not. You first have to eliminate all the water from the sponge before it can useful help mop up further water. The cells of the liver are the same. If each cell is full of toxic matter then these cells need to be regenerated first before any other detoxification activity is initiated. Cellular drainage works on detoxification at the level of each individual cell.

However, even good hydration will not necessarily eliminate all toxins. If blood circulation is sluggish and organs such as the kidney and liver are compromised for any reason then toxin loads may build up within cells. To help drain these toxins from the cells, certain herbs are used that help to stimulate blood flow and release toxins. These will be given as homoeopathic remedies.

Naturopaths and homoeopaths can advise you which drainage remedies might be suitable. Although there are a number of websites that sell products for those wishing to self-treat, it is strongly advised that you find someone who can do a meridian stress assessment using EAV (electro-acupuncture) equipment. They will then be able to assess the specific toxins that need to be eliminated and, in addition, also provide the remedies.

Liver Flush

The liver is the largest organ of the body. It processes all pharmaceuticals and supplements. However, the liver can be weakened by the overload of toxins. When the liver no longer is able to do its job, you will feel this in a number of ways: low energy levels, digestive problems, depression, headaches, dizziness, joint pain, sleeping disorders, dry skin or eczema, irritability, PMS – and cancer.

The purpose of a liver flush is to flush poisons out of the liver and so help its regeneration. Orthodox surgeons pour scorn on the idea that a poorly functioning liver has anything to do with the development of cancer, but most complementary health practitioners disagree. So, in fact, do some orthodox doctors. Dr. Harold Manner has absolutely no doubt that liver dysfunction is the root of the problem: "...the livers of cancer patients have become clogged with many of the poisons they were meant to eliminate...Cancer can be reversed and controlled only if we regenerate the liver. Fortunately for us, the liver is the one organ in the body capable of regenerating itself."

Herbalist, Christopher Hobbs, in his book *Foundations of Health*, recommends the following flush.

1. Squeeze oranges or grapefruit or other citrus fruit to make a cup of liquid.

2. Add 2 cloves of garlic freshly squeezed and a small amount of ginger juice—made by grating fresh ginger and squeezing it in a garlic press. *would not rec, this—*

3. Add a table spoon of good quality olive oil. *but ask a professional*

4. Shake it vigorously and drink. *about liver detox + load on liver when cancer cells start dying*

next pg.

5. Then drink one or two glasses of herbal tea made with the following: equal parts of fennel, flax, fenugreek and peppermint with one quarter parts of burdock and liquorice. Simmer in water for 20 minutes.

He recommends drinking this mixture first thing in the morning after some stretching exercises and then not eating for at least an hour. He suggests doing this for two cycles of ten days at a time separated by three days at least twice a year but more frequently as required.

Epsom Salts

Epsom salts are a more drastic way to flush the liver, specifically to eliminate gallstones. It is recommended that you have a bath in dissolved Epsom salts everyday for a week or more before taking them internally so as to allow the body to absorb magnesium – magnesium deficiency being very common. It is also recommended, by Hulda Clark among others, that you do a parasite purge before doing a liver flush, as parasites in the liver will interfere with the elimination of gallstones.

Herbs and Liver Support

A number of herbs are also specifically recommended to support liver function, particularly burdock, dandelion, and milk thistle. Of these, milk thistle is the most important. A number of herbal combinations are sold as specific liver cleanses.

Having said all this, there are many who think a liver flush is too extreme – and should not be done if there is any risk that the cancer has spread to the liver. Instead of a flush, a diet of fruit and vegetables – no meat, dairy or grain – will be naturally detoxifying in itself. Freshly juiced carrots and beetroot are also very beneficial to the liver. *these are good anyway,*

Liver Detox Using Coffee Enemas

The doctors who treated my wife found the concept of coffee enemas to be particularly worthy of ridicule. However, it is an established method favoured by many, if not most, alternative practitioners for helping to cleanse and stimulate the liver and so help it in its work in removing toxins. It is particularly associated with the Gerson and Kelley approaches discussed later in this book.

It is important to remember that if cancer tumours begin to break down they release toxins into the body and an already weakened liver may easily become overloaded. People have died in this way from the overly powerful healing effects of vitamins and herbs. There is a direct connection between the lower colon just before the rectum and the liver. Coffee that is taken in as an enema is held for as long as possible – 15-20 minutes. The coffee helps to cleanse the liver. Several enemas a day may be required. There are a number of re-usable enema kits on the market which come with clear instructions on how to use them. There are also special coffees designed to be used for this purpose. A Google search for 'coffee enema' will provide many sources of equipment.

Having said this, however, you should not do more than one or two enemas a day at most (unless directed by a practitioner). The rectum is very efficient at absorbing whatever is put in it – hence the value of suppositories. Coffee enemas can result in a sudden lowering of blood levels of sodium, potassium and chloride electrolytes. This can have very harmful consequences. Dr. Robert Buckman, in his book *Magic or Medicine*, blames over-zealous use of coffee enemas for two deaths. It was not the coffee but the water that had the negative impact. As with colonic cleansing, it is important to replace electrolytes, perhaps by drinking raw fruit and vegetable juices immediately afterwards.

Cleansing the Lymph System: Lymphatic Massage

Lymph is a clear fluid that travels through the body's arteries and tissues to cleanse them. It circulates through the lymphatic system.

Lymph nodes are the filters along the lymphatic system. Their job is to filter out and trap bacteria, viruses, cancer cells, and other unwanted substances, and to make sure they are safely eliminated from the body.

Lymphatic massage is a light touch technique used since the 1930s to promote health and aid recovery from illness. It is also called lymphatic drainage. Lymphatic massage is used to promote general wellness. It is a gentle technique which prevents or reduces fluid retention, and enhances the removal of toxins from body tissues.

The lymph vessels are just under the skin, so moving the lymph requires a very light touch. Lymphatic massage is widely available and is practised by most massage therapists.

However, for the cancer patient, lymphatic massage is best done with extreme lightness of touch–preferably under the guidance of a trained professional - as there is a danger - theoretical but not proven - of promoting the spread of cancer cells. However, this danger should not be exaggerated. Lymphatic massage promotes the movement of lymph towards the chest where it becomes exposed to highly oxygenated blood capillaries that surround the lungs – which in turn are likely to kill off any circulating microscopic metastases. The dangers of a static lymphatic system are far more serious.

Also, for those who have had some form of radiation or removal of lymph glands there is a danger of promoting or worsening any existing oedema – which is caused by lymph being unable to drain away so causing painful swelling.

Strong massage is contraindicated only in association with high-dose enzyme therapy, with melanoma or if someone is immune compromised from chemotherapy or radiation or suffers from a clotting disorder. But even those patients can have a light massage.

The importance of human touch is well-known. Babies die if they are not properly cosseted. Massage is an important therapy that should not be neglected.

The Benefits of Rebounding — Chris Wark did this

Bouncing on a rebounder – a mini-trampoline - is another good way of getting the lymphatic system moving and boosting the immune system. You don't have to bounce energetically, just raising and lowering the heels to set up a rhythmic bounce is sufficient. Some people do this for 30-60 minutes a day while watching television. Some have taken to calling this exercise 'lymphasizing' – exercising the lymph!

Oil Pulling

This is a simple Ayurvedic technique for which powerful long-term health benefits are claimed. Using only sesame or sunflower oil, take a tablespoon of oil into the mouth and suck, swirl and swish it round the whole mouth for around 15 minutes. Then spit the oil out (it has become toxic). This is particularly recommended for anyone with gum disease but is beneficial to everyone who is ill in any way. It is well accepted that oral infections and gum disease have a powerfully negative impact on the heart and may be implicated in cancer. This is a cheap and simple health promoting practice.

Skin Brushing

The Skin is the largest organ in the body, and is responsible for a quarter of the body's daily detoxification. Brushing the dry skin is a simple way of helping the lymph system to eliminate toxins. It also strengthens the immune system, stimulates the glands and even improves digestion. Skin brushing should be done with a long handled bristle brush made of natural materials. The skin should be dry, not wet, when brushed. Some practitioners recommend that the abdomen should be brushed in an anti-clockwise direction and other areas should be brushed towards the heart. Brush each part of the body several times vigorously–though breasts should be brushed lightly, avoiding the nipples which should not be brushed at all. Start with the soles of the feet because the nerve endings there affect the whole body, then the ankles, calves, and thighs, up across your buttocks stomach and chest. After the brushing session you can have a shower.

Hydrotherapy + hot & cold showers

Water is a powerful cleaning agent and the skin is an important organ for elimination of toxins. Putting these two together we get hydrotherapy. There are many forms. Saunas and steam baths are one form of hydrotherapy. Spend at least half an hour in the heat - but not continuously. 5-15 minute sessions are the norm. The purpose is not only to sweat out the poisons in the body. The heat itself acts as an immune system stimulator. Some health clinics will offer a hydrotherapy treatment involving wrapping the body in hot towels but a hot bath at home - as hot as can be borne - can work just as well. Add one pound of baking soda and one pound of sea salt or deep mine salt (not standard table salt which is totally ineffective). Rock salt is not so good. Stay in the bath for 20-50 minutes and then have a quick shower to rub off the soda and salt. This is known as a detox (detoxification) bath. It is important with all these forms of hydrotherapy to drink lots of water – distilled, reverse osmosis or natural spring/mineral water -- before, during and after the hydrotherapy sessions.

Water should also be drunk in large quantities everyday. Many health experts warn that many of our problems arise from the fact that we are semi-permanently dehydrated. We drink coffee and tea and beers and so on all of which are diuretic, causing water to be expelled from the body. Our blood and body's cells are absolutely dependent on an adequate supply of fresh, clean water. We need at least four pints a day. Some people think that many illnesses arise directly as a result of inadequate intake of water: asthma, allergies, diabetes, arthritis, angina, all intestinal problems and many degenerative diseases.

However, too much water can also be bad for us as that can dilute the sodium salts our cells need. Don't go overboard.

Water Massage

Most spas offer water massage treatments in which you are massaged by jets of water, There are also 'Dry Hydrotherapy' machines that claim to boost oxygenation of the blood, eliminate toxins, reduce pain and muscular tension.

Alternating Hot and Cold Showers ← *Chris did this @ Chrisbeatcancer.com*

This is not a detox regime but a way of stimulating the metabolism of the body. Isolate the area where the tumour is located and alternate showers of very cold and very hot water. Do this at frequent intervals.

The Water Question: What Kind of Water?

Up till now I have discussed a number of water-based procedures without confronting the elephant in the room - what kind of water? Let's look at the whole question of water.

First, it is strongly believed by many that tap water, chlorinated and/or fluoridated or simply heavy in calcium, is extremely unhealthy and interferes with the absorption of nutrients. The option generally argued for is pure distilled water. However, there are critics who say that distilled water leaches minerals from the system and would therefore lead to inevitable mineral deficiencies. The retort to this is that, yes, distilled water does leach out minerals but these are not the organic minerals that the body can use - they are inorganic minerals that are potentially toxic to the body and so distilled water is doing the body a favour by removing them. Most health systems in fact promote the use of distilled or ionized water as the only water that should be drunk. However, there are others who are vehement that distilled water should be taken regularly only for a short period of time, because it does deplete the body of organic minerals— nd also because distilled water is likely to be slightly acidic in its pH. There are also concerns that it is 'de-energized', unnatural and distorted in its molecular structure.

You see, there is no consensus. The danger of depletion of trace minerals is a serious matter – one proposed cure for cancer is to take in large amounts of trace minerals (see Percy Weston's story on p. 192). It has been pointed out that people who drink lots of bottled soft drinks (made with distilled water) are almost always mineral deficient.

Others recommend various mineral or bottled waters – however, the plastic containers they come in contaminate the water with infinitely small amounts of oestrogen mimics and the heavy metal antinomy – and that is very bad news. Also most mineral waters contain inorganic minerals that are of no use to the body. Bottled 'Spring Water' may be just tap water, or may come from a polluted source.

However, there are those who say that the answer is tap water fed through a simple home-based reverse osmosis filter, which filters out all the impurities. If this is the solution you opt for make sure you change the filter regularly. However, one kinesiologist I know has reported that reverse-osmosis water has been tested as dead and should be avoided. Perhaps better than a filter is to have an ozonating machine and run ozone through the water–this kills all microbes and at the same time substantially increases the oxygen content of the water–a big plus when we remember that cancer thrives in low environments characterized by low oxygen levels. Water heated in a microwave machine should be avoided at all costs.

To test the quality of water you are taking in you can plant seeds in two or more containers and water each container with a different type of water. Compare the health of the plants that grow from these seeds.

However, to leave the discussion there would be doing a great deal of disservice to water's potential as a healing agent in its own right. First of all we need to meditate on a simple truth: We are water. Or at least 70-80 percent of us is water. Yet we tend to think of water, if at all, as something simple. Water is very far from being simple. In fact it is unique in many of its characteristics: It is one of the few natural substances whose solid form is lighter than its liquid form. It is also an extremely powerful solvent. Without these two characteristics life on Earth would be impossible.

As our bodies are composed very largely of water, dehydration is a matter of some concern. And there is strong evidence that the majority of people are almost permanently dehydrated. This is the conclusion of Dr. Fereydoon Batmanghelidj, who argues in his book, *Your Body's Many Cries for Water*, that almost every ailment known to man can be cured by drinking half your body weight (as measured in pounds) in ounces of water. For example, a 200 lb man should drink 100 ounces of water a day, which is 12-13 standard 8-ounce glasses.

In addition for every cup of coffee or alcohol, you should drink two more of water. Further, for every four glasses of water you should take in a quarter teaspoon of unprocessed, mineral rich sea salt. In fact, you can use this salt liberally on food as well. That's it. It's free and according to those who espouse it, it works. Dr. Batmanghelidj claims that this can cure heart disease, asthma, rheumatism and many other conditions. He makes no claims with regard to cancer – but that is no surprise: cancer is a dangerous subject. In any case cancer cannot be cured in isolation from the health needs of the rest of the body.

Incidentally, Dr. Batmanghelidj thinks ordinary tap water is generally fine.

Not all agree, however, that simple tap water will do. The problem, they say, is that no amount of drinking tap water will prevent this dehydration. Tap water is not taken into the cells efficiently. However, researchers have discovered that the water melt from glaciers is an almost perfect form of living water containing suspensions of trace minerals but no mineral salts. In this form water is able to saturate cells very quickly.

Two types of water have been developed that also help saturate cells fast. The first, developed by an American scientist, Dr. Patrick Flanagan, is made by adding a microcluster of colloidal minerals to distilled water. This product has been patented under the name Crystal Energy. The result is a water that contains no mineral salts but contains a colloidal mix of many trace elements – just like the glacial melt waters on which it was modeled. For more information go to www.phisciences.com.

Another form of water that is capable of saturating cells is known as Willard Water. This was initially developed as an industrial cleaner but it was discovered incidentally to have powerful pain relieving qualities and an ability to speed up the healing process. This product is also known as catalyst altered water. For more information about this remarkable product go to www.dr-willardswater.com

Both of these waters are added to normal filtered water. They are relatively inexpensive but for the cancer patient they represent a miracle. For one thing, they ensure that nutrients are taken in by the cells very efficiently. In both cases users are warned that drugs will act faster when taken in conjunction with either of these two forms of water.

There is a third type of water that is also of interest to the cancer patient: electrolysed (or ionized) water. This is a product that has been widely used in Japan for more than 25 years. Essentially, water is passed through an electrolytic process which produces on one side an acidic form of water and on the other side an alkaline form. The acidic version is a general all purpose anti-microbial treatment which can be sprayed on food to keep it free of mold and can be gargled or rubbed on the skin to treat herpes, acne, athletes foot and so on.

Of more interest to us is the alkaline electrolyzed water which has an extremely high pH value. As we shall see when we come to the discussion of diets, an acidic body state is unhealthy. Conversely, an alkaline state is good. For those with cancer, one mode of thought is that a quick fix is to speedily raise the pH value of the body's tissues. Cancers, according to this theory (for which there is a great deal of evidence), cannot survive in a highly alkaline bodily terrain. Drinking electrolyzed water is one way to raise the pH very quickly. At the time of writing a 32 oz bottle costs around $20, which will provide about 5 days worth. For more information see: .www.mnwelldir.org/docs/water/electrolyzed_water.htm

It is possible to purchase an ionizing water purifier that will allow you to create your own ionized alkaline water. There are many models on the market costing from $500-$2,000. There is also a water vitalizing system which, according to the marketing blurb, creates hexagonal water which is more easily absorbed; see www.thewolfeclinic.com for details.

However, these machines are expensive. Another cheaper and simpler way of making sure your water is alkali is simply to dissolve some baking soda in it.

All of these different types of water demonstrate that what appears to be simple (what could be simpler than water?) is really a complex subject and one that is worth investigating. These different waters are options, each of which appears to solve the same problem, that of getting water into the cells to flush out toxins and to replenish the healthy cellular medium.

The issue of what water to drink has recently been enlivened by a Japanese researcher, Masaru Emoto, who has written several books extolling an almost mystical message. In his view water is the mirror of the soul. Emoto believes that, in addition to all its other unique qualities, water has another characteristic that has not yet been widely recognized. It carries in it vibrational information.

Emoto claims to have found that water will recognize the word 'love', for example, and will respond by producing a beautiful crystal shape. However, if we give the word 'hate' it will produce a very deformed crystal. Interestingly, he found that chlorinated tap water was incapable of forming crystals – he used distilled water for those experiments where he compared the effect of external influences (such as microwave ovens) on water's ability to make crystals – not good in the case of microwave ovens.

Emoto believes that we should respect water and show it respect. He believes that the words we use to address water will change it in a subtle way and make it more healthy for the body. He therefore recommends thanking the water to express gratitude to it before we drink it.

His interest was sparked when he decided to freeze water in order to study the crystalline shapes that appeared when it melted. He took photographs of these crystals. The results can be seen in the photographs in Endo's books - *The Secret Life of Water*, *The True Power of Water* and *The Hidden Messages in Water* – which have become international best sellers.

According to an article in *New Scientist* magazine (8th April 2006), scientists are taking a closer look at water and finding that it has interesting energetic properties which may explain why a homoeopathic solution which may be so dilute that not one molecule of the original substance remains and yet it retains its effectiveness. According to Cambridge University researcher, Felix Franks, genes and proteins cannot function without the presence of water. "Without water, it's all chemistry," he says. "But add water and you get biology."

If DNA needs water to function properly, we can see the necessity to ensure the proper hydration of every cell.

As a postscript to this discussion of water, an American company, Oculus Innovative Sciences, has developed a form of ion-hungry, super-oxygenated salt water that is extremely hostile to bacteria, viruses and fungal infections. Called Microcyn, it is hoped that it will prove to be an effective agent against hospital acquired infections. As fungal infections appear to be connected in some way with cancer—either as cause or effect—and as this water is super-oxygenated, it may also be beneficial for cancer patients. It is sold for external use but is non-toxic to animals or humans if ingested. For more information see www.oculusis.com

Infra-Red Sauna Therapy

Infra-red light is light that is invisible to us, at the opposite end of the visible light spectrum from ultraviolet light. Unlike ultraviolet light it is associated with health. (Factoid: Approximately 80 percent of the sun's rays fall into the infrared range.) Compared with a traditional sauna, the far infra-red sauna is much lower in ambient temperature, does not use water and is better at promoting whole body detoxification. The toxins are eliminated through sweat.

It is claimed that in addition to its detoxification benefits, infra-red saunas also directly help stimulate the immune system, improve oxygenation of tissues, and make cancer cells more vulnerable and so easier to kill. This is a long-term therapy. Ideally, one or two sessions a day for up to two years is suggested. After each session a shower is essential to clean off toxins that have been expelled and to prevent them from being reabsorbed.

Some claim that even better than far infra-red saunas are infra-red electric light saunas. These use a different way of emitting the infra-red light. Whereas far infra-red saunas use ceramic or metallic elements for heating that mainly emit radiation in the far infrared range, infrared electric light saunas use incandescent infra-red heat lamps for heating. These emit red and orange light and near, middle and some far infra-red light. Dr. Lawrence Wilson is a leading proponent of this therapy. For further information go to his website at www.drlwilson.com

Chelation

Chelation is a method by which unwanted metals are purged from a system by putting another substance through the system which binds to the metals and so flushes them out. The need for such a chelating substance was strongly felt before the war by industry: paint, rubber, petroleum and electro-plating industries: all needed substances that would bind to and eliminate corrupting substances. Research in pre-war Germany came up with an extremely good substance: ethylene-diamine-tetra-acetate, known since then as EDTA for short.

Its first use for medical purposes was in 1947 to clear the bloodstream of a cancer patient suffering toxic side effects of chemotherapy. It did the trick. In the early 1950s EDTA was used in a number of circumstances where workers were suffering in large numbers from heavy metal poisoning. In every case it worked marvelously, according to Harold and Arline Brecher who have written a number of books on chelation therapy. "The treated [men] spontaneously reported unanticipated health benefits. Among the varied improvements were increased endurance, improved stamina, better memory, enhanced vision, hearing and smell, clearer thinking, fewer headaches, less anxiety. Those with early signs of arthritis or atherosclerosis enjoyed even more extraordinary recovery - increased mobility, reduced leg cramps, easier breathing." (Brecher, 1992)

Since then hundreds of studies have consistently shown the benefits of chelation therapy particularly for atherosclerosis - a problem for which the heart bypass operation was designed.

Additionally, it appears that chelation therapy has a possible cancer preventative action. The evidence? A Swiss study investigating the link between lead-based gas fumes and cancer incidence by Drs. W. Blumer and T. Reich, based on the health records of 231 Swiss citizens living next to a heavily used highway. Blumer and Reich were in a position to compare long-term death rates in a matched population of chelated and non-chelated patients. They found a significant mortality difference between the two groups. Of the 231 people in the study, 59 adults had chelation; 172 matched controls did not. Only one (1.7 percent of the chelated persons) died of cancer, as compared with thirty (17 percent) of the non-treated. After exploring all possible explanations for this statistical disparity in cancer mortality, the authors concluded that chelation was the sole reason for the 90 percent decrease in cancer deaths.

This supports the experience of doctors who use chelation in their practices. One, Dr. E.W. McDonagh, founder member of the International Academy of Preventive Medicine, found that of 25,000 patients that he had treated with chelation only one of those who had not previously had cancer was later diagnosed as having cancer. Taking this as an interesting indication of chelation's merits, he looked for cases of Vietnam veterans who had been severely poisoned by Agent Orange. This group is known to suffer very high incidences of cancer. He found 63 cases who had also, later, had EDTA. Not one of them subsequently developed cancer. But a word of caution, chelation may not be so effective if cancer has already started to develop before the chelation treatment started.

How does chelation work, if it does, against cancer? First, by removing toxic metals, it is removing a source of free radicals. It is therefore a preventive measure. For patients who already have cancer, it improves blood circulation by clearing arterial obstructions and so allows greater supplies of oxygen to reach the cancer site. Cancer tumours do not like high-oxygen environments. Also, it is believed that EDTA strips away the protein coat that surrounds tumour cells - this protein shield is what protects the cancer cells from T-lymphocytes, the white blood cells whose job is to kill invaders. Because of the protein layer T-lymphocytes do not identify the tumour as an enemy to be overcome. Once the protein layer has been stripped away the T-lymphocytes can start to do the job.

During chelation, the patient is hooked up - for 2-3 hours per session - to an intravenous drip which contains not only EDTA but also megadoses of vitamins. Increasing numbers of people are undergoing chelation treatments as a general preventive health measure.

One caution is that chelation needs to be carefully administered as there can be kidney complications from the extraction of too much toxic metal in a short time. A careful graduation of chelation treatments is therefore required. A standard treatment will include 20 sessions. Also high supplementation of zinc and selenium is needed as good metals are taken out with the bad. Some infrequent effects of chelation may include: low blood calcium, cardiac arrhythmia, fever, headaches and inflammation of the vein. However, these side effects are not common. Chelation is contra-indicated in the cases of damaged kidneys, liver disease, TB, brain tumours and pregnancy.

It is also possible to self-administer a chelation programme by taking an oral chelation course of capsules. Karl Loren is a long time advocate of this and he sells his oral chelation Vibrant Life capsules from www.oralchelation.com. Calcium Disodium EDTA is available from www.naturodoc.com. Another product that has been recommended can be found at www.thedoctorwithin.com. Chelation can also be done using a suppository – see www.detoxamin.com

Ionising Footbaths

These are hydro-therapy devices in which you place your feet in a footbath containing a saline solution. The water is charged with negative ions which draw out the positively charged toxins from the body. The process gently detoxifies the body of excess heavy metals, toxins, and infectious agents. It also helps to reduce inflammation and improve liver, kidney and colon function. A 20-30 minute session will result in the initially clear water round your feet becoming murky as toxins are removed. By removing the toxins through the bottom of the feet, the detox sickness caused by most detoxification protocols is avoided. That, at least, is the claim.

There are a number of ionic footbath systems on the market: Aqua Chi, BioCleanse, Ion Cleanse and others. Many testimonials attest to their energising and health promoting effects. Most systems cost over $1,000 and there are parts that need to be replenished regularly, so this is not a cheap option.

Bentonite Clay

Bentonite clay is so named because it was first mined near Fort Benton in Wyoming USA. It contains high concentrations of a medicinal mineral called Montmorillonite, which comes from weathered volcanic ash. This name derives from Montmorillon, France, where the medicinal mineral was first identified. Sometimes mineralogists use the term smectite instead to describe the same substance.

Bentonite, then, is a powdered medicinal clay which happens to be one of the most effective colon cleansers available – it scrapes the interior lining clean so that it is capable once more of absorbing efficiently the nutrients that pass down it . At the same time it is a nutritional supplement in its own right as it contains many important minerals and trace elements. The clay itself passes through the intestines without being digested. It absorbs all types of toxin from heavy metals, pathogenic viruses, molds such as aflatoxin, and pesticide residues. One of the reasons it is so effective is that bentonite's minerals are negatively charged electrically and they bind with toxins which tend to be positively charged.

Bentonite has many general healing abilities: providing relief from both constipation and acute diarrhoea (no matter what the cause), ulcers and much else. A table spoon of dissolved bentonite clay taken two to three times a day for two to four weeks will have a strong regenerating effect on the entire body—as can be seen from the improved colour of the whites of the eye, improved vitality and emotional well-being.

The best way to drink clay is on an empty stomach, at least an hour before or after a meal.

The clay is also available as a thick, more-or-less tasteless, greyish gel, but this form is best avoided. It tends to come in plastic containers and there are fears that bentonite, being such a potent attracter of toxins, may leach out toxins from the plastic. However, it also comes as a powder, which is better.

Start with one tablespoon daily for a week, perhaps mixed with a small amount of juice, if this seems comfortable, then increase to two spoons a day. The maximum dose would be four table spoons a day. You can also sprinkle bentonite in a bath and let it soak in through the skin.

Zeolite (Clinoptilolite)

Zeolites are naturally existing, negatively charged minerals, formed by the fusion of glass-rich volcanic rock with either fresh water or seawater. They have a number of rare properties. Clinoptilolite, the zeolite that we are concerned with, has the demonstrated ability to capture and eliminate free radicals, heavy metals, carcinogenic chemicals such as nitrosamines, and even   viral particles.

So far so good and if this was all that claimed for Natural Cell Defence (NCD), it would be worth taking for these properties alone. And anyone taking it should know that it is generally recognized as having no ill effects whatsoever as long as it does not amount to more than 2 percent of total food intake. The only caution is that anyone taking it should make sure they are fully hydrated at all times.

However, the big buzz surrounding zeolite is not its detoxification ability but rather its anti-cancer effects. In animal studies conducted by Ljiljana Bedric, Ph.D., at the Faculty of Veterinary Medicine in Zagreb, Croatia, 51 dogs with various cancers were treated with zeolite. All the dogs improved some having a dramatic reduction or elimination of their tumors. In only one week, six dogs with prostate cancer were found to be completely tumour free. In human studies, 114 patients were given 10-20 grams or more of megamin capsules containing a specially processed form of zeolite.

The terminal brain cancer patients showed some improvement in their condition within 3 to 4 weeks. Almost all of the forty lung cancer patients experienced decreased pain and improved respiration within the same time frame. Another fifty-three patients with terminal gastrointestinal cancers improved but at a much slower rate.

Another group of 16 cancer patients were treated by doctors at the Svecnjak Polyclinic with only Megamin therapy for a period of three years. At the end of the three years, 13 (81 percent) of the patients were in complete remission. This patient group included: 3 liver cancers, 4 metastatic melanoma, 2 bronchial carcinoma, 1 bladder cancer, and 1 hepatocellular carcinoma. The other 3 patients had obtained partial remission and stabilization of their cancers (2 lung cancer and 1 breast cancer).

Megamin can be obtained from www.megamin.net

Zeolite is also available in liquid form from multi-level marketing company, Waiora, with their product, Natural Cell Defence. Destroxin is a powdered form, which has the further advantage of being much cheaper. This is available from www.cutcat.com. Another zeolite product called Denali Green is currently getting a lot of word-of-mouth support. Do an internet search for the latest info and for suppliers. There are testimonials relating to its ability to kill tumours over time. One indication of its power is the fact that many testimonials refer to a Herxheimer response (i.e., the onset of negative symptoms as the first sign of healing). As always, when this happens, cut back the dose or stop taking the product for a few days until the symptoms go.

Removal of Parasites

Are we harbouring many parasites? It depends who you talk to. But increasingly, among the alternative health community, it has become commonly accepted that 80-90 percent of us are carrying a load of parasites in the form of various worms and flukes.

To get rid of them Hulda Clark, the person most associated with this treatment recommends the following regime involving three herbs: Black Walnut Hulls, Wormwood and Common Cloves.

"These three herbs must be used together. Black walnut hull and wormwood kill adults and developmental stages of at least 100 parasites. Cloves kill the eggs. Only if you use them together will you rid yourself of parasites. If you kill only the adults, the tiny stages and eggs will soon grow into new adults. If you kill only the eggs, the million stages already loose in your body will grow into adults and make more eggs. They must be used together as a single treatment." (Hulda Clark, *The Cure for all Cancers*.

These will, she says, eliminate over 100 types of parasites with no side effects.

Eliminating Fungi and Yeasts

Another kind of parasite are the fungi and yeasts that live in our bodies and which, when the immune response is weakened, can take over. These, like cancer, live and thrive in tissues that are poorly oxygenated. They can therefore be seen as an early warning system. To eliminate them, we can attack them directly or we can eliminate them indirectly by making the tissue environment healthier. This is done by increasing oxygen levels.

It is important to eliminate fungi and yeasts not only because they are a sign of systemic ill-health but also because their by-products overload and weaken the immune system.

One way to eliminate them is through diet (see the anti-Candida diet on p. 149).

Like cancer, fungi and yeasts also thrive on sugars so the first step to elimination is to halt intake of all sweet foods. Secondly, yeast containing foods should be avoided: bread, fermented beverages (beer, wine, brandy, scotch, etc.) mouldy cheeses, processed and smoked meats, and so on. There are a number of herbs that have an anti-fungal effect: wormwood, garlic, grapefruit seed oil among others. These should be taken on a rotating basis. Acidophilus and the use of good digestive enzymes are also recommended. For infections on the skin, tea tree essential oil can be applied liberally directly on the infestation with good results – mixed with castor oil and propolis. Also colloidal silver can be useful. And then of course there are the anti-fungal drugs that your doctor could prescribe.

DIETARY APPROACHES TO HEALING CANCER

Introduction

The idea that food might have something to do with cancer prevention or cancer cure is one that has not always been encouraged by the U.S. National Cancer Institute: "There is no diet that prevents cancer in man. Treatment of cancer by diet alone is in the realm of quackery." Dr. Michael Shimkin wrote in 1975. For decades spokesmen for the leading American cancer institutions poured scorn on 'food faddists' who promoted 'wonder foods'. Yet, now, these voices are not so loud. It is now accepted, for example, that a high fibre diet is important for intestinal health. However, nutrition still plays a very minor role in the education of a doctor. Most doctors go through their medical training without touching on the subject. One doctor told me that the word 'vitamin' had never been uttered during his years as a medical student.

But this neglect of nutrition is a modern attitude. Two and a half thousand years ago, Hippocrates said: "Let food be your medicine and medicine be your food." Six hundred years ago, Paracelsus talked of curing cancer by natural means. "In the hand of the physician, nutrition can be the highest and best remedy," he said. Unfortunately, he didn't keep statistics. By the 20th century, this idea that nature does not need to be over-ridden by drugs had become derided - and still is derided by large numbers of doctors. But people are voting with their feet and scientists from the U.S. National Cancer Institute are belatedly finding evidence to support their concerns.

One American study published in 1994 reported a sharp drop in the incidence of colon cancer between 1985 and 1988 - 8 percent for men and 11 percent for women. "The most salient risk factor for colorectal cancer is diet," the authors reported; dietary fat, particularly animal fat, was associated with a high risk, and dietary fibre, particularly insoluble or grain fibre, was associated with low risk. Fruits, vegetables and vitamin D were also seen to have a protective effect while a sedentary life-style and obesity were correlated with a higher incidence of colorectal cancer. An 8 to 11 percent drop in incidence over three to four years. This is a very significant development.

Evidence that diet and environmental factors could be the key to all cancers is, of course, implicit in comparisons of cancer rates in different countries. We know it is not genetic because immigrant families, after a generation or two, develop the cancer profiles of their host countries. We can see this clearly by comparing the statistics of death rates from various cancers round the world. Look, for example at the statistics on the next page.

What do we find? Higher cancer incidences in northern Europe. Very low rates in poor countries where the diet will be largely cereals and vegetables. There is clear indication here that the diets of prosperous countries, high in animal fats, are to blame for significant numbers of cancer cases. Wealthy Hong Kong, for example, compares badly with neighbouring China. It can't be genetic. If it's not food-related, what else could it be? It might of course be climatic. Poor countries tend to be warmer countries. It may be the amount of food eaten rather than the type. Whatever the case the evidence is clear that cancer is caused by environmental factors.

Colon Cancer

	Men	Women
USA	16.7	11.4
England and Wales	20.2	13.7
Ireland	23.2	15.1
Scotland	20.6	15.2
Germany	21.1	15.2
Denmark	22.8	17.5
France	17.3	10.3
Spain	13.2	9.2
Italy	15.6	10.3
Greece	6.8	5.5
Japan	15.1	9.7
China	7.9	6.5
Hong Kong	14.8	10.7
Mexico	3.3	3.1
Argentina	13.7	9.3
Chile	7.0	6.0

[Age-adjusted death rates per 100,000 population for colon cancer (1988-91)

Colon cancer, of course, has obvious links to food. But what about other cancers? Do the death rates for these other cancers also support the view that diet is a major factor? The next two charts show figures for breast and lung cancers. As you can see, the same picture emerges.

Breast Cancer

	women
USA	22.4
England & Wales	28.7
Germany	21.9
Spain	17.1
Greece	15.2
China	4.6
Japan	6.3
Mexico	8.1
Argentina	20.9

[Age-adjusted death rates per 100,000 population (1988-91)

Lung Cancer

	men	women
USA	57.1	24.7
England & Wales	57.0	20.5
Germany	48.7	7.8
Spain	45.2	3.4
Greece	49.8	6.9
China	34.0	14.5
Japan	30.1	8.0
Mexico	16.5	5.9
Argentina	39.2	5.8

[Age-adjusted death rates per 100,000 population (1988-91)

The lung cancer figures, at first sight, may not appear to support the argument (certainly the figure for Chinese women is anomalous – the result almost certainly of the double whammy of a husband who smokes and low quality charcoal used for cooking) - but the Chinese, Japanese and Greeks are ferocious smokers and certainly a far larger proportion of the male population in these countries smokes than in the USA. Yet their death rates are much lower. How can this be? Diet is the obvious answer. If we compare the top five with the bottom five for all forms of cancer we get the following:

	Men	Women
1.	Hungary	Denmark
2	Czechoslovakia	Scotland
3	Uruguay	Hungary
4	Poland	Ireland
5	France	New Zealand
42	Israel	Mexico
43	Venezuela	Greece
44	Mauritius	Japan
45	Ecuador	Puerto Rico
46	Mexico	Mauritius

So relative poverty, a diet heavy with vegetables, olive oil or tofu - add in sunshine, music and laughter. These are, it has been argued, the ingredients for a cancer-free life. The Mediterranean diet of olive oil, pasta, vegetables with a little wine and lots of grapes has been put forward by some as a healthy diet that we should adopt. Certainly it is a tempting one.

These epidemiological comparisons of countries are one basis for the argument that diet can help protect against cancer. And given the impact of diet on cancer incidence it seems reasonable to suggest that the huge and continuing increases in cancer incidence are due to changes in the diet we eat or the quality of the food we ingest.

There is general agreement from all sides that 70-90 percent of all cancers are lifestyle and environment, and of this at least half are in some way related to diet and nutriti a further 30 percent are the result of cigarette smoking. Some studies supporting a nu approach to prevention are summarized here:

1. A large-scale study in New Zealand published in 1994 showed that vegetarians had less than half the cancer risk of their meat eating friends.

2. A 50-year study in England and Wales found that breast cancer mortality fell from the beginning of World War II because intake of animal fats and sugar fell due to rationing. In 1954, consumption of these items returned to pre-war levels. However, breast cancer rates did not return until about 1969, suggesting that there is a 15-year time lag between ingestion and development of the disease. This is close to the 20-year time lag reported between increase in smoking habits and increased incidence of lung cancer.

3. Seventh Day Adventists, of whom roughly half are vegetarian, have significantly lower cancer levels than average, 84 percent less cervical cancer and 30-44 percent fewer cases of leukaemia.

4. The Hunza people of northern Pakistan are renowned for their freedom from degenerative diseases. Dr. Robert McCarrison who visited the area from 1904-1911 said, "I never saw a case ... of cancer." He attributed their health and longevity to their diet of whole-wheat chapattis, barley, maize, green leafy vegetables, beans and apricots. Later experimenting on rats, he found that rats fed on the Hunza diet remained healthy and free of disease, while rats fed on the normal Indian diet contracted heart disease, cancer and other ailments.

But Can Diet Cure Cancer?

This suggestion is strongly condemned by the orthodox profession. The authors of *Everyone's Guide to Cancer Therapy* say flatly : "Following a certain diet or eating certain foods will not make cancer go away....None is known to be helpful. Many result in nutritional deficiencies... Moderation is still the best approach to diet for all medical problems."

This sounds authoritative but it is not. This is simply the unsupported opinion of surgeons and oncologists who have no training or experience in the nutritional sciences and who have done no research on the subject. The need for evidence and proof cuts both ways. We are free to make up our own minds on the matter.

Interestingly, one study of 200 cancer patients who had experienced "spontaneous regression" – that is, the inexplicable disappearance of cancer tumours without any obvious cause – found that 87 percent had made serious dietary changes, which were mostly vegetarian in nature, and many others had undergone some detoxification program or used nutritional supplements.

It is clear that proactive cancer patients are making dietary changes and that these are having an effect.

Fasting

Fasting is generally seen simply as a system of detoxification, but, for the cancer patient, it is also potentially a very powerful anti-cancer therapy.

Doctors, by and large, take it as an article of faith that it is important to eat well in order to maintain the health and vigour of the body. Even Max Gerson, whose dietary regime is discussed below, opposed the idea of fasting because it would result in vitamin and mineral deficiencies and so weaken the body further. However, there is a great deal of evidence that fasting, either voluntarily or involuntarily can have a positive effect on the body's health.

Fasting as a way of achieving physical and spiritual purification is a common aspect of religious life. Fasting is frequently mentioned in the Bible. Moslems fast at Ramadan. The ancient Greek philosophers were also frequent fasters. Before anyone could be accepted as a student by Pythagoras, he had to undergo a forty day fast. Jesus also underwent a 40 day fast in the wilderness. In addition to its therapeutic value it was, presumably, a means of determining who had the necessary discipline for study. Asclepius is the Greek God of Healing. Healing through fasting was a regular feature of life at his temples. All the great doctors from Hippocrates to Avicenna have recommended healing fasts. Even the non-medical Mark Twain approved of fasting: "A little starvation can really do more for the average sick man than can the best medicines and the best doctors. I do not mean a restricted diet. I mean total abstention from food for one or two days. I speak from experience. Starvation has been my cold and fever doctor for fifteen years."

The masterwork on fasting is Herbert Shelton's *The Science and Fine Art of Fasting*, which was first published in 1934. In a foreword to this edition, Shelton describes the case of Henry Tanner M.D., who, in 1877, felt he could no longer cope with the pains and illnesses that were plaguing him. It was an accepted fact at that time that to go without food for ten days was a certain way to enter the beyond. So Tanner, preferring to ease his way to the next world, rather than to commit an act of violence against his person, took to his bed and refused all food. So far from dying, he found that, by the 42nd day he had recovered. When he announced this to his colleagues, he was denounced as a fraud. To prove he was not a fraud, he undertook another forty-two day fast under the supervision of the United States Medical College of New York. He was placed in a fenced off area and a watch was kept on him by 60 volunteer physicians. "During the first fourteen days of the fast I drank no water and breathed air in the hall that would vomit an Arizona mule."

Amazingly, he didn't die of dehydration! He was eventually allowed access to water and fresh air. On the eighteenth day, he got into an argument with a medical student over which was the best source of food: oxygen or beef. He challenged the student to walk around the hall until one of them dropped out. The medical student dropped out puffing and panting on the eighteenth lap, leaving Dr. Tanner a clear winner.

Shelton describes the case of an overweight 53-year-old English businessman who was blind in both eyes due to cataracts, had no sense of smell and who had heart trouble. He went on a fast from October 31st 1932 to February 8th 1933 - 101 days. He lost 89 lbs, regained his sight and his sense of smell. His heart trouble was much improved. He had started the fast as an experiment, intending only to go on it for ten days. After that he had just continued from day to day, gradually feeling better. But those who go on fasts to lose weight should know that the weight lost is very easily regained especially if ravenous eating follows the diet.

Shelton argues that fasting, far from being an abnormal reaction to ill-health is actually a very natural one. He points to the fact that wounded or ill animals very often refuse food until they are well on the mend. When we are ill we very often feel no appetite at all for food. The obvious implication is that the body does not wish to have food - and since the body is credited with healing powers, what it wants is probably good for it. Animals will also go for months in hibernation without any food or drink of any kind.

Fasting works against cancer because of a process known as autolysis, self-digestion. This autolysis is a controlled process by which the least essential parts of the body are self-digested. This is also true in starvation. The body seeks to preserve the most essential organs and tissues by allowing the least essential to be digested first. This is very important when it comes to cancer. Cancer tumours are recognized as being the least essential tissues in the body and so are easy victims of the autolytic process.

Shelton gives a number of examples of people who were cured of cancer by means of a fast, but he cautions that there is a wide variation in response from person to person. In some people the tumour will be devoured quickly, in others slowly. In one case a cancer cure required a fast of 21 days followed shortly after by another of 17 days. This was considered by Shelton to be abnormally long. Another woman had a speedier response: "(after) exactly three days without food, the 'cancer' and all its attendant pain were gone. There had been no recurrence after thirteen years and I think that we are justified in considering the condition remedied."

Shelton does accept that, when a cancer tumour has grown very large it may take years of on and off fasting to absorb it - and even then it may not be possible. But on the whole he is extremely optimistic about the cancer curing potential of a fast.

Is fasting hard to do? Apparently not. After a few days, it seems that the hunger goes. Many fasters experience clear improvements in their mental abilities. Shelton says: "All of man's intellectual and emotional qualities are given new life."

Having said this, anyone undergoing a fast must expect to experience in the first week a number of unpleasant sensations: headaches, nausea, etc. which is the body's response to accumulated poisons that are being eliminated.

Is there any more modern evidence that fasting works? Certainly there is evidence that low calorie diets are health promoting:

1. In 1942, Albert Tannenbaum, cancer researcher at Michael Reese Hospital in Chicago, found that mice on a low calorie diet had substantially lowered incidences of induced breast tumours, lung tumours and sarcoma than mice on an unrestricted diet. He also found that mice on a high-fat diet had a significantly higher incidence of spontaneous breast cancer. Tumours also appeared much earlier in mice fed with a high-fat diet.

2. In 1944, cancer researcher J. Saxton reported that a special strain of laboratory mice having a high leukaemia rate fed only 40 percent of a normal diet reduced their leukaemia incidence from 65 percent to 10 percent. A 1947 study found that the opposite effect also occurred. A high-protein diet increased leukaemia incidence.

3. A 1982 study at UCLA found that mice fed 28-43 percent fewer calories lived 10-20 percent longer than their controls and had fewer tumours of the lymphatic system.

Dr. Virginia Vertrano, who took over Shelton's clinic reports: "I kept a lady alive for ten years longer than the doctors said she'd live by fasting her once a year and keeping her on an all raw-food diet between the fasts. She had a very malignant breast tumour." (quoted by Richard Walters, 1993). However, she cautions that some tumours return once the fast has finished.

At the end of the fast, you should not go for a sudden blow out. A juice diet should be the first step on the road to a normal diet with some thin oatmeal porridge or vegetable soup working slowly up to a vegetable stew.

As a postscript I would like to offer the following story. Shortly after the first edition of this book came out I was visiting a friend whose father, Dr. Solomon Bard, is well known in Hong Kong as a medical doctor, archaeologist and musician. He told me a story from his own experience in support of fasting. At that time he had been a medical student at Hong Kong University. In 1941 Hong Kong fell to the Japanese and he was interned. With him in the camp was a man that he knew only had weeks or months to live. This man had an aggressive testicular cancer which had been treated with radiation but which had returned and there was nothing more the doctors could do about it. Obviously, any kind of medical intervention was made impossible by his imprisonment. But the man didn't die. He was alive at the end of the war – and still alive ten years after that in perfect health. Dr. Bard rold me he had drawn the conclusion that if he had even been diagnosed with cancer he too would have gone on a Japanese camp diet of rice and vegetables (mainly cabbage) in quantities just sufficient to maintain life.

Even more interestingly, when I publicized this story in Hong Kong another correspondent told me he knew of two men who had been cured of syphilis by the Japanese prison camp diet!

Animal studies have also shown that a hunter-gather type diet, which involves long periods of famine between moments of glut, is also highly protective against cancer – and this may be because of the autolytic process described above.

Finally, Barry Sears, biochemist and author of *The Zone*, has this to say: "calorie restriction – coupled with the correct macronutrient composition – is far more effective than any drug in the prevention or treatment of cancer." Read that sentence again. It is very important. The correct macronutrient composition, according to Sears, involves low levels of insulin-producing foods (cakes, biscuits, etc.), low in total fat, high in activated omega 3 oil, EPA. One should take 3 grams of protein for every 4 grams of carbohydrate, with most carbohydrates coming from fruits or fibre-rich vegetables.

The Australian herbalist, Walter Last, promotes what he calls a urine fast in which nothing is eaten or drunk except one's own urine. For further details of urine therapy see p. 203.

Fasting for many people will seem to be problematic in that it will take great will power to refrain from eating. There is a South African plant called Hoodia which the Bushmen of the

Kalahari desert eat to keep away hunger pangs. This is available on the internet as it marketed as a useful weight-loss tool.

The Breuss Juice Fast

According to Rudolf Breuss, an Austrian healer, cancer can live only on the protein of solid food. He therefore advised cancer patients to drink nothing but vegetable juice and teas for 42 days — the length of time, according to Breuss, that it takes for a cancer tumor to die.

His 'Breuss Juice' consists of 50 percent red beetroot, 20 percent carrots, 20 percent celery root, 5 percent raw potato, 5 percent radishes.

For a daily juice requirement, he recommends the following amounts: 300 grams of Red Beets, 100 grams Carrot, 100 grams Celery root, 30-50 grams of raw potato, 30-50 grams Radish.

These should be juiced and strained to get rid of sediment. The juice should be eaten by the spoonful, and while sipping slowly and before swallowing you should salivate strongly. Half a litre of Breuss juice is considered appropriate for a day's intake.

This is the core of the Breuss cancer cure. In addition to the juice, you are recommended to drink special herbal teas. For the first three weeks of the six week program, a cold kidney-enhancing tea is recommended for first thing in the morning followed an hour later by two cups of warm tea containing the following herbs: St. John's Wort, Peppermint and Lemon Balm. This is followed an hour later by the drinking of a little juice – after a lot of salivating. You should then take the juice 10 to 15 times throughout the morning but only when you feel like it. Sage tea can be drunk throughout the day. Also one cup of cold Cranesbill tea (geranium robertianum) should be drunk every day throughout the 42-day juice fast. During the complete treatment you should not take any food other than the vegetable juice mixture.

According to Breuss, sage tea drunk everyday will keep you free of almost all illness. It is made by putting two teaspoons of fresh sage in half a litre of boiling water. This should be boiled for 3 minutes, left to steep for ten minutes and then drunk.

One person who followed this diet successfully commented that for several weeks during this diet he felt extreme weakness but that his strength recovered towards the end.

The Five-Week Juice Fast Cure

In her book *Cancer Battle Plan*, Anne Frahm describes how, for eighteen months, she went through every form of conventional therapy - surgery, chemotherapy, radiation, hormone therapy and finally, a bone marrow transplant. They all failed. She was told that she had at most a few weeks to live. Hers was a breast cancer that had metastasized to the backbone - and even to the bone marrow. A more hopeless case it is impossible to imagine. However, she refused to 'lie down and play dead' and instead went to see a nutritional counselor. Alongside her dietary changes, she had a daily enema and was forbidden by her nutritionist from taking in any animal product. By following a strict juice diet, she claims, all signs of cancer quickly left her. "Within five weeks after starting a strict programme of detoxification and diet under the guidance of a nutritional counselor, my cancer had packed its bags."

Her recovery was begun by going on a juice fast that looked like this:

8:30 am	grapefruit juice with olive oil. She brewed a pot of Jason Winters' Tea to sip throughout the day.
9:00 am	apple juice with fibre cleanse, plus enemas.
10:00 am	green-drink with vitamin C powder
11 am	apple juice with fibre cleanse
Noon	carrot juice, acidophilus
1:00 pm	green drink with vitamin C powder
2:00 pm	apple juice with fibre cleanse.
3:00 pm	carrot juice
4:00 pm	green drink
5:00 pm	apple juice with fibre cleanse
6:00 pm	carrot juice
7:00 pm	green drink with vitamin C powder
8:00 pm	carrot juice
9:00 pm	green drink with vitamin C powder
10:00 pm	apple juice with fibre cleanse

Jason Winter's Tea is a proprietary tea made from a number of herbs.

The ingredients for the juices were organically grown apples and carrots and they were mixed 50-50 with distilled water. No tap water was allowed. The juices have to be drunk soon after they are made as the nutrients quickly oxidize. (Eating two apples a day has been suggested as a good cancer preventative.)

As for the 'Green drink', in an interview she reveals that she used Kyo Green but there are a number of different green drinks on the market containing a mix of barley and wheatgrass sprouts, chlorella, spirulina and other green vegetable products. These are discussed on p. 161-162.

For Anne Frahm, this was the start of a programme that would lead on to a largely raw vegetarian diet supported by enzymes, amino acids and vitamin & mineral supplements; strengthened through morale boosting activities and exercise. And, if we believe what she says, by following this diet rigorously all signs of her cancer were gone in five weeks. Anne lived for another ten years.

Anne Frahm's story is enlightening. It is clear evidence that it is never too late. That even someone on the brink of death can return to full health. Anne Frahm's experience is clear evidence demonstrating that food alone can cure cancer in a person who is still prepared to fight despite gloomy medical predictions.

Schulze's 30 Day Incurable's Program

Richard Schulze is a prominent American herbalist who believes that even terminal cancer patients can cure themselves if they are prepared to stick to a 30-day raw-food diet or preferably juice programme supplemented with herbs, colonics every other day, hot and cold showers, warm castor oil packs, exercise and sunlight. To order his book and a month's supply of supporting herbs, superfoods and so on go to his website at www.800herbdoc.com/home_800x600.asp

DIETS

A large number of diets have been proposed for cancer patients. Here I will look at the best known. However, before looking at the diets, we should look at the act of eating itself

Chewing Food Slowly

As we saw with the Breuss Juice fast (above), the manner of eating may itself be an important fact to which we should focus attention. It is also a key tenet of the macrobiotic approach to health. The thinking behind it is very simple. First, the body has two basic modes: tense and relaxed. For most people the body is in a state of more or less constant tension from morning to evening. When the body is tense, adrenalin is released which triggers the fight or flight response. In this mode, the body is not prepared to absorb all the nutrients in the food. Rather it is ready for the speedy elimination and only partial digestion of the food. Even the food that is digested is not made use of because the body's cells have other priorities. A relaxed body, however, is able to benefit from the nutrients taken in.

It is advised that a little prayer of thanks to those around you and to the world and the forces that have produced the good food you eat will relax the body and harmonise the mind. Slow chewing maintains that state. Additionally, chewing food until it is completely dissolved – each mouthful should be masticated up to 200 times - allows the powerful digestive enzymes in the mouth to predigest the food before it hits the stomach. This allows much better absorption of nutrients. One last benefit of slow chewing is that the body becomes aware of its state of fullness in time to have an impact on the amount of food eaten.

With that point made let us now look at a number of diets that have been proposed as powerful healing strategies.

The Grape Diet

Basil Shackleton was a very ill man when he came, almost at the end of his tether, to the grape diet. His only remaining kidney was diseased and would not respond to drugs. He had been chronically ill for over 40 years, having caught bilharzias when a young boy growing up in Africa. In despair he turned to a cure that he had only vaguely heard about - a diet of grapes. In his book, *The Grape Cure*, he explained what happened: "There is magic in the world - and there are miracles !... after twenty-three days on the treatment... I came through ... looking and feeling twenty years younger - and I was completely and permanently cured!... My body became charged with a new vitality. I felt radiant and whole."

This grape cure is probably an ancient Mediterranean folk cure. It is nothing more or less than the eating of grapes - all of the grape (skin, pips and all) - and nothing but the grapes - for a period of four weeks or longer. No drugs, no other foods, no liquids other than hot or cold water - hot for those times when you will feel nauseated. The water may be drunk at all times but not within an hour after eating the grapes as this will only dilute the strength of the natural chemicals in the grapes. The grapes must of course be washed thoroughly - and soaked two or three times - to wash off any pesticides that might be on the skin. Organic grapes would of course be better but these are not so easy to get hold of. During the grape cure there must be at least one bowel movement every two days - if not, then an enema or colonic is necessary - because the faeces is the main channel for the elimination of toxic matter. Shackleton also recommends a glycerine suppository for the purpose of encouraging a bowel movement. However, he added that in his experience it wasn't necessary!

The importance of crunching the grape seeds needs to be emphasised. Seeds are designed to pass undisturbed through the digestive tract. The chemicals contained in the seed have been found to be powerful anti-cancer agents and these need to be released. It is possible to buy grape seed extract as a supplement. An article published in the October 18, 2006 issue of the journal clinical Cancer Research based on research at the University of Colorado Health Sciences Center in Denver reported that grape seed extract inhibits the growth of human colorectal tumors in cell cultures as well as in live mice. So remember, crunch those pips.

Anyone following a toxin-removing regime is likely to suffer badly in the first week from headaches, but these symptoms will gradually disappear. The headaches are a barometer of your condition. The worse they are, the more toxins you have in your body that need to be eliminated. Shackleton ate between four and five pounds of grapes a day and after four weeks - having started the diet near death's door was able to say, "All forms of irritability and frustration - from which I had suffered for so many years - had completely disappeared. It was quite impossible for me, it seemed, to get angry! All negative symptoms recorded before the treatment had completely vanished. I was [even] able to read a newspaper without glasses."

The idea of a grape cure has been around for many centuries but it is associated in most people's minds with the name of Johanna Brandt who, shortly after the World War 1, left South Africa for America to popularize her 'grape cure' which involves fasting, eating grapes, and drinking grape juice.

Brandt claims that she was diagnosed with stomach cancer in 1916. She treated herself by fasting but that the cancer came back each time she started to eat normally. Eventually she stumbled on the grape cure and this time the cancer was indeed cured. She also claimed that the grape cure had demonstrated effectiveness against arthritis, diabetes, gallstones, cataracts, ulcerated stomach, tuberculosis, and syphilis. Her story was published in book form in 1928 as *The Grape Cure*. In this book, Brandt wrote: "The grape is highly antiseptic and a powerful solvent of inorganic matter deposits, fatty degeneration, morbid and malignant growths. It acts as a drastic eliminator of evil while building new tissue."

Brandt noted that unsweetened grape juice may be substituted for grapes and weak patients, may be the treatment of choice. Where fresh grapes are not obtainable raisins may be added to the grape juice to give bulk to the diet.

Grape juice contains several major cancer killing nutrients, such as: ellagic acid, catechin, quercetin, oligomeric proanthocyanidins (OPC) or procyanidolic oligomers (PCO), originally called: pycnogenol (in the seeds), resveratrol (in the purple skin), pterostilbene, selenium, lycopene, lutein, laetrile (in the seeds), beta carotene, caffeic acid and/or ferulic acid, and gallic acid!

Modern proponents of Brandt's version of the Grape Cure say it is advisable to fast from 8pm to 8 am so that the cells are really hungry when they get their grape juice. The cells therefore gorge themselves on the lovely sugars they find in the grape and these sugars contain the arsenal of cancer poisons that kill the cancer.

During a grape fast no other food is allowed at all and only distilled or other form of natural, non-chlorinated water is allowed.

In general, the "Grape Cure" diet cannot be mixed with other alternative cancer treatments. However, some grape diet advocates say it is allowed, indeed recommended, to add chlorella and spirulina which contain many necessary nutrients that grapes do not have. These should be taken at the same times as the grapes.

Modern proponents of the diet also suggest that most grape juices now available are simply not acceptable—either because they have been pasteurized or because they have at some time come in contact with tap water.

One further warning: The first ten days on the grape diet produces some fairly toxic smells as the intestine and stomach are cleaned out. It is at this time that you may also feel some distressing symptoms as toxins are released into the system. These will not last long. Substantial weight loss is also to be expected in the first few weeks.

Contemporary practitioners of the grape cure talk of staying on the grape-only diet for six to ten weeks at a time, rather longer than Basil Shackleton recommended.

Not all grapes are the same. The muscadine grape is an older variety, closer to the wild original. Although lower in resveratrol than normal grapes, it is higher in other healthy phyto-chemicals and research has shown that muscadine grape skin extract has a powerful anti-cancer effect in the laboratory.

At the end of the diet you should ease off it by adding uncooked, whole vegetables and fruits to your diet.

Dr. A. Ferenczi and Beetroot Therapy — worth researching

From 1950, Alexander Ferenczi, M.D., a Hungarian cancer therapist, at the Department for Internal Diseases at the district hospital at Csoma, Hungary, began putting patients on a diet of red beetroot (raw or juiced) which they ate in addition to their normal diet. Patients ate up to 1kg daily. The patients he worked with had all previously received chemotherapy and radiation but were, at the time he started to treat them with beetroot juice, mostly at the final, cachexic, stage.

Brief details of this treatment were reprinted in the *Australian International Clinical Nutrition Review* in July 1986.

One case study he reported was a 50 year old man referred to as D. S., who had a lung tumor "After 6 weeks of treatment the tumor had disappeared...After 4 months of treatment he gained 10kg. (22lbs.) in weight...The improvement lasted for about 6 months." All other tests confirmed that he had the symptoms of a clinical recovery. However, he discontinued taking the beetroot, the cancer returned and no further treatment could save him.

Ferencsi worked with a number of patients and in all cases there was clear clinical improvement from the use of beetroot. Beetroot was, in one case, so successful in attacking the tumour that the patient died from the toxic overload that resulted. This suggests that anyone following this regime should accompany it with a daily detox–perhaps the coffee enemas that Gerson recommended. *toxic from dead cancer cells.*

From this, two lessons must be taken on board. People with cancer should start the beetroot therapy as early as they can, perhaps building up slowly from 250 grams a day to a kilo, reducing the intake in the event of nausea, but maintaining the beetroot intake for years as a maintenance regime. In fact, for those of us who do not yet have cancer, regular beetroot consumption is clearly to be recommended.

The active ingredient is believed to be the purple coloring chemical anthocyanin. Anthocyanins are widely present in fruit and vegetables particularly those that are dark red and purple and research is showing that they have many health benefits. In addition to being an anti-cancer agent, it is useful as a way of protecting the body from the damage caused by radiation and chemotherapy. *Liver overload*

However, a word of warning from the Cancer Nutrition Center (www.cancernutrition.com) "Beets clean up cancer faster than the liver is capable of processing all the wastes dumped into it at any one time. Consequently, the internal administration of beetroot needs to be staggered out somewhat, and closer attention given to detoxifying the liver and colon at the same time the beetroot therapy is commenced. Never drink beet juice by itself. Pure beet juice can temporarily paralyze your vocal chords."

The Gerson Diet – *chrisbeatcancer.com & courtney both juiced & vegan - not a 100% Gerson*

The story of what happened to Dr. Max Gerson is the kind of story that can break your heart. It demonstrates without a shadow of a doubt that when the medical authorities wish to crush someone they can – and that they will do so if they consider someone to be a threat to their interests.

Max Gerson was a Jewish doctor of rising eminence who fled Nazi Germany for America - only to find himself persecuted there for his methods of treating cancer. He had become well known in Germany for having cured a number of incurable diseases - lupus, tuberculosis - with the help of diet. Among his patients were Albert Schweitzer's wife whom he cured of tuberculosis by dietary means. On his death in 1959, Schweitzer said of him: "I see in him one of the most eminent geniuses in the history of medicine."

plus they used supplements.

Apparently, Gerson started looking at diets to treat his own migraines. A few years later, a migraine patient informed him that not only had his headache disappeared but so too had his 'incurable' disfiguring skin disease, lupus. This success brought him some recognition – even in the American medical journals. At first, when he was dealing with obscure diseases the American medical journals were happy to record his achievements. But when he claimed to be able to cure cancer by diet alone his articles were rejected by these same journals. Then he was accused of keeping his methods secret. When, frustrated with these obstacles, he went to the press, he was vilified.

Max Gerson then wrote his book: *A Cancer Therapy*. This was a summary of 30 years of cancer work using dietary means. The Gerson diet, because it aims at the healing of the whole body, can, it is claimed, heal many of the major chronic health conditions including coronary heart disease, diabetes and even premature senility. Gerson stated his fundamental principle in this way: "A normal body has the capacity to keep all cells functioning properly. It prevents any abnormal transformation and growth. Therefore, the natural task of a cancer therapy is to bring the body back to that normal physiology, or as near to it as is possible. The next step is to keep the physiology of the metabolism in that natural equilibrium."

Gerson's diet consists of fresh juices of fruits, leaves and vegetables; large quantities of raw fruit and vegetables; vegetables stewed in their own juice, compotes, stewed fruit, potatoes, oatmeal and saltless rye bread. Everything must be prepared fresh and salt must be completely excluded. After six to twelve weeks, animal proteins can be added in the form of pot cheese (saltless and creamless), yoghurt made from skimmed milk, and buttermilk. The original Gerson diet also included raw veal liver juice. This, however, has been discontinued at the Gerson Institute because modern farming techniques have destroyed the value of the liver and calves are being born with diseased immune systems.

One underlying principle is to exclude sodium as far as possible and to enrich the body's tissues with potassium - "to the highest possible degree". Gerson was in favour of Lugol solution (half strength) to provide potassium and iodine. Developed by the French physician, Jean Lugol, in 1829. It is a transparent brown liquid consisting of 10 parts potassium iodide (KI), 5 parts iodine and 85 parts of (distilled) water. It is an effective bactericide and fungicide and general antiseptic.

"High potassium/low sodium environments can partially return damaged cell proteins to their normal undamaged configuration," he wrote. Potassium deficiency has been shown by others to be present in the following diseases: cancer, leukaemia, diabetes, glaucoma, chronic arthritis, acute and chronic asthma and sinusitis.

This aspect of the Gerson diet needs to be stressed. The high-potassium, low-sodium balance is well accepted as being one of the key cornerstones of good health. But before you reach for your potassium capsules, you should be warned that there are real dangers associated with sudden potassium overload – dangers to the heart, the muscles and the kidneys. You should only take potassium supplements under the guidance of a nutritionist. The best way of taking in potassium is through foods: almonds, apricots, avocados, bananas, lima, mung and pinto beans, dates, dried figs, hazelnuts, raw garlic, raw horseradish, kelp, blackstrap molasses and brewer's yeast. In fact brewer's yeast, on its own, is considered to be a powerful anti-cancer agent.

On the Gerson diet, the following are forbidden: Tobacco, salt, spices, tea, coffee, cocoa, chocolate, alcohol, refined sugar, refined flour, candies, ice cream, cream, cake, nuts, mushrooms, soybeans and soy products, pickles, cucumbers, pineapples, all berries (except red currants), avocadoes, all canned foods, preserves, sulphured peas, lentils and beans, frozen foods, smoked or salted vegetables, dehydrated or powdered foods, bottled juices, and all fats (except flaxseed oil), and oils.

Some food items are forbidden at the beginning but may be introduced to the diet later. These include: milk, cheese, butter, fish, meat and eggs. When cooking, aluminium pots must not be used - only stainless steel, glass, enamelware, or earthenware pans and containers. In addition to diet, hair dyes are also forbidden.

Almost everyone following this diet will suffer some degree of nausea, headaches, gas, depression and even vomiting. Gerson recommends peppermint tea served with some brown sugar and a bit of lemon as a cleansing drink to take away any bad tastes or inability to stomach the diet.

Patients also have to expect 'flare ups' - a sudden incidence of unpleasant symptoms - which do not last more than a few days. These are in fact essential to health as they indicate that the body is expelling toxins. It was, and remains, a key aspect of the Gerson approach that without these flare ups the patient will not be cured. The more poisoned the body was prior to treatment, the more serious the flare ups. These flare ups are the result of a toxic release and the body must be detoxified with the use of coffee enemas to ensure that the patient is not damaged by them. It has been argued that it would be very dangerous to combine the Gerson diet with any other effective regime as this might bring on an unexpectedly quick flare up of dangerous intensity.

Beata Bishop is one person who has been cured by strictly following the Gerson regime. In her case, it took about eighteen months before she was certain she had beaten the disease. Her book: Triumph over Cancer starts with these words:

"I should have died of malignant melanoma, one of the fastest spreading cancers, around June 1981. Today I am healthy in the full sense of the word; not just not-ill but enjoying great well-being and energy."

In April 2008, Ms. Bishop sent me an email to confirm that at the age of 75 she was still very much alive and active – she was just off on a lecture tour.

Gerson also recommended Niacin 50 mg, six times daily, for six months. As for vitamin B12, he was undecided but he was against the administration of other vitamins because he noticed they sometimes had the effect of causing a tumour to grow back. This is because, he says, non-cancerous tissue in a cancer patient does not react in the same way as normal healthy tissue. That is to say, vitamins may normally be very healthy - but they can have negative effects in people with cancer.

And what evidence did Gerson put forward to support his claim that his diet was effective as a cancer treatment? In his book, *A Cancer Therapy*, he provides case histories of 50 patients that he cured.

One of these cases, Case No. 46, was a Mrs E.B. Aged 48, married with two children. She presented with a cervical carcinoma which was showing signs of invading neighbouring tissues. The biopsy showed clear malignancy. By the time she reached Gerson she had already had radiation treatment but the tumours had returned. He started her on the diet and she kept to it faithfully for 18 months. At the end, she had no sign of cancer. She slowly weaned herself off the diet and eleven years later was still cancer-free.

How successful is the diet? Various estimates have been given–ranging from as low as 5 percent to as high as 80 percent. One of the problems is that the Gerson diet is extremely rigorous and the extent to which ex-patients of the clinic have maintained the diet is unknown. But in one small retrospective study of melanoma, the results were extremely good: 100 percent of the stage I and II melanoma cases surviving for five years–in fact none of them died of melanoma and one was still alive 17 years later. For stage III cases the results were 82 percent compared with 39 percent reported by the American Cancer Society. It appears that the Gerson diet is particularly helpful for people with melanoma. There are suggestions that it is less successful with other types of cancer. For further information contact: The Gerson Institute, P.O. Box 430, Bonita, California 91908. USA Tel 1-(619)-685-5353 www.gerson.org or Gerson Research Organization www.gerson-research.org

The Moerman Diet

In 1938, Dr. Cornelis Moerman developed a diet that he used to treat those cancer patients that came to see him. He had to suffer professional ridicule for several decades but eventually, in 1987, the Dutch Ministry of Health publicly recognized the Moerman therapy as an effective cancer treatment. Moerman, like many others favouring nutritional health, lived rather longer than most of his colleagues. He was 95 when he died in 1988.

Moerman first became involved when a man by the name of Leendert Brinkman came to him seeking his help. He had a stomach tumour that had spread to his groin and legs. The doctors had given up on him. Moerman told him to eat as many oranges and lemons as he could. He ate them "by the truckload until I was up to my eyes in vitamin C" - a year later he was free of tumours. He went on to live to a healthy old age, dying at the age of 90.

This success led Moerman to develop his nutritional ideas. Eventually he came to believe that there were eight substances of vital importance to ideal health. These should be taken in supplemental form as well as through dietary means. The required doses of the eight substances were as follows:

Substance	Dose
1. Vitamin A	50,000 IU - 100,000 IU
2. B-complex vitamins	2 large dose tablets
3. Vitamin C	as much as can be tolerated
4. Vitamin E	400-2,200 IU
5. Citric Acid	3 tablespoons (of solution: 10-15g Acidum citricum in 300 g of water)

6. Iodine	1-3 drops of 3percent iodine solution in 300 g of water
7. Iron	
8. Sulphur	1,000 mg

Citric acid helps the blood flow, iodine is important for stimulating the thyroid gland. It also works with sulphur to help oxygenate cells. Iron is needed to prevent anaemia. It should be noted that Moerman's liking for iron is not universally accepted among the vitamin and mineral supplement crowd today. Iron has also been implicated, in other studies, as a cancer-promoting agent. Cancer tumours have a great need for iron and some approaches to cancer are based on depriving it of this mineral – so with the regard to the iron, caution is strongly advised.

Moerman's diet allows selection of any of the following:

Grains: whole-grain breads and pastas, brown rice, barley, oat bran, wheat germ, what or corn flakes

Dairy: butter, buttermilk, cream cheese, cottage cheese, egg yolks, plain live yoghurt

Vegetables: most vegetables lightly steamed. Highly recommended: beet juice and carrot juice, limited intake: Brussels sprouts, cauliflower, parsley

Fruit: most fruits. Most recommended: mixed fresh orange and lemon juice.

Others: bay leaf, garlic, herb tea, nutmeg, cold-pressed olive and sunflower oil.

Prohibited foods: All meats, all fish and shellfish, alcohol, animal fats, artificial colourings, beans, peas, lentils, mushrooms, potatoes, red cabbage, sauerkraut, cheeses with high fat and salt content, margarine and other hydrogenated oils, coffee, cocoa- or caffeine-containing teas, egg whites, sugar, salt, white flour and tobacco.

As we can see there is a great deal of overlap with the Gerson diet. Of the two, Gerson's is clearly more rigorous in that it stresses that the intake must be raw - but if even the lighter regime of Dr. Moerman is considered to be effective then some leeway is clearly permitted.

Is there any proof that it is effective? A number of doctors sympathetic to Moerman's diet set up a research project which followed 150 patients who had used the Moerman diet either alone or in combination with other therapies. They found that 115 (76.66 percent) of the patients were cured – 60 (40 percent) using the diet alone.

Results of small studies like this are open to many objections but the result indicate that further research should be done. The Dutch Ministry of Health accept Moerman diet is a bona fide and effective cancer treatment. The American Cancer Society to say, disagrees.

The Macrobiotic Diet

Our vet's father had lymphoma & lived 10yrs on macrobiotic diet and 'other wierd stuff"

Modern macrobiotics was developed in Japan at the turn of the century. Two educators, Sagen Ishitsuka, who was himself a doctor, and Yukikazu Sakurazawa cured themselves of serious chronic illnesses by changing their diets to one consisting of brown rice, miso soup, sea vegetables and other traditional foods. Sakurazawa went to Paris in the twenties and - using the name George Ohsawa - began to spread the word.

Ohsawa's Macrobiotic diet is based on Eastern philosophy and takes its starting point in the idea of Yin and Yang, the dark passive female and light active male forces which must be maintained in a state of harmony. The body, as with everything else in the universe, must also maintain a healthy balance between these two forces. As each person is unique, the point of balance will be different for each person. Individual cancer tumours also have yin and yang characteristics. For example, while cancer of the tongue is yang, all other tumours of the upper digestive tract are considered to be yin.

From a macrobiotic point of view, cancer is simply a sign, one among others, that the body is in a disharmonious state. The objective, then, is simply to restore the harmony. The only way we can achieve this is through dietary means, such as that recommended by Michio Kushi and Alex Jack, in their book: *The Cancer-Prevention Diet.*

Food item	Percentage of daily intake

Whole Grains   50-60 percent

These should be eaten in whole form - and not cracked. Brown rice should be pressure cooked rather than boiled. Breads should not contain yeast, so chapattis and tortillas and sourdough bread are recommended.

Soup   5-10 percent

One or two bowls of miso or tamari soup. Miso is a kind of fermented soybean paste. Miso should have aged more than 1½ year and be made of organically grown soybeans.*

Vegetables   25-30 percent

These should be fresh. Up to a third can be eaten raw.

Beans and Sea Vegetables   5-10 percent

next pg →

Oils:

Unrefined sesame, corn or mustard seed oils are best. Unrefined safflower, sunflower, soy and olive oils can be used occasionally.

Others

Sea salt - though meals should be neither too salty nor too bland. Salt should be used in the cooking and not at the table.

(* Note: It is known that miso contains a number of anti-angiogenesis substances that interfere with tumour growth)

One of the surprising features of the macrobiotic diet is its avoidance of fruits. This avoidance isn't absolute but fruits are advised only occasionally and only in the proper climatic zone and in the proper season. A person in Europe in winter should not be eating bananas or even oranges. Also to be avoided, in addition to red meats, are dairy products and any form of processed food, are cooking spices and herbs, butter or margarine, iodized salt, ginseng, eggs and yoghurt. Another surprise is the ban on any kind of vitamin or mineral supplement.

Is there any evidence that the macrobiotic diet is effective? Kushi and Jack offer a number of stories of people being cured. One was Jean Kohler, a 56-year-old pianist and professor of music. One summer, he suddenly became aware of an itch that spread up his leg. After several tests were conducted the doctors discovered a massive tumour on his pancreas. Pancreatic tumours are almost always fatal. He was told nothing could be done and that he had anywhere from one month to three years to live. He accepted chemotherapy but after a few days decided that he didn't want to continue with the treatment as it was too debilitating. He started to look for an alternative therapy and was referred to the Kushi Institute in Boston. He started a macrobiotic regime and within six months all signs of cancerous activity had ceased. This was confirmed by medical tests.

Kohler lived another seven years and died of something else entirely. He publicized his case whenever he could and even wrote a book about it.

In another case, Dr. Vivien Newbold, an emergency care doctor in Philadelphia, became interested in macrobiotics when her husband had a metastatic cancer of the colon. He reduced the cancer by 70 percent by going on a macrobiotic diet. She subsequently wrote an article detailing the effect of a macrobiotic diet on six cases in which the five cases who stuck with the diet went into total remission for over five years. This article was rejected by three professional magazines. She was also told by the American Cancer Society's director: "It is of no interest to us."

In 1993, however, the *Journal of the American College of Nutrition* published a study of the effects of the macrobiotic diet on people with pancreatic cancer. After one year, 52 percent of those on the diet were still alive compared with only ten percent of the controls - a 500 percent increase in one- year survival rates.

For further information contact: Kushi Institute, PO Box 7, Becket, MA 01223, USA.

Barry Sears, a biochemist and pioneer in biotechnology who wrote a best-selling book, *The Zone*, analyzed the macrobiotic diet and praised it for the fact that it has low overall fat, especially bad omega 6 fats, but is rich in the activated omega 3 fatty acid EPA (fish and sea vegetables), but he faults it for being too high in grains. He characterizes the diet as being 'like taking two steps forward and one step back'.

The Alkaline pH Diet   *I've heard a lot about this*

The foods we eat, once they have been digested and the useful food elements extracted, leave a residue, or an ash, in our bodies and this ash will either be acid, alkali or neutral. The acidity or alkalinity of any substance can be determined by comparing it to a pH scale. If it tests at below 7.0 on the scale then the substance is acid. If it tests above 7.0 then it is alkali. A healthy state of being is slightly alkali (7.35-7.45). Unfortunately, for most people living on convenience foods, the body's tissues are increasingly tending towards an acidic, disease-vulnerable state.

In a famous analysis, which was to lead to a Nobel Prize, Dr. Otto Warburg described the environment of the cancer cell. A normal cell uses oxygen to convert glucose into energy by the process of oxidation. When there is insufficient oxygen around the cell to be used for this purpose, the cell reverts to a more primitive process, converting glucose by fermentation. This fermentation process produces lactic acid as a by-product and the acid lowers the cell's pH (i.e., it makes the cell more acidic) and this in turn makes the cell unable to control its own cell division processes. The result is cancer. At the same time, the lactic acid causes intense local pain and destroys the cell's enzymes. From this we can see that an acidic state is essentially cancerous and an alkali state is healthy. We can also see that a cancer cannot continue to exist when the surrounding tissues are highly alkaline (that at least is the theory).

The following two lists show the foods that leave an alkali ash (good) and those that leave an acidic ash (bad).

Alkali-Ash Foods

Almonds, apples, apricots, avocados, bananas, dried beans, beetroot, blackberries, broccoli, Brussels sprouts, cabbage, carrots, cauliflower, celery, chard leaves, cherries (sour), cucumbers, dried dates, dried figs, grapefruit, grapes, green beans, green peas, lemons, lettuce, goat's milk, millet, molasses, mushrooms, onions, oranges, parsnips, peaches, pears, pineapples, sweet potatoes, white potatoes, radishes, raisins, raspberries, rutabagas, sauerkraut, green soybeans, raw spinach, strawberries, tangerines, tomatoes, umeboshi vinegar, watercress, watermelon.

Acid-Ash foods

Bacon, barley grain, beef, blueberries, bran (wheat and oat), bread (white and whole meal), butter, cheese, chicken, cod, corn, corned beef, crackers, cranberries, currants, eggs, flour (all types),

next pg

147

haddock, lamb, dried lentils, lobster, macaroni, oatmeal, oysters, peanut butter, peanuts, dried peas, pike, pork, rice (white and brown), salmon, sardines, sausage, scallops, shrimp, spaghetti, winter squash, sunflower seeds, turkey, veal, walnuts, wheat germ, yoghurt.

Refined sugar and olive oil are neutral ash foods that nevertheless have an acidifying effect on the body.

The pH of the body is also affected by emotions and activity–stress and aggressive sports create a more acid environment; relaxation and relaxed exercise create a more alkaline environment.

Drinking a teaspoon of sodium bicarbonate in a glass of water at night is also recommended as a way of raising alkalinity. In fact sodium bicarbonate has been used as a cheap and effective way of attacking cancer cells by introducing it as close to the tumour as possible by intravenous injection or vaginal flush. An Italian doctor, Dr. Tullio Simoncini, has claimed a high degree of success using this method.

Another approach, recommended by an Appalachian folk healer in the 1930s, is to heat one part of baking soda with three parts of pure maple syrup for five minutes, stirring briskly. When this mixture is consumed, the theory is that the cancer cells suck up the glucose along with the baking soda that is bound to it. The sudden increased alkalinity in the cell kills it. Some critics point out, however, that maple syrup cannot chemically bind with sodium bicarbonate. However, Bill Henderson, who has experimented on himself, says he experienced clear and indeed powerful demonstrations that this mix had a healthy impact on his bowel movements. Whether it also has an anti-cancer effect is still very much in the realm of anecdote and folk lore.

Oxalic Acid Diet

This is a diet whose aim is to increase the oxalic acid concentration of the blood, according to the man whose inspiration this is: Colonel Joe Hart, a retired American army officer. This will, he claims, help cure you of cancer and a number of other health conditions. Before starting this discussion, however, it is important to note that oxalic acid is a powerful poison and should never be ingested in its purified chemical state. Half an ounce of oxalic acid will kill you within an hour.

Col Joe – Francis J. Hart – has noted first that a healthy body has a high oxalic acid presence in the blood – an odd fact given that it is supposedly poisonous. Also he notes that the foods that are most commonly focused on as being beneficial against cancer – carrots, cabbage, beetroot, etc.– are precisely those that are highest in oxalic acid – and he believes that oxalic acid is what keeps the blood clear of cancer cells.

His diet consists of eating vegetables selected from the following list: Snap beans, Brussels sprouts, beets, carrots, cassava, chives, collards, garlic, lettuce, parsley, purslane, radish, spinach, sweet potato, turnips and watercress. Nuts – especially walnuts - are also a good source and contain fatty acids (oleic & linoleic), which will increase the intestinal absorption of the acid. He also advises that all cooking be done with olive oil (cold pressed extra virgin is best). Chocolate is also good – but not the milk and sugar that goes with it.

Unfortunately, the benefits of oxalic acid can be blocked by other dietary and items such as citric acid, calcium, cow's milk (and milk based products), vitamin B6 (pyri[...] alcohol – though if you like a tipple then choose a cheap red wine which is high in oxa[...] danger of citric acid comes not from ingesting too many oranges but from its use as a preservative in most processed foods (all of which must be avoided). The non-dietary blocker that most concerns Col Joe is radiation – from cell phones, irradiation of food and from every other source of radiation. For further information and for testimonials go to Col. Joe's website www.coljoe.com

The Anti-Candida Diet

hmmm – note lot of veg. & dairy & processed a common element in these diets

Fungi and yeasts are associated with cancer and can themselves harm the body with their toxins. To get rid of them, Philip Day, author of *Cancer: Why We're Still Dying to Know the Truth*, suggests the following diet.

Eliminate: All cow's milk products and derivatives including yoghurt;   all yeast-containing products: including alcohol, bread, vinegars; mushrooms; processed and smoked fish and meats; all sugar products including honey and artificial sweeteners; nearly all fruit; root vegetables with a high sugar content: carrots, parsnips, sweet potatoes, potatoes, beetroot.

Other foods to be eliminated are: all pastries, cakes, cereals, fast food snacks, white rice, corn, pasta, chick peas, dried beans, lentils and pinto beans, coffee, all soy products, all sauces, all hydrogenated oil products.

Instead you should eat plenty of the following foods:

Vegetables: Bean sprouts, bell peppers, broccoli, Brussels sprouts, cabbage, cauliflower, celery, Chinese greens, cucumber, endive, fennel, garlic, green beans, hot chilli peppers, kale, lettuce, onions, parsley, radishes, spring onions, spinach, Swiss chard, turnips, yellow beans.

Meat, etc.:   Free-range eggs, fresh fish (deep sea, wild), lamb, veal, chicken, turkey.

Herbs: Culinary herbs and spices are permitted.

Oils: Avocado oil, cod liver oil, fish oil, flaxseed oil, grape seed oil, hemp oil, olive oil, evening primrose oil.

Fruit: You are allowed one apple, pear or kiwi fruit a day.

next pg.
Raw Food diet

3 Doctors cured their cancer w/ raw Food diet

they eat organic & occasionally eat organic meat - still eat lots of veg. & veg juice

Raw-food Diet

Chris Wark @ Chrisbeatcancer.com & courtney cured their cancers by going raw for several months

The main problem with cooking food is that not only does it destroy some of the vitamin and nutrient qualities of the food, it also destroys the enzymes that help to digest that same food. (If you are going to cook, remember that steaming food is the best way.) Raw food is therefore generally much healthier than cooked food.

Vegetables and fruit can be eaten either raw or as a juice. The foods that have been identified by the other dietary regimes above are all suitable for this diet. A number of people claim to have cured their cancers simply by turning to an all raw-foods diet–among them a number of doctors. This diet was promoted by the Danish doctor Kristine Nolfi. She cured her own cancer with a hundred percent organic and vegetarian raw-food diet, and then continued to cure cancer patients in the same way on her health farm.

When she discovered that she had cancer, she wrote: "I started immediately, going to a small island in the Kattegat where I lived in a tent, ate raw vegetables exclusively and sunbathed from four to five hours a day when weather permitted. When I felt too warm, I plunged into the sea. My fatigue continued throughout the first two months, and the tumor in my breast did not diminish. But then my recovery began. The tumor grew smaller as I regained strength, and I felt better than I had for several years."

She eventually lost her medical license for using 'dangerous' and unapproved methods but her fame nevertheless spread throughout Scandinavia. It should be noted that after a year she went back to a diet that was only 75 percent raw vegetables, and soon afterwards she felt the tumor return.

A New Zealand doctor, Eva Hill, successfully treated her basal carcinoma following a raw-food diet – becoming a well known advocate in the antipodes. She had to overcome a few legal barriers before it became accepted that she should be allowed to treat cancer patients in any way likely to be successful. And, in Britain, Dr. Barbara Moore successfully cured herself of Leukemia in the same way. She subsequently went on to publicly demonstrate the health of her vegetarian diet by walking the length of Britain from John O'Groats to Lands End.

Lactic Acid Diet

Lactic acid is a natural preservative in that it inhibits pathogenic bacteria. It is a by-product created by the breakdown of sugars and starches by lactobacilli–a family of bacteria that includes the well-known acidophilus. These living lactobacilli produce many helpful enzymes, antibiotics and anti-carcinogens. Lactic acid, their by-product, promotes the growth of healthy flora throughout the intestine as well as preventing the growth of harmful bacteria. It is also an extremely fast fuel that is vital for ensuring that our bodies get a steady supply of carbohydrates. Athletes use drinks containing lactates.

In the 1950s, German cancer therapist, Dr. J Kuhl, used a diet high in lactic acid fermented foods with good results. It was Dr. Kuhl who discovered that there was an important difference between 'healthy' lactic acid and the lactic acid produced by cancers. He noted that Lactic acid

note

Chris ate alot of sauerkraut on his salads & veg juice

produced by a tumour rotates light to the left and enhances tumour growth. Lactic acid produced by lactic acid bacteria, on the other hand, rotates light to the right and inhibits tumour growth. ?

A lacto-fermented diet consists of foods like sauerkraut, olives, pickles, vegetable juices, dairy and naturally fermented soy products like miso. But note that not all soy sauces are good - some commercially produced soy sauces contain dangerous chemicals.

To make your own fermented vegetable preparation: shred green or red cabbage, grated beetroot, diced Brussels sprouts, red peppers, chillies, cucumbers and add either sea salt or, if you prefer not to use salt, add some strong alcohol and water (but not tap water as chlorine interferes with the process). Mash the mixture for several minutes and then bottle it in sealed glass containers. Leave some space between the top of the mix and the top. Leave for at least three days at room temperature before refrigerating—but the longer the better. Do not open at any time as oxygen interferes with the fermentation. When it's ready eat it.

The Dries Cancer Diet

Dr. Jan Dries is a leading Belgian naturopath and active promoter of a vegetarian diet. His starting presumption is that wild animals do not get cancer, that we are a monkey and that wild monkeys live mainly on a diet of fruit and nuts—and this answers all their nutritional needs. Another basic principle behind his anti-cancer diet is that the consumption of natural foods is, in effect, the consumption of sunlight – the more sunlight a food has absorbed, the more powerful it is as an enhancer of the immune system.

The Dries cancer diet, unlike almost every other anti-cancer diet, promotes the consumption of large quantities of raw fruits, particularly tropical fruit such as pineapple and mango. In addition, the diet includes some raw vegetables, seeds, yoghurt, buttermilk and some oils. These foods are chosen on the basis of their bio-energetic value measured in bio-photons.

All chemicals whether they are preservatives, fertilizers or pesticides, undermine what he calls the 'bio-energetic value' of food. So too does cooking. The Dries cancer diet promotes the eating of raw, preferably wild or organic, fruits. The Dries diet divides foods into seven groups of decreasing bio-energetic value. The first group consists of the foodstuffs that, according to Dries, have the greatest bio-energetic value. But food from all seven groups should be eaten.

Group I: Pineapple, Cactus fruit, Avocado, Raspberry, Honeydew melon, Pollen, Comb honey

Group II: Bilberry, Kiwi, Cherry, Persimmon, Apricot, Melon, Mango, Papaya, Almonds, Chervil, Mushrooms, Honey

Group III: Feijoa, Red currants, blackcurrant, Strawberry, Lychee, Passion fruit, Red and green grapes, Medlar, Peach, Sunflower seeds, Pumpkin seeds, Wheat germ, Germinated wheat, Sprouts, Liquid brewer's yeast, Panaktiv*

Group IV: Banana, Gooseberries, Green melon, Brazil nut, Coconut, Vegetables, Dairy products

Group V: Oranges, mandarins, apples, pears, plums and grapefruit.

Group VI: This group consists of common vegetables

Group VII: Avocados, nuts and seeds

(*Panaktiv is a liquid brewer's yeast developed by a Dr. Metz—see www.drmetz.de for further details.)

Group 1 foods should be eaten at every meal. Foods from the other groups should be eaten with decreasing frequency depending on their place in the hierarchy. It is recommended that you follow the Dries diet exclusively for three months.

The result, according to those who have undergone this diet, will be a very obvious detoxification of the body – bad smells and so on for a few weeks. But once this is complete there are no further negative impacts. Personal testimonials refer not only to the healing potential of the diet but its ability to help patients undergo radiation and chemotherapy with very much reduced levels of side effects. You can expect substantial weight loss.

If there is an issue with this diet it is the apparently high intake of sugars. However, while refined white sugar will cause a sudden leap in blood sugar levels – it is known as a high-glycaemic food - fructose, despite being a sugar, is in fact one of the lowest-glycaemic foods there are. Its glycaemic index rating of 20 compares with 31 for skim milk, 59 for refined sugar, and a whopping 98 for the same amount of mashed potatoes. While there is some dispute among nutritionists as to the healthfulness of a fructarian diet, some cancer studies have shown that high fructose intake is correlated with lower rates of prostate cancer.

Dries is not alone in advocating a raw fruit and/or vegetable diet. It has been pointed out that such diets are high in water and bulk fiber content and result in low nutritional intake. Since cancer growth appears to be directly related to food intake, this is good news. In experiments using mice fed on raw fruits and vegetables, the benefits of the raw diet were lost when soy protein or other dietary 'improvements' were added. So this diet, in the guise of being a diet, may be just another way of fasting.

Contact details: Jan Dries, Avicenna Health Ctr, Schepersweg 112, 3600 Genk, Belgium, Tel: 32 89 396 169 Fax: 32 89 355 307

Since different diets are based on different principles and have different objectives it is not necessarily a good idea to mix and match.   *very important*

OTHER FOOD BASED THERAPIES

The Budwig Protocol

This is the most highly regarded of all dietary approaches and supporters of the Budwig Protocol claim a 90 percent success rate against all forms of cancer. Dr. Johanna Budwig, an eminent German biochemist, was the first person to promote the health benefits of flaxseed oil.

Budwig was among the first scientists to take a close look at an area that had previously been lumped together and ignored – the fats. She soon discovered that although some fats, the saturated fats, were harmful, others the 'natural electron-rich, vital, highly unsaturated fats' had enormously beneficial properties. The saturated fats tended to clog cells and organs and the result of this process, eventually, is diabetes, arthritis, heart disease and cancer. The most highly unsaturated fats are those Budwig grouped together under the heading 'linoleic acids'. By this she meant both linoleic acid (an omega 6 oil) and alpha-linolenic acid (an omega 3 oil). It is now known that omega 6 oils, in excess, promote inflammation and cancer, while omega 3 oils are healing.

These so-called 'essential' fatty acids are vital for the proper oxygenation of the body. For Budwig the key element that made these unsaturated fats life promoting was their electrical charge created by a surrounding field of electrons. Unfortunately, industrial handling of these fats strips away this field of electrons and destroys their vitality. She likens them to a battery that has run flat.

These de-activated unsaturated fats along with the saturated fats are no longer able to travel through the small capillary network of the blood system. The result is that they clog the capillaries and as a result the tissues these capillaries serve become de-oxygenated. As cells accommodate themselves to this new low-oxygen environment, cancer can be the end result.

The solution, according to Budwig is to take in Flaxseed oil (also known as linseed oil) which contains an excellent mix of 4 parts alpha-linolenic-acid (ALA) to one part linoleic acid. However, in its pure form it is not so easily absorbed by the body. Looking around for a protein-based substance in which to dissolve the flaxseed oil and allow it to become water soluble (and so more easily absorbed by the body) she found in succession skim milk, quark and low-fat cottage cheese. Some nutritionists are now proposing that yoghurt or whey concentrate might be equally good.

One tablespoon of flaxseed oil (liquid, never capsules) should be hand blended, very thoroughly, with one or two spoons of soft low-fat cottage cheese or, preferably, quark. This can be taken once a day for normal health maintenance and six to ten times a day to cure cancer. Cayenne pepper and garlic can be added for taste (and because they are also beneficial). People with advanced liver cancers may not be able to tolerate such quantities straight away so dose levels will have to be built up slowly. *Can mix in berries for Breakfast. Bill Henderson's Book uses as part of his program*

This is the core of the Budwig Protocol which should be supported by a diet that contains fresh, preferably raw (and consequently enzyme-rich) fruits and vegetables, unprocessed cereals, and fresh cold water fish, 6-8 glasses of bottled distilled water and herbal teas. Starting the day with freshly home-made sauerkraut is a key recommendation. Foods to avoid include all processed oils, fried foods, sugar, artificial sweeteners or any processed food containing preservatives, or chemical

Lactic Acid diet on pg 150 promoted saurkraut

note similarities in a next pg bunch of these diets ⟶

additives. In addition, as much time as possible should be spent being exposed to the sun's rays without sunblocks. In her booklet, *Flax Oil as a True Aid Against Arthritis, Heart Infarction, Cancer and Other Diseases*, she discusses in great detail the electromagnetic benefits of light on the body.

She also recommends a number of oils, called EL-DI (short for Electron-Differentiation) oils, that can be rubbed on the skin. They are available from: Gesundheitsprodukte-Reformwaren, Tel: 07441-2877 (011 49 7441 2877 from USA & Canada); email: Wolfgang.Bloching@t-online.de

However, as some people have discovered, it is not a good idea to take powerful anti-oxidants like vitamin C or ellagic acid at the same time as the Budwig Protocol, as these tend to deactivate the benefits of flax oil. Even too many citrus fruits should be avoided. In fact, Budwig was opposed to the taking of any man-made supplements.

In most cases, according to Dr. Budwig, this protocol will be sufficient to cure cancer, arthritis and heart disease. What's more, there are large numbers of testimonials to support this claim. She and her supporters claim a 90 percent success rate with all forms of cancer. However, in a small number of cases the body lacks certain enzymes and nutrients and so the body is unable to process the flaxseed oil. In this case, fish oils should be added to the diet along with Brewer's yeast. (In fact there is a record of a 78-year-old man who recovered slowly – it took him six years - from a widely spread lung cancer by taking 15 grams of fish oil a day. This was reported in an article by Dr. Ron Pardini of the University of Nevada)

It has been said that strictly speaking the Budwig Protocol, as it is known, does not attack cancer, it merely corrects a previous deficiency in omega 3 oils. Armin Grunewald, M.D., Dr. Budwig's nephew has commented, "Dr. Budwig's approach is not a method of healing cancer but a technique which strengthens the body's own immune defence against cancerous cells." In 1990, oncologist, Dr. Roehm concluded: "this diet is far and away the most successful anti-cancer diet in the world". This Budwig Protocol has claims to be a very powerful anti-cancer tool as the many testimonials on the Yahoo health groups flaxseed oil page demonstrate. For more information go to:

www.health.groups.yahoo.com/group/FlaxSeedOil2/files/

Another very useful information site is

www.healingcancernaturally.com/budwig_protocol.html

It should be noted, as a postscript, that flaxseeds are one of nature's more potent anti-cancer plants and not just because they are the richest plant source of omega-3 fatty acids. Flax has at least 100 times more lignan precursers than any other known edible plant. Lignans are natural plant compounds that possess strong anticancer properties. One of these lignans is Secoisolariciresinol Diglycoside (SDG) which on its own has been shown to inhibit metastases.

However, lignan-enriched flaxseed oil is not advised by Budwig purists. The process of adding lignans to the already lignan-rich flaxseed oil has negative consequences for the quality of the oil.

Also, there is a new flaxseed strain called Linola that has been developed to provide oils for the food industry. Sadly, this form of flaxseed oil is very low in ALA and so it too should be avoided. In the USA, Barleans brand flaxseed oil is highly regarded and I am informed that if you contact them directly and tell them you have cancer, they will give you a substantial discount. To enquire, call them at 1-800-445-3529. www.barleans.com. Flaxseed oil is sold at most health food shops. It must be kept in dark bottles and kept in cool places. It quickly loses its potency in light conditions.

As a postscript to the flaxseed story, Steve Martin, who runs a very interesting site at www.grouppekurosawa.com, quotes the case of an 83-year-old man who had terminal prostate cancer. Taking a flaxseed product, he saw his PSA score drop from 155 plus to 14.5 over a few weeks. According to Martin, the lignans in flaxseed oil cause cancer cells to die through apoptosis. The product he recommends is Jarrow Formulas Omega Nutrition Cold-Milled Flaxseed, which is organic, and provides 105 mg of lignans per tablespoon.

Controlled Amino Acid Therapy (CAAT)

This is a combination dietary regime, accompanied by supplements and a specially formulated amino acid mix. The regime is customized for each patient.

Formulated by Dr. Angelo P. John, this therapy is offered exclusively by the AP John Institute for Cancer Research. The object of the therapy is to create a diet that deprives the cancer tumour of certain amino acids and carbohydrates (which are converted into sugar during digestion – and cancers love sugar). This approach has a great deal of experimental support.

The whole therapy program lasts six to eight months and costs approximately US$1,200 a month. For further information go to www.apjohncancerinstitute.org

The Dairy-Free Diet

Wow – note again vegetarian she went back to eating meat – read next page

Prof Jane Plant was diagnosed with breast cancer at the age of 42. At the time she was a successful geochemist (she subsequently became chief scientist of the British Geological Survey). She went on a vegetarian diet. She had a mastectomy. She had radiation. But the cancer kept coming back. At its fifth recurrence, she underwent a course of chemotherapy but was told that she had at most a few months to live. She had by this time an egg-sized tumour on the side of her neck.

All this time she was researching and looking for answers. Then, one night, brainstorming with her husband about why breast cancer rates in the west were so high and yet were extremely low in China, it suddenly occurred to them both that one of the key differences in diet was that the Chinese don't eat dairy products.

Plant immediately eliminated all dairy products (including goat and sheep) from her diet. Six weeks later, the tumour had disappeared. Since then she has stayed on her dairy-free diet and has remained clear of cancer.

Giving up dairy products was only part of a health regimen she has followed since then. She now advocates taking folic acid and zinc supplements, drinking filtered water and never consuming anything that had been packaged in plastic (phthalates, harmful carcinogenic chemicals, leak from soft plastic into food).

next page →

cancer promoter per Blaylock book

She is not alone. Hearing of her success, over 60 other women decided to follow her regime and also recovered. As a result of these experiences, Plant wrote her book: *Your Life in Your Hands.*

The reason for milk's deadly effects is that it contains insulin-like growth factor (IGF-1). This chemical occurs naturally in women to help their breasts develop. Plant found that pre-menopausal women with the highest IGF-1 concentration in their blood had a far higher risk of developing breast cancer (other studies have found a link between IGF-1 and prostate cancer).

This correlation of breast cancer, in particular, with increased use of dairy products has a lot of support from epidemiological studies. Plant has also found that pasteurization appears to result in the production of free oestrogens—and these may stimulate IGF-1 activity resulting in long-term tumour growth. Milk also contains dioxins and other environmental toxins that come down the food chain as they are fat soluble and end up particularly concentrated in milk.

Instead of dairy products, Plant recommends soya milk, herbal tea, humous, tofu, nuts and seeds, non-farmed fish, organic eggs and lean meat (not minced beef, which tends to be dairy cow) and plenty of fresh organic fruit and vegetables (in salads, juiced, or lightly steamed). Below, we will see that not everyone agrees with her that soy products are good. *note*

no

Traditional Chinese Medicine (TCM) & Diet

TCM encompasses a number of different practices: diet, herbs, acupuncture and qigong. Here we will look at the dietary aspect.

TCM views the body in a way that is hard to reconcile with Western perceptions. First it has a concept of 5 elements: fire, earth, metal, wood and water. Then there are the 5 bodily systems: heart, spleen, lungs, liver and kidney.

Each person varies in the extent to which these elements influence their bodily systems. The elements are in dynamic relationship with each other as are the bodily systems.

In addition there are opposed pairs of dynamic forces: Yin (female) and Yang (male). All of this is infused by 'qi' energy, blood and other bodily fluids; and then there are the pathogenic factors: the bodily systems can be hot or cold, damp or dry. TCM assesses these systems and forces to determine whether there is a state of deficiency, balance or excess.

The bodily systems—heart, lung, etc.—are not the same as the Western organs of the same name. When the TCM doctor talks of kidneys, for example, he is not referring to the physical organ that we know as the kidney but to a range of functions.

All of this can easily sound bizarre but we should remember that the Chinese are among the most pragmatic people in the world. If something doesn't work, they don't persevere. TCM has been around for well over three thousand years. We must therefore assume that it has been at least moderately successful at what it does.

However, in relation to cancer we must understand that TCM does not, generally speaking, recognize cancer, it only recognizes the imbalance of the bodily systems. The one exception to this is breast cancer which was isolated several hundred years ago as a specific ailment with a specific cause: liver qi (pronounced 'chee') stagnation. This is interesting in that many (if not all) alternative practitioners point to poor liver function as a major contributory factor of cancer.

The TCM doctor's approach is to seek to bring the body back into a harmonious state of health. If he can manage that, it is possible the cancer will depart. However, the general consensus is that, in relation to attacking cancer tumours specifically, TCM is not particularly effective. TCM doctors that I have talked to see the role of TCM as supportive of other therapies and as a way of protecting the body, or particular organs or eliminating specific symptoms: nausea, for example.

There is no such thing therefore as a TCM anti-cancer diet (though there are websites that put forward supposedly TCM anti-cancer diets). There are only patient-specific diets. These diets need to be specially formulated depending on the specific signs and symptoms that the particular patient exhibits. For some people, raw foods may be beneficial, but for others, they may be harmful – similarly grapes will be appropriate for some but not to those who have a hot constitution).

Since the assessment of the situation is crucial to deciding what particular diet should be followed, it follows that you need to be careful in selecting an appropriate TCM doctor. The minimum requirement is that they have completed a five year full time university course.

In China today all proper TCM doctors have to study for 5 years followed by a year of practical work. This then is followed by advanced training of about 3 years. Each province in China has a specialist TCM university but the best is the China Academy of Traditional Chinese Medicine in Beijing. Anyone wishing to go to Beijing can contact the Guang An Men Hospital which is affiliated to the Academy (Email: gamhkycy@netchina.com.cn for details).

Dr. Luke Tian, a TCM doctor practicing in Rockville, Maryland, specialises in treating cancer, and he has a number of testimonials from patients that he has helped with Chronic Lymphocytic Leukemia (CLL). For further details see www.lukeacupuncture.com.

See also the interesting website at www.tcmtreatment.com

Ayurvedic Medicine and Diet

There are many similarities between TCM and Ayurvedic medicine. Ayurvedic medicine also has a five element concept (air, fire, water, earth and ether) but it also has a concept of three basic body types or doshas: Kapha, Pitta or Vata. If you are more drawn to an Indian dietary approach then you should seek out an ayurvedic practitioner to develop a dietary strategy which may be your central anti-cancer therapy, or a support for other therapies.

Much of the discussion of TCM also applies to Ayurvedic medicine. Any diet that is formulated will be specific to each patient.

Again, the question of how you can assess the professional ability of an Ayurvedic doctor needs to be asked. First of course there is the normal personal assessment. However, for many people, it is a surprise to learn that Ayurvedic doctors, like doctors of TCM, are not folk healers but are university trained. In India today there are close to 200 undergraduate colleges of Ayurveda offering a five-year degree course in Ayurvedic Medicine, including one year internship, part of which is spent in conventional medicine departments. In addition there are 55 postgraduate colleges of Ayurveda offering a 3 year M.D. PhD in Ayurveda.

The pre-eminent institution is the All India Institute of Medical Sciences (AIIMS) (address: Ansari Nagar, New Delhi 110029, Ph: +91-11-660110,6864851 Fax: +91-11-6862663 Email: pkdav@medinst.ernet.in).

Another centre in Kerala, the Athulya Ayurvedic Medical Research Centre, has a website with details of patients whose cancers have been successfully treated using Ayurvedic medicine. For further details go to www.ayurvediccancertherapy.com

THE HEALING ATTRIBUTES OF INDIVIDUAL FOODS

Vegetables

Beetroot

From 1951, Alexander Ferenczi, M.D., an Hungarian cancer therapist, at the Department for Internal Diseases at the district hospital at Csoma, Hungary, began putting patients on a diet consisting almost entirely of eating large amounts of red beetroot (raw or juiced). Brief details of this treatment were reprinted in the *Australian International Clinical Nutrition Review* for July 1986.

One case study he reported was a 50 year old man referred to as D. S., who had a lung tumour "After 6 weeks of treatment the tumour had disappeared...After 4 months of treatment he gained 10kg. [22lbs.] in weight." All other tests confirmed that he had the symptoms of a clinical recovery. The active ingredient is the purple coloring chemical anthocyanin. Anthocyanins are widely present in fruit and vegetables particularly those that are dark red and purple and research is showing that they have many health benefits.

Bitter Melon

This is a light-to-medium-green Chinese melon recognizable for being 6-8 inches long with knobbed ridges - a very bumpy vegetable! Its botanical name is Momordica Charantia. In Cantonese it is known as Fu (bitter) Gwa or Leung (cooling) Gwa. When lightly fried or steamed it has a sharply tart but not unpleasant taste. It is very popular in summer months when it is eaten to cool the body down. This 'cooling' effect may be felt as a cleansing or purifying process. It is not recommended for pregnant women as it can have the effect of inducing spontaneous abortion (and as we know, anything that can cause spontaneous abortion can also help eliminate tumours—and vice versa). For cancer patients it is suggested that the bitter melon fruit and leaves are eaten together in large daily quantities. The bitter melon fruit (i.e., the part that is normally eaten) has a powerful ability to lower blood sugar—and as sugar is cancer's main fuel, this is very good news.

Bitter melon is being recommended by a number of AIDS activist groups as an immune support for people infected with HIV. For these purposes, the fruit of the bitter melon is not used. A 'tea' is made from boiling a pound of leaves and vines with two litres of water, brought to the boil and then simmered for 60-90 minutes (stirring every 20 minutes) and then cooled. Alternatively leaves and water can be put through a blender. In both cases the resulting 'tea' is strained to remove solid particles. It is then taken into the body through the colon in the form of a retention enema.

This way of taking bitter melon may also be beneficial for cancer patients. Bitter melon tea appears to be, like garlic, a powerful anti-viral agent and is also effective against the Herpes Simplex virus. One source of bitter melon tea is www.charanteausa.com

Cayenne Pepper

Cayenne Pepper is known to be very effective for heart problems and can even stop a heart attack. Herbalist, Dr. Richard Schulze also claims that it has powerful anti-cancer effects. He tells the story of a man who had an inoperable brain tumor. He went home, did a colon/liver detox and then started a regimen of ten cups per day of cayenne pepper tea. In three months he returned to his doctor and his X-rays showed a dried up, dead tumor in his head. In countries that have some very hot cuisine, Thailand for example, you find significantly lower cancer and heart disease rates.

In March 2006, the journal Cancer Research published the results of a study undertaken at Los Angeles' Cedar-Sinai Medical Center demonstrating that capsaicin, the ingredient that makes peppers hot, has the effect of causing cancer cells to die by inducing apoptosis (natural cell death)

Schulze recommends one teaspoon of organic cayenne pepper, or an equivalent number of drops of a good cayenne pepper tincture, in a glass of hot water three times a day for almost everything. It may, however, be necessary to build slowly to that level if you are not used to hot foods. Capsules should be avoided as the interaction of the cayenne in the mouth is an important feature of its benefits.

Cayenne has an immediate impact in widening the blood vessels, which allows more blood and oxygen to reach distant sites—this means that besides being effective in itself it will also speed the delivery of other drugs and herbs you take at the same time. If cayenne is not immediately available then chillies will be good, but sweet paprika is an extremely weak substitute – having a heating potential of less than 1,000 Scoville units compared to Cayenne's 50,000 units.

Cruciferous vegetables

This vegetable family which includes broccoli, cauliflower, cabbage, Brussels sprouts, collards, kale, mustard greens, turnips and turnip greens contains a number of compounds that have shown inhibitory action on cancers in animals. Communities that eat higher amounts of these vegetables show reduced incidence of cancer. Large amounts of cabbage and broccoli are particularly recommended.

The potential of cabbage as an anticancer treatment was known over 2,000 years ago. The Roman statesman, Cato the Elder (234-149 BC), in his treatise on medicine wrote: "If a cancerous ulcer appears upon the breasts, apply a crushed cabbage leaf and it will make it well."

A key compound that has been isolated from broccoli and cabbage is indole-3-carbinol and this is available as a supplement. Recommended minimum dose 300-400mg. This supplement must not be taken by any woman who is pregnant. It has been shown to have anti-cancer effects for a number of cancers—particularly cervical and breast cancers.

Garlic

Garlic is a very potent anti-pathogen. Recent tests at the University of Alabama Medical School suggest that it is as powerful as many modern anti-bacterial and anti-viral drugs - with minimal toxicity - "The only toxicity is social" said one commentator wryly. To beat the social side effects chew on parsley leaves or take garlic in de-odorized pill form. Kyolic ® brand garlic pills are highly regarded because of the quality of attention paid to the soil that the garlic is grown in and the quality of the cold-aging process that the whole cloves of garlic undergo. In China, garlic extract is used in IV infusions to treat systemic fungal infections.

One or two cloves a day can be sure to keep the doctor away. Garlic is also a potentially useful protective agent for the liver. It may be relevant that garlic is a very good source of selenium, germanium, amino acids and enzymes among other things. Garlic is the most potent member of the onion family but the other members are also associated with good health. Apart from garlic and onion, this family includes asparagus, chives, leeks, and sarsaparilla.

Garlic can also be applied externally with good effect. A poultice of finely chopped or juiced garlic, slippery elm, pokeroot - a wild plant common to the southern states of America whose leaves appear in salads - castor oil, vinegar, water and, on open wounds, cayenne pepper. Place this mixture with any additional herbs desired on a gauze pad and apply it to the skin closest to the tumour site. The poultice should be washed off in a shower every 12 hours and the area under the poultice allowed to breathe for 1-2 hours before a new poultice is applied. The result will burn the skin and may even raise a blister. These burns can be treated with lavender essential oil, aloe vera or comfrey. DMSO can be added to the poultice to aid absorption through the skin. This is claimed to be a very powerful anti-tumour treatment.

Sea Vegetables (Seaweed)

We call them seaweed but the Japanese, in particular, have a liking for these edible plants that grow in the sea. One seaweed extract marketed under the name Viva Natural has been found to be active against lung cancer and leukaemia. There is also some evidence that these vegetables may be active against breast cancer. Kelp and dulse are widely available seaweed extracts. Kombu, however, should be eaten in moderation as it contains very high iodine levels and can induce temporary hyper-thyroidism which stops when levels of iodine are reduced.

U-Fucoidin, also marketed as Modifilan, is an extract of various brown seaweed (kombu, wakame, mozuku, and hijiki) that contains a polysaccharide known as Fucoidan. Japanese researchers have found in laboratory studies that it causes cancer cells to self-destruct. For more information see www.modifilan.com and www.glycoscience.org.

Limu Moui is essentially the same product but coming from Tonga rather than Japan. For what it is worth, Tongans and Okinawans both eat a lot of brown seaweed extract and have low cancer incidence rates. There are a number of other fucoidan products available on the internet.

Tomatoes

The humble tomato has been found to be a rich source of lycopene which has been shown to have strong anti-cancer effects. Interestingly, the lycopene levels of cooked tomatoes are over ten times higher than their levels in raw uncooked tomatoes. No one understands why this should be the case.

tercress

Watercress has recently come to the fore as an anti-cancer superfood. It is the richest natural source of a compound called PEITC (phenylethylisothiocyanate) which has been shown to have powerful anti-cancer properties. PEITC is not just a potent inhibitor of cancer, it also has the ability to kill cancer cells. As if this wasn't enough it has also been found to prevent cancer-causing agents being metabolised into carcinogens and also has the ability to stimulate the enzymes involved in the detoxification of carcinogens.

An American scientist, Stephen Hecht, demonstrated that smokers eating only 2 oz of watercress with each meal were protected from a key carcinogen (known as NKK) which is associated with tobacco and implicated in lung cancer. It is now known that watercress also contains another compound—methylsulphinylalkyl glucosinolate - more usually found in broccoli and Brussel sprouts, and that together these compounds form an extremely powerful anti-cancer weapon.

Super Greens

There are a number of words used to describe this group of food products: Phytofoods, Green Foods, Superfoods.

These terms have been applied to a number of plant sourced whole foods that are 'nutrient-dense' (i.e., they are packed with vitamins, minerals and a lot more). No matter what else you plan to do as part of your anti-cancer strategy, you should make sure these foods play a part.

Barley Green Essence and Wheatgrass *Bill Henderson Book recs. Barley tablets*

Barley Green Essence is the concentrated extract of young barley, rye and oat shoots which have been allowed to grow until the leaves have become dark green. This was developed by a Japanese scientist Yoshide Hagiwara to support his own health. Wheatgrass is a variation which was developed independently in America by Ann Wigmore. Both consider their products to be effective components of a holistic anti-cancer dietary regime. There are now a number of similar products on the market containing additional herbs, enzymes and so on.

Hagiwara believes "the leaves of the cereal grasses provide the nearest thing this planet offers to the perfect food." Green Barley Essence is available as a powder and in capsule forms though he personally recommends the powder form as better. The potassium content of this product is very high, which makes it a good food for people working under high stress - when blood potassium levels will show a marked tendency to fall. Potassium is therefore being used up at a high rate and needs to be replaced. If it is not replaced then the result is fatigue. Green Barley Essence is also very high in vitamins. It has six times as much beta carotene and three times as much vitamin C as spinach. It is high in folic acid and nicotinic acid (important B vitamins) as well as biotin, chlorophyll and choline. Chlorophyll, which in plants is the substance that transforms sunlight into food, is very close in chemical structure to the haemoglobin in our blood - the only difference being one of its mineral components. Blood is bonded with iron while chlorophyll is bonded by magnesium. Hagiwara believes that the blood can be reinvigorated by eating chlorophyll.

Barley Green powder is also a very powerful alkalising agent, which as we have learnt is a good thing. Finally, it contains all the enzymes the body needs.

Cancer survivor Bob Davis believes that dried green barley leaves – in pill form (he takes 20 x 200 mg a day) cured him of his cancer within ten days. His story can be found at www.cancer-success.com.

Chlorella and Spirulina

It is believed that these two freshwater algae contain every single nutrient required by the human body. They have been called 'the perfect whole food'. It is also claimed that they can reverse a wide range of diseases including all types of cancer.

The range of health benefits claimed for chlorella is extensive: it supports and reinforces the immune system; it detoxifies the body by ridding it of heavy metals and pesticide residues; it improves digestion and helps elimination; it normalizes blood sugar and blood pressure and it balances the body's pH—and it fights cancer by stimulating the body's own anti-tumour resources.

Marine Phytoplankton

The surface waters of the oceans of the world contain vast colonies of microscopic plant life, marine phytoplankton. These are at the bottom of the food chain for all ocean life. They convert the sunlight, water and minerals of the sea into nutrients—using chlorophyll in the same way that other plants do. In short, they are a complete food source. As with their fresh water cousins, chlorella and spirulina they have a strong alkalizing, detoxifying effect. These too can very usefully be added to the diet. There are claims of very rapid healing benefits for a wide range of chronic conditions including cancer.

Green Drinks

There are a large number of formulas containing a mix of chlorella, spirulina, wheatgrass, barley sprouts and many other ingredients: herbs, vitamins, enzymes, and fruit and vegetable extracts. You should compare the ingredients of the various products as they are all significantly different. Some of the more popular formulas are: Barleans's Greens, Green Defense, Kyo-Chlorella and Barley Power .

I would personally recommend that you take one of these as they have a very powerful alkalizing effect which is essential for anyone seeking to maintain or regain good health.

Medicinal Mushrooms

Mushrooms are well known for their potent medicinal qualities. Here are the ones most useful for the person with cancer.

i. Agaricus Blazei Murill (ABM).

This Brazilian mushroom, discovered only in the 1970s by Western scientists near Sao Paulo, has demonstrated remarkable anti-cancer properties. Normally, the polysaccharides found in fungus only affect solid cancers; however, the polysaccharide in Agaricus (also known as ABM) is effective against almost all cancers. The polysaccharides appear to activate white blood cells known as macrophages which filter the blood by destroying viruses, bacteria, and perhaps even cancer cells. Shiitake, Maitake and Reishi (see below) also contain these polysaccharides. In one Japanese study, ABM was found to eliminate all cancerous tumors in 90 percent of the experimental mice. In another study the mice were fed Agaricus as a preventative and then injected with a very powerful cancer-causing agent 99.4 percent of them showed no tumor growth.

ABM contains much higher levels of beta glucans than the other medicinal mushrooms (Maitake, Shiitake, and Reishi) and it stimulates NK (Natural Killer) cell activity at a rate higher than MGN-3. Japanese oncologists are in no doubt as to its benefits and Japan is now buying over 90 percent of the available ABM from Brazil.

RAAX11

One extract from ABM is RAAX11. It is currently being studied in Brazil and has demonstrated some astonishing results for breast cancers.

Daily dosage for normal body maintenance and prevention is about 6 grams (about a quarter of a dry mushroom) or 40 grams (aprox. 2 mushrooms) for serious illness. Tea is also a popular way of taking the mushroom. Use about 1 mushroom per liter (1 quart) and simmer it for an hour. Drink a cup a day, warm or cold. Taking vitamin C promotes absorption.

OPC

OPC is a combination of ABM with Oleander, Cat's Claw and Pau D'Arco. It was developed in South Africa and anecdotal reports trestify to its effectiveness. Note that although dramatic long-term effects have been seen with OPC, there may be some short-term negative side effects. Marc Swanepoel, who is the patent holder, gives the following list: slight nausea and vomiting, diarrhoea, pruritus, pain at a tumour site, tachycardia and arrhythmias. Because of its blood-thinning properties, people on medical blood-thinning preparations should consult their doctors before using the OPC. People on heart-active drugs, such as digoxin (Lanoxin®), digitoxin or anti-arrhythmics should also speak to their doctors before using the mixture. No other drug interactions have been reported. Pregnant women should preferably not use the mixture due to its anti-angiogenesis effect. Other short-term detoxification symptoms like a slight rash, runny nose, pimples and slightly painful joints, may be experienced.

Recent research conducted at M.D. Anderson Cancer Center has shown that oleander attacks cancer in a number of different ways: it inhibits angiogenesis, promotes apoptosis, stimulates the immune system, reduces the power of cancer cells to defend themselves and promotes autophagy, a process where cells consume themselves. So, all in all, a very powerful weapon.

Sources: Agaricus and other mushrooms can be obtained from www.mitobi.com. ABM freeze dried extract in capsules is available from www.hplus.com and to order mushrooms in bulk, wholesale from China go to www.abmcn.com. RAAX11, along with branded mixtures RF1000 and are available on wholesale terms from: www.takesun.com or www.agaricus.net. OPC is also available at less cost from Marc Swanepoel who can be contacted at www.sutherlandiaopc.com

ii. Maitake

This mushroom is arousing a great deal of interest as it appears to have powerful anti-cancer effects, as well as being helpful to people with AIDS, diabetes and high blood pressure.

Maitake has been found to contain grifolan and beta-D-glucan, two important beta-glucan polysaccharides - molecules composed of many sugar molecules linked together. These have been shown to have a strong effect in activating microphages, which have been described as the heavy artillery of the immune system.

Laboratory studies have shown that maitake extract can block the growth of cancer tumors and boost the immune function of mice with cancer. It has also been shown to reduce tumours in people with stomach cancer and leukaemia. Cancer research on this mushroom is still in a very early stage but the initial signs are encouraging.

iii. Reishi (Ling Zhi)

The Japanese call it 'reishi', the Chinese call it 'Ling zhi', the Russians call a closely-related mushroon 'chaga' (mentioned in Solzhenitsyn's great novel *Cancer Ward*). It was highly revered by Taoists in search of the elixir of immortality. Of course, any herb associated with long life is very likely to have shown clear evidence of general medicinal value. There are a number of varieties, the most potent of which is considered by the Chinese to be the red fungus - but this may simply be because the colour red has very positive symbolism in Chinese culture. Reishi mushrooms are very high in polysaccharides and these may be responsible for its immune system stimulation effect. The Chinese view it as a tonic that boosts the vital life energy they call 'qi' (pronounced: chee).

Studies have shown that reishi mushroom extracts can kill stapphylococci and streptococci bacteria. This makes it a very useful treatment for pneumonia and hospital acquired infections. Interestingly, low doses of the mushroom appear to be more effective than large doses. The optimal dose appears to be 4 grams a day. One Japanese cancer surgeon, Dr. Fukumi Morishige, stumbled on this by chance when a woman who was dying of cancer suddenly appeared to be cured. He discovered that her husband had been giving her fresh reishi mushroom tea everyday. Morishige now prescribes a daily intake of 4 grams of reishi tea with 10 grams of a special form of vitamin C known as nucleic acid ascorbate. Morishige discovered that large doses of vitamin C prevented the diarrhoea caused by taking in too much reishi. He therefore reasoned that the vitamin C was having the effect of increasing its absorbability. In this way he was able to increase the dose of reishi to 9 grams a day. Reishi can also be taken effectively by intravenous injection. Morishige has treated and cured a number of cancer patients using nothing else but this combination of vitamin C and reishi mushrooms.

Studies undertaken by the National Cancer Research Centre shows that mice injected with reishi extract showed tumour regression between 50 and 100 percent, depending on the dose.

People who take reishi mushrooms show a marked increase in blood oxygenation levels, and for this reason it is also used as an antidote to altitude sickness. The importance in cancer treatment of having high tissue oxygen levels has already been mentioned and this may be one of the ways in which reishi has an anti-cancer effect.

Some healers use it in combination with shiitake mushrooms and astralagus. It is used to treat asthma, allergies as well as insomnia. It can have a few unpleasant side effects: dizziness, light-headedness and itchiness. These can be dealt with by lowering the dose and then slowly increasing it. There have been no signs of toxicity in many studies - even up to levels equivalent to a human taking 350 grams a day.

Reishi is very bitter and not eaten as a food. It is cut into pieces and brewed in hot water: 5 grams/litre. The water is simmered until it is reduced to a third of a litre. It is then drunk. The vitamin C has to be taken separately as it is destroyed by heat. Reishi is also available in capsule form. At present it is quite expensive and as a result a great deal of fake ling zhi has made its way on to the market.

Apart from its claimed anti-cancer effects, it is recommended in Japan as a way of reducing side effects for patients undergoing radiation and chemotherapy.

iv. Shiitake

The shiitake mushroom (Lentinus edodes) is the other well-known Japanese medicinal mushroom. Among its many excellent qualities is the fact that it contains ergosterol, which can be converted by sunlight into vitamin D–a potent cancer fighter in its own right.

In traditional Chinese and Japanese medicine shiitake is considered to have a powerful and positive impact on qi energy. It is also considered to be a food that promotes longevity, protects the immune system, promotes good circulation and prevents liver disease.

Scientists are now studying an extract of shiitake known as lentinan for its potential anti-tumour effects. It works by stimulating certain types of white blood cells important in immune function rather than by directly attacking cancer cells.

RM-10™ Combination mushroom product

This is a combination of 10 certified organic medicinal mushrooms (including Agaricus, Reishi, Shiitake, Maitake, Cordyseps sinensis, and Coriolus versicor, among others), extracted through an enzymatic enhancing process and combined with aloe vera and the herb Uncaria tomentosa (Cat's claw).

It was developed by Jordan Rubin, who was motivated to help his grandmother who was diagnosed with advanced metastatic disease. She agreed to follow his regime and is now cancer free. Independent researchers and alternative therapists have confirmed that it is highly effective – and is very helpful in minimising the toxic effects of chemotherapy. It is sold by Garden of Life vitamins as helpful for a number of immune-compromising illnesses. There are a number of internet suppliers.

Sun Soup

Sun Soup is a product containing shiitake and other mushrooms, soy, and a number of Asian herbs. Developed by Alexander S. Sun, PhD, a biochemist from the University of California, Berkeley, who did research at Mt. Sinai Medical Center, New York, and Yale University, in order to help his mother survive cancer. Despite poor prognosis she did indeed recover with the help of this soup. Independent research indicates that it does have tumour inhibiting qualities. For further details see www.sunfarmcorp.com

Fruit
The following fruits are considered to be particularly rich in healthy nutrients.

Apples

We all know that 'an apple a day keeps the doctor away' – and there is good reason for that. Sadly, many of the commercial varieties of apple found in our supermarkets are not so good as the old 'heritage' varieties. Apples contain many phytochemicals that are medicinally beneficial and some reports suggest that eating two or more apples a day could help prevent cancer. Apples contain one chemical, Phloridzin, indeed they are the only major source of it, which modulates sugar transport in the intestine and has the effect of slowing the absorption of sugar. Given the huge need for sugar that cancer tumours have, this could be very good news. The varieties that have the best phyto-chemical content are Hetlina and Monty's Surprise but if you take a rough and ready guide that four or five Red Delicious equal one of the above, you will not go far wrong. Note that half the benefit of the apples is in the skin.

Oranges

You may remember that Dr Moerman's first patient (see p. 143) ate oranges until they were coming out of his ears. It's not just the vitamin C but also the citric acid that is effective. But the benefits of the orange are not restricted to the juice of this fruit. The peel also contains a potent chemical, D-limonene, for which there is strong evidence of anti-cancer activity. Researchers at the University of Wisconsin found that when D-limonene was added to the diets of rats who had developed tumors, 90 percent of them had their tumors disappear completely. So make sure you juice the peel as well as the (organic) fruit.

Finally, an interesting point: Citrus fruits, although acidic outside the body, have a very alkalising effect once they are consumed.

Exotic Fruits

Besides grapes and apples, a number of fruits – usually exotic – have been promoted, often by multi-layer marketing companies, as being enormously beneficial to health. However, although it is reasonable to be somewhat cynical, most of these fruits and their juices do have health supporting qualities. It is very unlikely that any on their own will cure cancer but they will help move the body to a place of nutritional health and may very well support someone who is undergoing chemotherapy or radiation.

Any dark coloured red or blue nutritious fruit grown in a place where there is strong sunlight will have many beneficial qualities. However, the quality of the purchased product may be affected by many factors such as sweeteners, fillers, preservatives, colouring agents and other additional ingredients. Use your common sense when purchasing. Read the labels carefully.

Here are some fruits that have attracted recent attention.

Noni

Noni fruit has been used in general folk healing wherever it grows. There is strong anecdotal and experimental support for its anti-cancer effects.

In 1997, Dr. Stephen Hall, author of a book on noni, reported: "A 75 y/o male with metastatic prostate cancer, most recent PSA of 55, I added ... Noni to his conventional treatment regimen and within 2 weeks, his PSA was 1.1." There is simply nothing else I am aware of that could possibly reduce Prostatic Specific Antigen from 55 (indicating uncontrolled cancer) to a normal 1.1, and do it in just two weeks" (www.cnw.com/~timo/scien/cancer.html).

Noni juice has been the subject of some controversy because interest in this product has been driven by a powerful multi-level marketing scheme operated by the Morinda Corporation, which has dominated information relating to the noni fruit. The problem has been to what extent we can accept statements like Dr. Hall's. It appears that everyone touting noni juice is also profiting from it.

Nevertheless, Japanese researchers have conducted independent animal experiments that clearly show a strong anti-cancer effect for noni juice.

Whether or not Tahitian noni is better than Hawaiian noni or noni from other sources is a matter for debate.

Acai, Goji, Mangosteen and Pomegranate

Acai: (pronounced "ah-sy-ee") is a small purple fruit that grows in the Amazon rainforest and tastes 'like a cross between blackberries and chocolate'. Its concentration of anti-oxidants is greater even than the blueberry (itself one of nature's healthiest fruits). Studies on the Acai fruit have found that it enhances the immune system, helps protects the heart, controls cholesterol and can reduce prostate enlargement.

Goji: The berries of this Himalayan fruit, cousin of the American wolfberry, are rich in polysaccharides. It has a role in traditional medicine against inflammation and one of the polysaccharides has demonstrated anti-cancer effects in the laboratory. It also has anti-coagulent properties so anyone taking blood thinning drugs should treat this fruit with caution.

Mangosteen: This is a fruit common to SE Asia. However, it is the rind of the fruit that contains the highest concentration of xanthones, the chemicals that are considered most active medicinally. There is some evidence that it has anti-bacterial, anti-fungal, anti-tumour effects and that it promotes the healing of wounds. This fruit product is available as a drink (which has a high fruit content) and as capsules (which have a high rind content).

Pomegranate: This fruit is native to the Middle East. Pomegranates are known to possess anti-inflammatory agents, which make them very interesting as potential anti-tumour agents. And in fact research has shown that it has a strong anti-cancer effect as well as supporting heart health. The BBC reported a senior researcher, Professor Hasan Mukhtar as saying: "Our study... adds to growing evidence that pomegranates contain very powerful agents against cancer, particularly prostate cancer." (BBC 28th Sept. 2005) A glass a day could be very beneficial both as a preventative and as a treatment. Of all the heavily touted fruits, the pomegranate has the best supported claims and is also the cheapest as it is not part of a multi-level marketing scheme.

Miscellaneous

Vinegar

Acetic Acid is a natural ingredient found in all vinegars. It is also the product of the normal metabolism of fats and carbohydrates when they are broken down in the body. It is calculated that the human body derives more than 80 percent of all its energy from acetic acid. Interestingly, while acetic acid is necessary to fuel the activities of normal cells it interferes with the process of glycolysis, which is the process by which cancer cells get their fuel. Acetic acid effectively blocks the glycolic process. Citric Acid can also shut down glycolysis. The most favoured type of vinegar is apple cider vinegar as it contains some of the benefits of apples along with the benefits of the vinegar. Personally, I take a splash of vinegar diluted with water as a regular thirst quenching drink. Bragg's organic unpasteurised vinegar is the most highly regarded – and they have a special deal for people with cancer. Enquire to www.bragg.com.

Food Controversies

Food, like religion and politics, is a subject about which there are opposing views and it is up to each individual to assess for him-or-herself where the truth lies. Are fruit to be eaten? No, say some, because they contain lots of sugar. Yes, say others, because - although they contain sugar , that sugar is fructose – and they are rich in other important health giving nutrients. Here then are some other key areas of disagreement.

i. Sprouts: Good or Bad?

Here I refer to the freshly sprouted seeds of a number of plants such as adzuki, alfalfa, clover, fenugreek, lentil, mustard, radish, sunflower, watercress and others including wheat, rye, millet and oat seeds. Simple sprouting equipment can be set up at home to ensure a regular and extremely cheap supply of sprouts. These can be eaten as they are or juiced with garlic.

The value of sprouts is that they are extremely rich in vitamins, minerals, enzymes and amino acids. In addition, according to advocates, they are 'biogenic' (i.e., capable of transferring their life energy to the bodies of those who eat them).

"When you eat a sprout you are eating a tiny, easy-to-digest plant that is at its peak of nutritional value. The seed releases all of its stored nutrients in a burst of vitality as it attempts to become a full-sized plant" (Wigmore, 1986).

Experiments with mice show that injections of sprout extracts have a strong inhibitory effect on cancer cells and are completely non-toxic at even large doses. Lentil, mung bean, and wheat sprouts were those tested with positive results.

However, there is an opposing view on the subject of sprouts. According to Charlotte Gerson, daughter of Dr. Max Gerson and the force behind the Gerson Clinics: "Sprouted alfalfa and other bean or seed sprouts are high in L-canavanine, an immature amino acid that is responsible for immune cell suppression. Also, patients with no prior history of chronic joint pain have developed the sudden onset of arthritic symptoms upon ingesting alfalfa sprouts. Healthy monkeys have developed lupus erythematosus from alfalfa sprouts in their diet." The main culprit appears to be alfalfa.

ii. The Soybean: Good or Bad?

Throughout the 80s and 90s the soybean was lauded widely, as many things from the East were. It was noted that in China and Japan, where tofu was a major part of the diet, that cancer rates were much lower. However, more recently, there has been a strong backlash. The soybean has been attacked for containing a large number of dangerous substances called phytates, one of which is phytic acid. Soybeans contain very high levels of this organic acid. These acids block the body's ability to take up essential minerals like calcium, magnesium, iron and especially zinc. Soybeans are very resistant to phytate-reducing techniques, such as long, slow cooking.

Soybeans also contain a number of potent enzyme inhibitors which block the uptake of trypsin and other enzymes that the body needs for protein digestion. Cooking does not completely de-activate inhibitors.

Soybeans also contain haemaglutinin, a clot promoting substance that causes red blood cells to clump together. This has the effect of preventing proper absorption of oxygen for distribution to the body's tissues.

However, these concerns relate to unfermented soy products. Fermented soy products do appear to be healthy, as the fermentation process neutralises the phytic acid. The fermentation also creates good bacteria – 'probiotics' – which help assimilation of important nutrients. In fact miso soup, a fermented soy product, has been shown to be highly protective against breast and prostate cancer – 3 bowls a day cut cancer risk in half.

Some doctors recommend fermented soy products for hormone-dependent cancers such as prostate, breast and some others for the reason that the soy products block the hormone receptors. Other researchers have noted that soy products contain genistein, which has been found to reverse some cancers.

Haelan and Soy Essence are fermented soy drinks for which strong anti-cancer claims are made. These are discussed on p. 244.

For further information see www.mercola.com/article/soy/index.htm

iii. Coffee: Good or Bad?

Almost all the anti-cancer diets ban coffee while at the same time espousing the benefits of coffee enemas – which cannot help but lead to the absorption of caffeine. This schizophrenic attitude now needs to take into account the results of a new study published in May 2007, conducted at the University of Ferrara in Italy, which has found that caffeine inhibits three factors -- VEGF, HIF-1 and IL-8 -- all of which are associated with the development of the blood supply that cancers need to develop if they are to grow. This process is known as angiogenesis. This means that caffeine is an anti-angiogenesis factor. This is very good news for coffee drinkers. It was already known from other studies that caffeine was associated with reduced levels of colorectal cancer.

VITAMINS & OTHER NATURAL SUPPLEMENTS

In this chapter I will look at the main supplements that are recommended as well as those which are contra-indicated or about which there is some controversy. But first let us look at the most basic disagreement of all. Even if we need a vitamin or mineral should we take supplements or should we try to get what we need through the food we eat?

To Supplement or Not to Supplement

Among health conscious people there is a debate as to whether supplements are a good thing. Those who argue against supplements put forward the following views:

1. We should be able to get all the nutrients we need from a healthy diet. So rather than take supplements we should concentrate on making sure we eat a properly balanced diet.

2. Supplements themselves have gone through some form of processing - and therefore suffer from the defects attributed to other processed foods. Also we cannot be sure that supplements contain the levels of vitamins that they claim to contain.

3. Vitamins and minerals work best when they are in organic combinations with other vitamins and minerals. In this form they work synergistically and so the resulting beneficial effect is maximized.

4. Some synthetic supplements block the body's access to natural sourced vitamins (notably Vit. E)

Those who favour supplements argue as follows:

1. We need to take larger quantities of most vitamins and minerals than we can easily find in the food we eat. Vitamin C is an obvious example.

2. We know that the food we eat is depleted of vital nutrients by the use of artificial fertilizers and pesticides and irradiation. In fact, given the wide use of pesticides, it is likely that most vegetables are poor in minerals (pesticides leach minerals from the soils). Since the mineral content of vegetables comes from the soil, diet is unlikely to provide what we need. In the case of animal husbandry, intensive farming techniques combined with the use of antibiotics and hormones make the resulting food a poor source of wholesome nutrition.

3. Much of the food we eat has had most of the vital nutrients destroyed by heating during the cooking process.

4. Pollution depletes our body's vitamin resources. The more polluted our environment the greater our need for higher levels of vitamin intake.

All these arguments on both sides of the dispute are good. Each of us has to weigh them up to arrive at a compromise that makes sense.

My own view is that we cannot rely on synthetic supplements alone – nor can we rely on fresh vegetables and fruit alone. Eating organic vegetables and fruit, preferably from a local producer, coupled with some supplements seems to me to be the necessary compromise. And although I see no way round the need to take synthetic vitamin C in large doses, I recognize that the 50 mg of vitamin C in an orange is very likely equivalent to much higher quantities of synthetic vitamin C measured in terms of biological activity.

Free Radicals and the Need for Supplements

There are many processes within the body that help us to remain healthy and resistant to disease. Attacking the body are a wide range of enemies: bacteria, viruses, fungi, many kinds of poisons, etc. In addition, the body is being damaged by the effects of free radicals.

What are these free radicals? Basically they are molecules that have been deprived of an oxygen atom and are therefore hungry for oxygen. They find this oxygen in the fats embedded in the walls of normal cells. They therefore have to attack the cell walls to get the oxygen they require. This damages and can even kill the cell. Free radicals are themselves the normal by-product of the body's chemical reactions - particularly those processes involved in eliminating potentially toxic cellular waste materials. The more toxic waste materials there are the more free radicals are created. And although free radicals are often seen as baddies, there are circumstances when they play a useful role in combating bacterial infections.

Free radicals are being formed all the time but their impact is controlled by the body in a number of ways. One is by having the means to repair the cell wall damage. Vitamin C is important for this process.

Another way is to intercept the free radicals before they do any harm. Vitamins A, C and E and the mineral, selenium, are called antioxidants because they help the body to protect itself in this way. They neutralize the free radicals before they reach the cells walls. Vitamin E works synergistically with selenium and also works with vitamins A and C by protecting them from oxidation.

Vitamins are of extremely low toxicity. It takes months on extremely high doses before the body begins to react negatively to those that are fat soluble – which can therefore be stored – such as vitamins A and E. (Vitamin C is not fat soluble and therefore is quickly passed out of the body.) This indicates, on its own, that the body welcomes these vitamins. When the body ceases to be able to tolerate them it indicates this by creating, almost always, a sensation of nausea. This should be sufficient warning to desist. An overdose of vitamin A will not take you by surprise in the same way as an overdose of any pharmaceutical or recreational drug.

What is also interesting is that, even before physical signs detectable by blood tests appear, the mind responds to low levels of vitamins: vitamin B complex deficiency can lead to mental illnesses. Depression is also a very common response to vitamin C and B deficiency. If we accept some arguments, most cancers and many heart diseases are completely explicable as being the result of inadequate vitamin intake.

Minerals are a slightly different matter. For some there is very little if any toxicity, while for others there are known limits beyond which it would be unwise to go. Details of these are given below.

How Do We Know What to Take and How Much to Take?

Anyone reading around the subject will discover that there is very little agreement as to how much of any vitamin or mineral we should be taking. British writers tend to be quite conservative, while Americans tend to be much more aggressive. This book takes the view that a risk-benefit analysis favours taking too much rather than too little. People with cancer should be more aggressive than people wishing to provide themselves with some protection. However, very large doses should be built up slowly - and also tapered off slowly.

Measurements of What Is Adequate

For most vitamins and minerals there is an RDA (Recommended Daily Allowance) value. This is usually an extremely low figure set by some authority. For example, the RDA for vitamin C was for many years 60mg. This was a measure of the amount an average person should take to ensure that he or she did not suffer from deficiency. In the US this has been replaced by the terms Reference Daily Intake (RDI) or DRI (Dietary Reference Intake). This is defined as representing "the upper tolerable limit of vitamin and mineral intakes that the U.S. Food and Drug Administration recommends for adults and persons 4 or more years of age," with little change in values – for example the RDA for vitamin C is now 75-90 mg. Tolerable? To whom? Do 4 year olds have the same needs as 75 year olds? Since many people comfortably take several thousand milligrams of vitamin C, we clearly have a problem.

Individuals Vary in Their Needs

Setting a measure such as RDA or DRI assumes we are all more or less equal in our needs. This apparently is not the case. The Nobel Prize winning biochemist Linus Pauling remarked: "Human beings differ from one another; they show a pronounced biochemical individuality." Indeed, according to his calculations, it is extremely unlikely that anyone on Earth is 100 percent average, that is to say, sharing characteristics with 95 percent of the population for every biochemical process in the body.

So it may be that some people are suffering deficiencies even though they are receiving much higher than RDA/DRI intakes. Modern nutritionists now work with another term: ODA (Optimal Daily Allowance). There is some variation from nutritionist to nutritionist as to what constitutes an ODA level - but in all cases it is significantly higher than the RDA or DRI level.

Can A Multi-Vitamin/Mineral Strategy Cure Cancer?

There are no 100 percent guaranteed cures for cancer. However, a study by Albert Hoffer and Linus Pauling compared two groups of cancer patients. Those who continued eating as they had done before they got cancer had an average life expectancy of 5.7 months. Those who changed their diets and took high-dose multi-vitamin and mineral supplements had an average life expectancy of six years! Women with cancers of the breast, ovaries and cervix did better, averaging ten years. So, on the basis of this result, there appears to be a very strong argument for taking supplements.

The Safety of Vitamins

From time to time there are scare stories implicating this or that vitamin or mineral. You should know that over the years 1983-2005 in the USA there were a combined total of exactly ten deaths associated with vitamins. More people died from eating soap. The safety record of minerals is almost as good – most fatalities coming from gross over-ingestion of iron supplements. Compared to the hundreds of thousands each year who die as a direct result of their standard medical treatment this is small beer.

Vitamins

We will now look at the evidence put forward supporting, or casting doubt on, the value of the main vitamins and minerals identified as being important in the fight against cancer. The most important vitamin is vitamin C so we will look at that first and in some detail.

Vitamin C

For anyone seeking to survive or prevent cancer, large doses of vitamin C are highly recommended. However, before starting to take so-called 'megadoses' (doses of 1,000mg and up) of vitamin C, you should read this section carefully.

The Vitamin C Controversy: Science and Politics

The vitamin C controversy is one of the best publicized and most fiercely argued in the annals of non-orthodox cancer treatments. Its most famous proponent was Linus Pauling, a double Nobel prize winner: in 1954 for chemistry and in 1962 for peace. It was Dr. Pauling's view that daily megadoses of vitamin C could prevent cancer - and could also cure cancer.

The Independent newspaper's obituary of Linus Pauling, who died in 1994, ended with these words: "His theories on vitamin C have now been largely discredited." This chapter will show that this is not, in fact, the case.

Pauling wrote three books putting forward the evidence in support of vitamin C: *Vitamin C and the Common Cold*, *Vitamin C and Cancer*, and *How to Live Longer and Feel Better*. In these books he quoted extensive experimental support for his conclusion that vitamin C has a general anti-viral effect which protects against any virus including influenza, polio, hepatitis, mononucleosis, and herpes.

In addition, "[G]ood intakes of vitamin C and other vitamins can improve your general health in such a way as to increase your enjoyment of life and can help in controlling heart disease, cancer and other diseases and in slowing down the process of aging" (Pauling, 1986).

This is a big claim to make. So what proof or evidence or theory did he put forward? First he pointed out that patients with cancer usually have very low concentrations of vitamin C in the blood plasma and in the blood leucocytes. This lack prevents the leucocytes from doing their job of engulfing and digesting bacteria and other foreign cells, including malignant cells, in the body. He felt that it was reasonable to suppose that the low level of vitamin C indicated it was being used up in the effort to control the disease. By giving patients a larger amount of vitamin C, their bodily defences should therefore be strengthened. This then was his starting point. Further evidence came from epidemiological studies that showed higher cancer incidence among people whose vegetable and vitamin C intakes were low.

He then established a professional relationship with the Scottish doctor, Ewan Cameron. Cameron had come to vitamin C by another route. His starting point was the known fact that malignant tumours produce an enzyme that attacks the intercellular cement of the surrounding healthy tissues. This weakens the cement to such an extent that the cancer is able to invade. Cameron suggested that one way of defending against the cancer might therefore be to strengthen the intercellular cement. Since vitamin C is known to be involved in the synthesis of collagen - the material of which the intercellular cement is composed, high doses of vitamin C should have the effect of strengthening these defenses by allowing faster synthesis. This should protect against the spread and growth of a tumour.

Cameron and Pauling started to experiment with vitamin C on terminal cancer patients at Vale of Leven Hospital in Scotland over the next few years. The results were so exciting that when Pauling suggested they do a double blind clinical trial, Cameron refused. He believed in the value of vitamin C. To deprive any of his patients of this treatment would therefore be unethical. So instead they carried out a controlled study, comparing the outcome of 100 patients who were randomly assigned to Dr. Cameron's care to the outcome of 1,000 patients assigned to doctors who did not believe in or use vitamin C therapy. The result? The patients treated with a daily 10 grams (10 x 1,000mg) of sodium ascorbate had a survival time 4.2 times longer than for patients who did not take such large doses. Some continued to survive, and survive, and survive.

A small but significant percent of the 'terminally ill' cancer patients for whom death was considered inevitable within a matter of weeks or months went on to long-term survival. In short, for some patients, admittedly a very few, vitamin C cured their cancer. (We must remember that Pauling did not give any patients doses higher than 10 grams. What would have happened if he had given them 20 or 30 grams, the levels that most advocates now consider to be the minimum necessary if a cure is to be obtained?)

These are exciting results and one would have thought the cancer associations would have been leaping over themselves to replicate the results. Nothing could be further from the truth. Pauling took these results back to the National Cancer Institute in America. They were only interested, they said, in animal studies. But when Pauling applied for grants to conduct this animal-based research he was turned down eight times. Eventually, he made a point of what was happening by publishing an advertisement seeking private donations to help him continue his research.

In this 1976 *Wall Street Journal* advertisement, he wrote: "Our research shows that the incidence and the severity of cancer depends on diet. We urgently want to refine that research so that it may help to decrease suffering from human cancer. The U.S. Government has absolutely and continually refused to support Dr. Pauling and his colleagues during the past four years."

Eventually sufficient pressure built up and the Mayo Clinic was asked to conduct clinical trials of vitamin C. One of these was conducted by a Dr. Moertel in 1985. His conclusion, which was widely reported in the press, was that there was no evidence that vitamin C had any beneficial effect on cancer patients. He had conducted a double-blind clinical trial that showed no difference between the survival of those who had been given vitamin C and those who had been given a placebo. Pauling was severely critical of the conduct of this trial.

"[Moertel] suppressed the fact that the vitamin C patients were not receiving vitamin C when they died and had not received any for a long time (median 10.5 months). [This misrepresentation] has done great harm. Cancer patients have informed us that they are stopping their vitamin C because of [these] 'negative results' ..." (Pauling 1986).

The question raises itself as to why the U.S. National Cancer Institute was so keen to ally itself to a negative result for vitamin C and so slow to support positive findings. Critics point to the fact that the pharmaceutical industry is well represented in the committees and subcommittees of all of the leading cancer-related institutions. If it were ever found that vitamin C was indeed a powerful anticancer agent, then the pharmaceutical companies could say goodbye to their lucrative business. Simply put, there is no money to be made out of selling vitamin C.

Pauling summed up his experiences thus: "Everyone should know the war against cancer is largely a fraud."

Postscript: In 2007 researchers at Johns Hopkins found that vitamin C did have another anti-cancer effect in that it helped diminish levels of a protein, hypoxia-induced factor (HIF-1). This protein helps oxygen-starved cells to convert sugar to energy without using oxygen and it is also important in initiating the development of new blood vessels which the cancer tumour needs to support its growth.

Other Benefits of Vitamin C

We should note in passing that benefits of taking large doses of vitamin C have been claimed for a wide variety of ailments ranging from wasp and snake bite to heart disease, meningitis, shock, schizophrenia and diabetes. In fact the list is so long that it would not do any harm to take large doses of vitamin C whatever the problem. Certainly, children with Down's Syndrome, who have higher leukaemia rates, should be put on vitamin C supplements (and also green tea). People with skin cancers can make a paste by adding a few drops of water to vitamin C powder and rubbing this on exposed cancerous areas several times a day, leaving it to dry. There are anecdotal reports that this has caused surface cancers to heal over.

How Much Vitamin C Do We Need?

Clearly vitamin C has a wide range of functions within the body and is an important nutrient. But why do we need such large quantities? The official RDA (Recommended Daily Allowance) for vitamin C is 60 mg per day. Most people assume that the RDA is an average intake that they should aim for, or an amount which should not be exceeded by too much. In fact, this is wrong. 60 mg a day is the quantity needed to ensure we do not get deficiency diseases like scurvy. So the RDA is a minimum amount. Vitamin C is a food substance or nutrient. Does it make sense to take in only the minimum amount of a food substance that will stave off deficiency diseases? Applied to food intake as a whole, does it make sense to take in only the amount of food that will prevent us from dying of starvation?

Once we have established that the RDA is a minimum amount, we should try to find out what the Optimum Daily Allowance (ODA) is. This will presumably be somewhere between the minimum and the maximum amount. But what is the maximum amount? The maximum amount obviously will be that amount that will lead to toxicity or ill-health. Taking this as a guideline we discover an interesting fact: there is no maximum level of vitamin C that will cause ill-health or toxicity! One suggestion that it could lead to kidney stones has never been validated.

It appears that no matter how much we take, we can never reach a dose that is toxic. There are two reasons for this. First, the body welcomes vitamin C in large quantities. Secondly, if the body gets more vitamin C than it can handle at any one time it dumps the excess vitamin C by causing diarrhoea, which stops as soon as vitamin C levels become manageable again. This diarrhoea-causing amount will vary from person to person. Known as the bowel-tolerance level, it will normally be in the region of 10-20 grams a day for a healthy adult but it will increase sharply to 30-60 grams or even more if there is a viral infection. Going back to Pauling's argument: this increased ability to tolerate higher levels of vitamin C during periods of ill-health suggests that the body is capable of using more vitamin C at times of ill-health. This leads, in turn, to the conclusion that the body is using the vitamin C to fight the illness. So one measure of ODA would be an amount slightly less than the bowel tolerance level.

We can approach this question from another angle. Humans are one of a small group of animals that don't produce vitamin C in their bodies. We share this defect with the other apes and, curiously, with that archetypal experimental animal, the guinea pig. For us, vitamin C has to be taken in from outside (i.e., in the food). Most mammals, however, manufacture vitamin C in their livers through the action of a particular enzyme. So how much vitamin C do these animals produce? It varies from species to species. A goat for example produces approximately 13 grams a day per 70 kg of body weight under normal conditions but if it gets stressed it will produce up to 100 grams or more. Mice produce 275mg of vitamin C per kilo of body weight a day under normal conditions. A mouse the size of a 70 kg man would therefore be producing 19 grams a day. These amounts can increase ten-fold when the animal is under stress.

This is, for me, the clinching evidence that large quantities of vitamin C are beneficial - and are indeed the 'normal' levels we should be taking in for optimal health. First, since man is a mammal, he almost certainly needs vitamin C in quantities similar to other mammals of the same size and weight. Secondly, if animals produce more vitamin C when they are under stress then presumably, the vitamin C is useful to help the body cope with stress - and illness is a form of physical stress. Interestingly, dogs and cats, which produce relatively low amounts of vitamin C have, after man, the highest cancer rates in the animal kingdom.

This leads to an interesting question: Why is it that man doesn't create his own vitamin C? The Encyclopaedia Britannica gives one possible explanation. Our inability to produce vitamin C may be the result of some genetic disease that wiped out the enzymes that perform this task in the liver. It is simply an accident of history that we have somehow been able to overcome.

Many people in America and Australia are taking ten or more grams a day just to maintain their health. For children, one advocate recommends that they can - and should - take 1 gram per year of life. An eight year old could take 8 grams a day. This is perhaps an extreme point of view but it is clear that a couple of grams will not cause an overdose.

Expensive Urine?

Finally, to deal with the argument that large doses of vitamin C merely lead to 'expensive urine' (i.e., to wasted vitamin C), experts have made the following points:

1. The urinary system is very prone to infection and so it actually makes sense to direct an anti-viral and anti-bacterial agent like vitamin C through this system. People who don't have 'expensive urine' may be more prone to urinary infections.

2. The presence of vitamin C in the urine does not indicate tissue saturation. Tissue saturation causes diarrhoea. The amount needed to get a urine reading is very much lower than the amount needed to cause diarrhoea.

3. The level of vitamin C in the urine is a good indication of the level in the tissues. If urinary levels are low, then so to will the tissue levels be low. High levels of excreted vitamin C are indications that the body's defences are in good shape.

How to Take Vitamin C

Having established the credentials of vitamin C, it is now necessary to explain that there are a number of different forms of the substance and that they are not all equal.

As straight ascorbic acid, it is slightly acidic. Usually, however, vitamin C is sold in tablet form as 'buffered' vitamin C, which means they are in a non-acidic form. This means that they are sold as a salt (i.e., as calcium ascorbate or sodium ascorbate) and so on.

Most pro-vitamin C advocates warn that the calcium ascorbate form is not recommended when a cancer tumour is present. Unfortunately, most on-the-shelf vitamin C pills are calcium ascorbate, including the Ester-C form of vitamin C. For cancer patients, L-ascorbic acid, sodium ascorbate, magnesium ascorbate, potassium ascorbate and zinc ascorbate are the preferred forms. For further information on vitamin C, the following websites are recommended www.vitamincfoundation.com, and www.orthomed.com

Pauling does warn that anyone going on a megadose regime of vitamin C to fight a cancer should not start with large doses - there is a danger of the tumour haemorrhaging - which can be fatal. Large doses should be gradually built up over a period of weeks, starting with say 3 grams a day and increasing by 1 gram every day, continuing until the bowel tolerance level has been established. A dose slightly lower than this should then be maintained. Pauling also warned that one should never suddenly stop taking it - instead it should be tapered off. He warned that a sudden stop might result in 'rebound scurvy'. Not everyone believes that this is a danger - but it may be and it would be wise to take precautions.

There is one final caution. If the cancer patient taking the vitamin C is in a defeated-defeatist frame of mind, the vitamin C may not be effective. This is because the vitamin C may be harnessed by the body for other purposes. This point is discussed on pp. 81-82. It is important that the cancer patient taking vitamin C should be encouraged and helped to take on a positively resisting frame of mind.

Vitamin C, in a buffered form, can also be taken intravenously. This allows the intake of very high doses of vitamin C directly into the blood plasma so getting much higher blood plasma levels of the vitamin than are possible by taking it orally. In fact this can be done at home if you follow the instructions at www.canceraction.org.gg/inext.htm#top.

It is also offered by most alternative clinics. In Britain it is offered by the Dove Clinic at www.doveclinic.com. Practitioners can contact http://bioimmune.com

Alternatively, you can dissolve the vitamin C desired in DMSO and rub it on the skin. DMSO is a powerful solvent that will take the vitamin C directly into the blood stream. I imagine this procedure would be very uncomfortable but would be perfectly safe – as long as the normal precautions associated with handling DMSO are observed – namely, very clean hands and skin and no gloves or jewelry of any sort (see p.243 for more information about DMSO).

Taking mega-doses of vitamin C intravenously (100+grams at a time) makes use of vitamin C in an entirely different way – it becomes a pro-oxidant rather than an anti-oxidant - and it is recommended that oral ingestion of vitamin C to bowel tolerance level should continue at the same time. A number of clinics are offering IV vitamin C therapy and it does seem as if this has a greater anti-cancer effect. For further information you can go to the following websites: www.canceraction.org.gg/inext.htm, www.maryclinic.com, www.orthomed.com/cancer.htm, and www.brightspot.org/cresearch/ivccancer.html

For people with brain cancers the fat-soluble form of vitamin C, Ascorbyl palmitate, is recommended. Not only can it be stored in the body longer than normal water-soluble vitamin C but it can cross the blood-brain barrier. However, in capsule form this supplement is useless. It needs to be dissolved in flax oil first.

Another, easier, way of getting vitamin C into the brain is to change it into DHA (dehydroascorbic acid – not to be confused with the other chemical DHA [docosahexaenoic acid]

that is found in fish oils). One way of making this is to dissolve as far as possible say 5 grams of vitamin C (a teaspoonful of powder) in a small amount of water. Then add the same amount of fresh 3 percent hydrogen peroxide. Wait until the foaming reaction has completed and consume. This combination is not acidic to the stomach.

Finally, a new form of vitamin C has recently hit the market. Lypo Spheric Vitamin C claims to be far more bio-available than other forms so that very little is 'wasted' in urine. For more information go to www.livonlabs.com. I have read a number of testimonials in free discussion groups of how easy this form of vitamin C is to tolerate and how quickly it has an effect. It may be that if the claims that 100 percent of the vitamin C gets through to the cells that Lypo-spheric Vitamin C taken orally may have the same impact as vitamin C taken intravenously.

Summing Up

I have nothing against Dr. Moertel personally but the chart below makes a point that cannot be made in any other way. It is not scientifically valid, it may even be considered in very bad taste, but it has a poetic immediacy that is unassailable.

Name	Age at death	Other information
Linus Pauling	93	Advocate of vitamin C
Albert Szent-Gyorgyi	93	Discovered vitamin C
Dr. Charles Moertel	66	Anti-vitamin C researcher, Died of cancer

It is perhaps fitting that Moertel and Pauling, arch enemies in life, should die within months of each other. It should be admitted that Linus Pauling's death has often been sniggeringly attributed to prostate cancer (and therefore by implication invalidating his vitamin C theories) — but it is my view that anyone who dies at the age of 93 actually dies of old age, no matter what the death certificate may say. Until a few months before his death, Linus Pauling was alert and in good form. He was still working! Clearly, he was living proof of the value of the regime he was recommending. Pauling's own recipe for a happy, healthy, long life, which he published in 1986, is as follows:

1. Take 6-18 grams of vitamin C everyday. Do not miss a single day.
2. Take 400-1,600 IU of vitamin E a day.
3. Take 1-2 high-dosage vitamin B tablets a day
4. Take 25,000 IU of vitamin A a day.
5. Take a multi-mineral supplement everyday which should include calcium, iodine, copper, magnesium, manganese, zinc, molybdenum, chromium and selenium.

6.   Keep intake of sugar to below 50 lbs a year.
7.   Apart from sugar, eat what you want - but not too much of any one food. Don't get fat.
8.   Drink plenty of water everyday.
9.   Keep active and do exercise but never excessively over-exert
       yourself.
10.   Drink alcohol only in moderation.
11.   Don't smoke.
12.   Avoid stress. Work at a job that you like. Be happy with your family.

When it comes to living longer, I prefer to take the advice of the longer lived.

In case anyone still has doubts about Pauling's stature as a scientist, James Watson, Nobel Prize winner and co-discoverer of the DNA double helix structure, referred to him as being an intellectual giant on a par with Einstein and Newton. Watson believed Pauling was only weeks or months away from solving the DNA problem when he himself found the solution.

Vitamin A (and/or Beta Carotene)

Note that beta carotene is known as the precursor of vitamin A. Vitamin A is obtained from animal sources while beta carotene comes from vegetables. Beta carotene is changed to vitamin A in the body only when it is needed, so vitamin A is best taken in the form of beta carotene. In that way the negative effects - possible toxicity - can be eliminated.

In a controlled study with people who chew betel nut and who therefore have a higher incidence of oral cancer, the group who received vitamin A (200,000 IU per week) had a pronounced remission from precancerous lesions and had fewer new lesions. One 1985 study, showed that cancer spread was much lower among mice fed with vitamin A supplements.

Another study has shown that women who take vitamin A during chemotherapy report a much lower incidence of unpleasant side effects - no doubt because of its important role for the growth of epithelial tissue.

Sources: Active vitamin A is found in fish oils, liver, eggs and dairy products. Yellow vegetables and fruits like mangoes contain beta carotene In both forms it is very susceptible to oxidation and can be destroyed by heat and light - so carrot juice has to be freshly pressed and drunk quickly to be effective.

ODA: 10,000-50,000 IU per day though higher amounts up 100,000 IU can be taken for extended periods - three to four months - in the case of patients fighting cancer.

Dangers: Vitamin A may cause birth defects or be toxic to infants so pregnant and lactating women should keep their vitamin A intake low. (5,000 IU or less). Also women who wish to become pregnant should reduce their vitamin A intake well in advance of conception.

Vitamin A is stored in body fat and is not water soluble so there is the potential for toxicity. However, you must take at least 100,000 IU of vitamin A daily for a period of months in order to display any signs of toxicity. Beta carotene, on the other hand, can be given for long periods of time virtually without risk of toxicity.

Signs of toxicity: Yellowing skin, fatigue and nausea, blurred vision and loss of hair.

Vitamin B Complex

These vitamins are not all - or even mainly - antioxidants. However, there are some strong anti-cancer effects associated with the B vitamins.

Thiamine, Vitamin B1, is recommended by some as a key component in a cancer cure as low levels of this vitamin prevent cell apoptosis (cell death)–see p. 240 for further details.

Riboflavin (B2) deficiencies, for example, have been shown clearly to lead to high levels of oesophageal (throat) cancer in animals. Also, niacin (B3) is known to be good for the liver. Vitamin B3 helps promote the transport of oxygen by dilating the blood vessels. More importantly, it is required for the production of NADH (Nicotinamide Adenine Dinucleotide), which is absolutely essential in a number of different ways for enabling aerobic metabolism. Since aerobic metabolism is exactly what we want to encourage if we want cancer cells to return to normal status, large doses of vitamin B3 should in theory be very helpful in the fight against cancer.

Lastly, B3, niacin, is known to have positive effects on mood, so can be taken as an anti-depressant.

It should be noted that niacin in large doses has the effect of causing a temporarily uncomfortable intense flush which is not at all pleasant but not in any way harmful. There is an alternative form of B3, niacinamide, which does not cause this sudden flush. However, since the sudden flush may be an important effect it is not known whether non-flush vitamin B3 is as good as niacin.

Vitamin B6: High intakes of this vitamin are associated with low rates of colorectal cancers. Studies on mice have also shown that, at high doses, it can eliminate colon cancers.

Vitamin B12 appears to have a strong synergistic relationship with vitamin C. In one study in which mice were implanted with tumour cells, only two out of fifty receiving the combination developed tumours. All fifty of the controls developed tumours.

Folic acid deficiency is widespread and this lack has been shown to be associated with cervical and breast cancers. Cervical cancer will respond to treatment with high doses of folic acid. A Japanese study has shown that large intakes of folate (10-20 milligrams) in combination with 750 micrograms of B12 had a very impressive protective effect. However, that said, there is increasing concern that folic acid in the form that is found in supplements and added to food is an artificial chemical and much that is taken in is not metabolised in the body but remains in its unmetabolised form– with worrying consequences. It is therefore much better to get folates in their natural form from foods. A cup of cranberries and blackeye beans, one and a half cups of pinto and garbanzo beans would supply a minimum day's needs. Other folate rich foods are: most beans, fruits, fruit juices and green leafy vegetables. Note that new evidence is showing cranberries to be very powerful inhibitors of cancer cell division.

Generally speaking, individual B vitamins should not be taken on their own in large doses for any length of time as this can lead to deficiencies in the other B vitamins - because they compete. The general rule of thumb is that you can take individual B vitamins up to three times their normal value in comparison with the intake of B complex as a whole. Folic acid is a possible exception to this rule.

Sources: widely available in dark green leafy vegetables, beans, brown rice and brewer's yeast but cooking reduces bioavailability.

ODA: B2: 50-500 mg - -B3: 500-1,000 mg - -B12:10-500 mcg - -Folic acid: 800-2,400 mcg

Toxic effects: There are no known toxic effects for B2 and B12 but for niacin there is the potential for a hot flush or itchy effect. There has been some recent concern that high intakes of folic acid are associated themselves with higher incidences of cancer. But these concerns need to be balanced against decades of research which have shown that high intakes of folic acid have healthy consequences.

Vitamin D

The RDA for vitamin D is 200 IU for those under the age of 50 and 400 IU for those over 50. However, new research has demonstrated that these levels are laughably low. The average person gets about 10,000 IU from sunbathing for about 20-30 minutes under a hot sun. And, as far as vitamin D is concerned, the more sunlight exposure you have the better. (For a more detailed discussion of sunlight see below under energy medicine). Food sources of vitamin D are poor sources in comparison to sunlight. A teaspoon of fish oil contains about 400 IU.

What are the dangers of too much vitamin D? None. Only one person in the world has ever been found to be suffering toxicity, and he was taking in 2.5 million IU a day (How he managed that, I have no idea). And he recovered quickly when this level of intake was stopped. In fact current research indicates that deficiency probably starts at intakes of less than 4,000 IU a day. Vitamin D can be stored in the body for about 60 days.

Until recently, this vitamin was seen simply as being necessary for the absorption of calcium. But it is now known to be a potent anti-cancer weapon in its own right. It has been found that vitamin D stabilizes chromosomes, repairs DNA damage, triggers programmed cell and inhibits angiogenesis (the development of a blood supply that the cancer needs to grow). It has been estimated that long-term high exposure to sunlight could prevent around 60 percent of cancers.

One scientist, Steve Martin of the Grouppe Kurosawa, believes that vitamin D 5,000 IU mixed with 6mg of melatonin powdered and dissolved in warm coconut milk (which itself is loaded with Lauric acid, a healthy fat even if it is a 'saturated fat') and taken at night on an empty stomach is as good a cancer preventative as any and that higher doses might even be curative. Grouppe Kurosawa (www.grouppekurosawa.com) is an interesting group that posts informative blogs on a number of health issues and they are willing to work as consultants with individuals who want a scientifically formulated approach to using natural supplements.

Other research has found that a metabolite of vitamin D (i.e., one of the chemical compounds that is produced as vitamin D is broken down in the body) called calcitriol (which is available on prescription) combined with a non-steroidal anti-inflammatory drug such as ibuprofen can significantly reduce the growth of prostate cancers by 70 percent. Both inhibit the production of prostaglandins which, among other effects, cause inflammation. Taken together they have an effect about three times greater than each taken alone.

Vitamin E

Vitamin E is often touted as the vitality vitamin. It has the unique characteristic that there are no known deficiency illnesses associated with it. What we call vitamin E actually comprises two closely related chemical families: the tocopherols (alpha-, beta-, gamma-, and delta-) and the tocotrienols (alpha to delta). Some vitamin E sold in stores is actually a synthetic form of only one of the tocopherols. Natural sourced vitamin E containing both tocotrienols and tocopherals is best.

It is not at all clear what the benefits and drawbacks are of vitamin E. Some say that vitamin E can protect cancer cells. On the other hand, it appears to help people to retain their hair during chemotherapy. New research has now found that the tocotrienols are more interesting for cancer patients than the tocopherols. They appear to have a dampening effect on cell proliferation, and so can help reduce cancer's ability to spread.

A number of studies have shown low vitamin E levels in the blood of people with lung, breast, bladder, cervix, and colorectal cancers. In a study of mice exposed to cigarette smoke, those supplemented with vitamin E and selenium suffered 8 percent deaths compared with 51 percent for the ones fed a diet deficient in these two substances. One study showed that the group of women with the lowest vitamin E levels had five times the risk of breast cancer compared with the group with the highest vitamin E levels. Some studies have also shown that vitamin E may help to reduce the side effects of chemotherapy. Having said that, there is also a body of opinion that believes that vitamin E both protects the tumour and can even promote tumour growth.

There are fears that synthetic forms of vitamin E provide little or no benefit but will block the ability of cells to absorb and make use of natural vitamin E. It is known that the body's ability to absorb one of the most important dietary forms (gamma-tocopherol) is hindered by high doses of synthetic vitamin E. Natural source vitamin E, providing a mix of tocopherols and tocotrienols, or any supplement with a high tocotrienol content is best.

Having said all this there does appear to be a man made variation of vitamin E that has a notable anti-cancer effect. This is alpha-tocopherol succinate. It has been shown to have a strong inhibitory effect on cancer cell growth with a number of different cancers. Life Extension (www.lef.org) markets a dry powder form of vitamin E alpha-tocopherol succinate.

Food Sources: vegetable fats and oils, whole grains and dark green leafy vegetables, nuts and legumes. However, food processing eliminates most of its vitamin E content. Unrefined or cold-pressed oils are best.

ODA: 200-800 IU per day (some advise up to 1,600 IU per day)

Toxicity: It is not advised for those with high blood pressure. However, no toxic effects have been clearly shown for doses below 3,000 per day. Signs of toxicity include nausea, flatulence, headache and fainting.

Vitamin K

Vitamin K was discovered in 1929 by Danish scientist, Dr. Henrik Dam. He called it "K" for its 'Koagulation' properties. It is sometimes referred to as "the forgotten vitamin". There are three types of vitamin K, known as K1, K2 and K3. Vitamin K3 is man-made and not normally recommended by most alternative practitioners (for exception see below). Vitamin K is required in large quantities and is associated with anti-ageing and for its antioxidant qualities (it is more powerful than vitamin E).

However, Dr. Jonathan Wright, a highly respected American doctor who favours alternative approaches, recommends a combination of vitamin C and vitamin K3 with a ratio of 100:1 - with a minimum vitamin C intake of 6,000 mgs. A dietary supplement, ProsStay, developed according to this protocol is available from Life Enhancement (www.life-enhancement.com). Dr. Wright is a consultant to Life Enhancement Inc. ProsStay is, as its name suggests, mainly targeted at prostate cancer, but there are reports that it is beneficial for other cancers too.

Sources: The richest natural source of vitamin K2 is natto, a fermented soybean product. Otherwise it is found in dark green vegetables—in sufficient quantities to interfere with anti-coagulant therapies.

ODA: 100 micrograms

Cautions: It is not recommended for pregnant women or nursing mothers.

Minerals

Everyone knows the importance of vitamins. But minerals, including trace minerals, are at least equally important for the healthy transfer of oxygen in and out of cells and for the other necessary bio-chemical operations required to maintain the good functioning of the body. Unfortunately, the vegetables that we depend on for our minerals are grown in increasingly mineral-depleted soils. However, as we shall see with calcium, not everything mineral is necessarily to be applauded.

Calcium

In relation to cancer, there is a big dispute over the question of calcium's potential for good or harm. There are two questions. First, is supplementing with calcium beneficial? And secondly, is it potentially dangerous?

The most famous advocate for calcium is Robert Barefoot, an American self-styled chemist, who is famous for promoting calcium from coral reefs – so-called coral calcium – as a cure all for cancer and many other conditions. His claims regarding the benefits of coral calcium are, however, heavily disputed by other leading alternative health advocates.

Ralph Moss reviewed the scientific literature and could find no support for the claims. Indeed he found that there may be a slight tendency for calcium to promote cancer – particularly prostate cancer.

In relation to prostate cancer, there is clear evidence that the calcium in dairy products inhibits the absorption of vitamin D and thereby promotes the growth of prostate cancer. Men who consume more than 600 mg per day of dietary calcium had a 32 percent higher risk of prostate cancer than those who consumed 150 or fewer milligrams per day.

It is important for cancer patients to keep this in mind in the face of claims by coral calcium proponents that one should increase calcium intake to very high levels. An overdose of calcium can lead to hypercalcaemia, a dangerous excess of calcium in the blood. Many patients with cancer already have a disturbed calcium metabolism - caused by the tumour itself - so that they are in any case hypercalcaemic. The symptoms of this are constipation, nausea, vomiting, abdominal pain, loss of appetite, and the production of abnormally large amounts of urine. Very severe hypercalcaemia often causes brain dysfunction with confusion, emotional disturbances, delirium, hallucinations, and coma. Muscle weakness may occur, and abnormal heart rhythms and death can follow.

A number of doctors have found that calcium has seriously negative consequences for patients with advanced cancer. One, Dr. Forbes Ross, reported: "On another occasion I had reason to administer calcium salts...to cases of cancer...I was appalled at the rate of growth of the cancers." (Dr. Forbes Ross, author of *Cancer: Its Genesis and Treatment*)

Dr. Max Gerson also believed calcium to be dangerous and blamed a number of cancer deaths on his use of calcium. It is now known that intracellular calcium is higher in cancer patients than in the normal population and is associated with rapid cell division. My advice therefore remains to be cautious.

Even when calcium is desired, not everyone agrees that calcium supplements or a diet of meat and dairy products is a good way to take it. Calcium, they say, should be taken in vegetable form. Their argument is that milk and meat - the sources of calcium with which we are most familiar - make our systems acidic and the body releases calcium from our bones to neutralize this effect. The best non-meat sources of calcium are seaweed like kelp, all leafy greens, figs, dates and prunes. In support of this view, some studies have shown that vegetarians have a significantly lower incidence of osteoporosis than meat eaters.

Milk, it should be noted, is contra-indicated for another reason. It has high concentrations of IGF-1 (Insulin Growth Factor) which has been found to promote breast and prostate cancer.

However, having said this, there is a calcium product on the market that is beneficial. This is Calcium D-glucarate. In this case, it is not the calcium but the D-glucarate that is significant. This is a naturally occurring substance that attacks an enzyme, glucoronidase, which interferes with the body's attempts to rid itself of cancer. It is considered to be a highly effective preventative of cancer – one that anyone who has already been treated for cancer should consider. It is inexpensive and can be obtained from www.lef.com.

Finally, it should be noted that calcium has poor bioavailability without the co-presence of magnesium, boron and vitamin D (sunlight). In fact, where they exist, low calcium levels may be caused not by inadequate calcium intake but by poor magnesium intake and lack of exposure to the sun.

Germanium

There are two forms of this mineral: organic and inorganic. Some cases of kidney failure have occurred with the latter. But water-soluble, organic germanium does not have these problems. Indeed it is considered to have an extremely powerful anticancer effect as well as being able to normalize the whole body's chemistry. The discoverer of organic germanium, Dr. Kazuhiko Asai, a coal engineer, wrote of the organic germanium that he had synthesised: "My organic germanium compound has proved effective against all sorts of diseases, including cancers of the lung, bladder, larynx and breast." He believed the reason for this ability was that germanium enriched the oxygen levels in the body. "I should say that all diseases are attributable to deficiency of oxygen. The dangers of an oxygen deficiency in the human body cannot be over-emphasised."

Food sources: It is very high in medicinal plants notably shelf fungus (Trametes cinnabarina) but garlic and ginseng also contain significant amounts.

ODA: None but recommended dose in case of need: 30-150 mg

Toxicity: At levels below 500 mg no toxic effects have been reported. Skin rashes and stool softening have been reported for doses of over 2 grams a day.

Iodine

Iodine is vital for good health but the Western diet has become depleted of food sources that contain iodine. In addition, baked goods that used to contain iodine now contain bromine, which competes with iodine within the body. The result is that we are getting inadequate supplies. Iodine is known to be antiviral, antibacterial and an important anti-cancer agent. In addition, it helps raise the pH of the body and helps to convert toxic estrogens into less toxic metabolites. This makes it particularly important for anyone with a hormone based cancer. The low incidence of breast cancer in Japan is often attributed to the high iodine intake in the Japanese diet. It has also been noted that prostate cancer in Japan rarely goes beyond the prostate – and one can live with a cancer that doesn't spread for a very long time! This too is associated with the high iodine intake in the standard Japanese diet.

Iodine can be taken in the form of seaweed or in a more concentrated form as potassium iodide solution or Lugol's solution, both of which are available on the internet. Iodoral is a potassium iodide formulation in the form of tablets. Atomic iodine is an iodine product with enhanced electrical activity – 7 percent solution is required.

Sources: Seaweed, Potassium iodide solution, Iodoral, Atomic Iodine

ODA: 500-1,000 mcg/d

Toxicity: Signs of an iodine overdose can range from a persistent metallic taste in the mouth, coughing, shortness of breath, diarrhoea, thirst, fever and even shock. However, it is now known that concerns about iodine over-dosing have been exaggerated in recent decades. Dr. Albert Szent Györgi, the Nobel Prize winning biochemist who isolated vitamin C wrote: "When I was a medical student, iodine in the form of KI (Potassium Iodide) was the universal medicine. Nobody knew what it did, but it did something and did something good." In those days the standard dose was 1 gram, which contains 770 mg of iodine.

Iron

It is now generally accepted that cancer patients should not take iron supplements. There is mounting evidence that excess iron is associated with lowered immunity and higher incidence of cancer. Also cancer cells have a high need for iron. Depriving them of this mineral will therefore impede growth of the tumour.

Anaemia, the well-known iron-deficiency symptom, may not in fact be caused by iron deficiency. It can be caused by a deficiency of vitamin B12 and/or folic acid as well as by the presence in the bloodstream of drugs or toxins. It is not therefore automatic that iron needs to be taken when anaemia is diagnosed.

However, there is an anti-cancer strategy that takes into account the cancer cell's hunger for iron. When artemisinin comes in contact with iron a reaction takes place, releasing a burst of free radicals. Although it is normally not advisable to take iron supplements in the case of cancer, when taking artemisinin, the reverse is true, as we wish to flood the cancer cells with iron. The free radicals then kill the cancer cell. For further details see p..235

Magnesium

Magnesium is a largely neglected mineral but one that is required in fairly large quantities by the body. Over 300 enzymes that influence the metabolism of carbohydrate, amino acids, nucleic acids and proteins require magnesium. In relation to cancer, it is known that there is a direct inverse relationship between soil content of magnesium and cancer incidence. Where magnesium content is higher, cancer incidence tends to be lower.

It is also known that for most Western countries, magnesium deficiency is the norm. One recent Swedish study showed that less than 20 percent of the 66,000 women it was following had a daily intake above 225 mg (350-500mg is recommended). The study also found that colon cancer incidence was inversely proportional to the intake of magnesium.

Magnesium is an important healing agent and it helps to mediate the potassium and calcium levels of the body's tissues.

The problem is how to increase magnesium levels in the body. One difficulty is that low tissue magnesium levels reduce the ability of the body to absorb more magnesium from the diet. One solution is to take the magnesium transdermally (i.e., through the skin). One way of doing this is to spend a lot of time in the sea, which contains high levels of magnesium chloride. An oil based form of magnesium chloride that you can spray on is available from Global Light Network (www.globallight.net). Dr. Mark Sircus is a strong proponent for this approach and his book Transdermal Magnesium Therapy is recommended (go to www.magnesiumforlife.com).

Another option is to have regular baths with magnesium oxide or magnesium citrate powder which is also easily absorbed. Finally, magnesium can be taken in by means of a homeopathic strength tissue salt: magnesium phosphate.

Substantially increased intakes of magnesium also benefit the heart, blood pressure, bowel cleansing, relaxation, back pain and sexual potency. Anyone who suffers from incapacitating back pain will also find magnesium extremely beneficial. It relaxes the muscles.

ODA: 400-800 mg (1,000+ mg a day if needed)

Toxicity: Toxicity is rare as most people have the problem of too little magnesium rather than too much. However, a daily intake of 8,000 mg or more is likely to be excessive.

Potassium

Sodium and potassium tend to compete within the body. If the body's tissues are high in sodium then the tissues will not take up proper amounts of potassium. The problem is sodium is 'bad' and potassium is 'good'. It is important to maintain a low sodium-high potassium balance in the body. Good amounts of vitamin B6 are also important to help regulate the balance.

Cells that lose their ability to regulate the proper balance of potassium and sodium quickly become unhealthy – a condition known as toxic tissue syndrome. The consequences are serious if not quickly corrected. That is why a high potassium and low sodium diet is necessary to correct many health issues including both cancer and problems associated with heart disease, high blood pressure, etc.

Potassium-rich foods are almonds, apricots, avocados, bananas, lima, mung and pinto beans, dates, dried figs, hazelnuts, raw garlic, raw horseradish, kelp*, blackstrap molasses*, raw parsley, rice bran, soybeans, full fat soybean flour, sunflower seeds and brewer's yeast*. (* These sources are extremely rich in potassium.)

While high potassium levels are generally recommended it is very possible to have too much potassium and this can have dangerous consequences for the kidney and can also put the body into a state of shock. Supplementation with potassium pills should therefore be avoided where possible. Potassium should be taken only in the form of food unless under close medical supervision.

ODA: 300-500 mg

Toxicity: Any intake above 1,000mg should be carefully monitored. Anyone with kidney disease or heart problems in particular needs to take care.

Selenium

Selenium is needed by all the tissues of the body. Selenium deficiency is quite common because in many parts of the world the soil is low in selenium and the result is that animals and vegetables grown on this land contains very little—and since this is what we eat and where we get our selenium from we too are deficient.

There is very strong evidence that selenium deficiency is implicated in heart disease, AIDS and cancer - and that these problems can be rectified by adding selenium to the diet in the form of supplements. Vitamin E and selenium work together synergistically - that is, their combined effect is greater than the sum of their effects when taken separately. However, vitamin C interferes with selenium absorption so there should be a gap of an hour between taking one or the other.

People exposed to environmental pollution may become deficient as selenium is used up fighting the heavy metals. For our purposes, selenium is known to help protect cells from damage from free radicals. The best natural source of selenium is Brazil nuts – which have such a high selenium content that an ounce a day is the most that should be eaten.

Also, a highly recommended selenium supplement is Se-methylselenocysteine (MSC) a naturally occurring selenium compound which has been demonstrated in animal and laboratory tests to cause apoptosis (natural cell death) in cancer cells.

ODA: 200-400 mcg per day.

Toxicity: Anyone taking in more than 2,000 mcg per day may suffer the effect of a garlicky odour in the breath, urine and sweat. Interestingly, birth defects may also occur at long-term intake at these levels. If you are not pregnant very high levels of selenium can be taken and these will likely have a beneficial impact on tumour growth. Long-term intake of 500-750 mcg has not turned up any sign of toxicity in humans.

Vanadium

Vanadium is a trace element that has recently been discovered to have a powerful anti-cancer effect, causing cells to undergo apoptosis (natural cell death). Vanadium appears to be non-toxic at even high doses when taken as a supplement. It is cheaply available from a number of sources as it is marketed as a dietary aid. One good source is Rainbow Minerals at www.rainbowminerals.net

Zinc

Zinc has acquired a good reputation as an immune system booster – particularly when accompanied by magnesium.. However, high zinc supplementation (100mg/day) has also been associated with higher levels of prostate cancer. It is therefore best not to take more than 30mg per day.

That would have been all I could say about zinc had my attention not been drawn informally to a study that was apparently published in the *Medical Press* (details unknown) in 1953 - and ever since largely neglected. This study showed that an injection of zinc and magnesium ascorbates in aqueous solution had a very profound effect on seven women with terminal cancer of the uterus. Five years later, four of them were still alive. In all, 200 terminal cancer patients received the substance and 90 percent were free from pain within ten days - the majority being free from pain within two days. Many demonstrated tumour regression. In addition to vitamin C, the patients all received a 3cc injection every other day. Each cc of the solution contained 1.5mg of zinc and 0.3mg of magnesium (both calculated as metal and both complexed with ascorbic acid). It is possible to find vitamin C in the form of zinc and magnesium ascorbates but, if taken orally, these would have to be taken in much larger quantities.

ODA: 30-50 mgs

Toxicity: Zinc toxicity only occurs when intake exceeds 1-2,000 mg per day. The result is gastric irritability and vomiting.

Multi-Mineral Formulas

Whereas most off-the-shelf multi-vitamin formulas are wholly inadequate as sources of vitamins, the same is not true of minerals – particularly the trace minerals.

CAA capsules

These are multi-mineral and vitamin capsules formulated by a New Zealand farmer, Percy Weston, who was diagnosed with cancer at the age of 39. He was also at that time crippled with arthritis. He blamed these problems on the superphosphate fertilizers that he and other farmers had begun to use on their farms. The initial result was improved yields but gradually the mineral content of the soil became seriously degraded. "At the end of 5 years [of using superphosphates] we had a plague of cancer lesions coming up on the ears of the sheep. It is the same condition that afflicts humans, and has the same cause."

He discovered that the highly acidic chemical superphosphates also killed the soil bacteria and earthworms necessary for the healthy regeneration of the soil. The result was—and remains - that the majority of our food contains excessive phosphorus, and is deficient in calcium, magnesium, selenium, zinc, cobalt and trace minerals.

When his animals exhibited cancerous lesions, Percy Weston went back to using natural rock phosphate and salt containing the missing minerals. The result? His sheep healed. When he himself was diagnosed with cancer, he decided to mix together a mineral formula based on his experiences with his sheep. His cancer left him, as did his arthritis, and he went on to live to the age of 100 – he was still farming at the age of 97. He was free of cancer, arthritis and heart disease to the end. He wrote an extremely important book, *Cancer: Cause and Cure*, that details his clear demonstration that one major cause – if not the main cause - of cancer is the way we grow our food. To test his theories, Weston found he was able to cause cancer in his animals at will, and he was also able to cure them every time, simply by giving his animals a diet without any trace mineral content – and then providing them with the missing trace minerals..

His multi-mineral mix (which does not, by the way, include vanadium, so this will need to be supplemented separately) should be accompanied by a diet that is low in phosphates. This largely means a diet of organic fruit and vegetables and no meat, eggs or dairy. Weston also produced another book, *Cancer Fighting Foods*, in which he lists the mineral content of most foods. His books and the multi-mineral mix are now marketed by a New Zealand company and can be ordered from www.zealandpublishing.co.nz

Beres Drops

Formulated by a Hungarian scientist, Dr. Jozsef Beres, Beres Drops is a liquid formula containing a patented combination of the following ingredients: Distilled Water, Glycerol, EDTA, Glycogen, Iron, L-Tartaric Acid, Zinc, Sodium, Succinic Acid, Magnesium, Manganese, L-Ascorbic Acid, Potassium, Copper, Molybdenum, Vanadium, Nickel, Boron, Fluorine, Chlorine, Cobalt.

On September 15th 1991, the Sunday Sun carried the story of a Mrs. Wendy Cook who claimed that three months on the drops had had the effect of shrinking a malignant tumour in her groin from 4 inches to one inch. Beres Drops are widely available from internet suppliers.

Liquid Mineral Complex

The sea contains a perfect blend of minerals and this product is essentially 'purified sea water'. This is a liquid blend of 84 ionically charged ocean minerals and trace elements. It is easily available from internet suppliers.

OTHER SUPPLEMENTS

The following supplements are, generally speaking, natural products that help to maintain the body's natural state of health which have also been shown to have a positive effect in helping the body combat cancer—one of which is freely available in your own home.

Acidophilus and Other 'Friendly' Bacteria

Did you know that you have more bacteria in your body than you have cells (and you have 75 trillion cells)? Most of these bacteria are in the gut. They are vital for the breaking down and digesting of food. They also keep other microbial predators at bay - specifically unfriendly bacteria, viruses and fungi. In fact, if you have any fungal or inflammatory attack of the urino-genital system then taking some capsules of lactobacillus acidophilus should go some way to solving the problem. Athlete's foot is also amenable. There is a healthy balance between bacteria and yeast (there are friendly yeasts too) but any sign of a yeast attack should be dealt with by taking acidophilus. They also have antibiotic properties that keep viruses under control. Polio viruses, for example, cannot survive in the presence of high concentrations of acidophilus.

Also, these bacteria help protect against cancer and even have an anti-tumour effect. Mice receiving acidophilus supplements showed 400 percent greater macrophage activity. Macrophages are the blood components that attack cancer tumours. Animal studies show that acidophilus helps to slow down and even stop tumour growth.

A Bulgarian doctor, Dr. Ivan Bogdanov, using a highly concentrated form of other bacteria, lactobacillus bulgaricus, obtained a complete remission in one patient suffering from terminal multiple myeloma. In fact the patient was sinking into a terminal coma when treatment started. Six months later there was no sign of the disease. His only treatment was with the bacteria.

In the Bulgarian study similar results were obtained with people suffering from many types of cancer. The amounts they took on a daily basis were equivalent to eating 40-60 kilos of Bulgarian yoghurt. The bacteria-rich product used was called 'Anabol'. However, I have not been able to source this product. The recommended daily dose is 10-15grams. More than this results in the possibility of tumour disintegration: a process which floods the body with toxic products and can kill the patient if detoxification procedures are not started immediately.

Products containing L. acidophilus and L. Bulgaricus are widely available – Natren, for example, (www.natren.com) has an L.bulgaricus powder and combination capsules – but. in all cases, they should be kept refrigerated in the shop and at home. Potency of capsules is highly variable so buying direct over the internet from a good supplier is strongly advised.

Alpha Lipoic Acid (ALA) (with Acetyl L-Carnitine)

Alpha lipoic acid is a powerful antioxidant that promotes the effects of the other vitamins. Acetyl L-carnitine is a naturally occurring amino acid. In combination, these two chemicals have an established ability to counteract the effects of ageing in cells. Any substance that promotes healthy cells will work against cancer. It is particularly beneficial at repairing the damage caused by chemotherapy and radiation. ALA also helps to reprocess vitamin C.

Amino Acids

Amino acids are the molecular bricks from which proteins are built. The body contains something in the region of 50,000 different proteins and 20,000 different enzymes. These are all built up by combining 29 known amino acids in different combinations. Most of the amino acids are synthesised in the liver–another reason why a healthy liver is vital for good health. There are eight amino acids, however, known as essential amino acids, that must come from our diet. Amino acid supplementation is strongly indicated for any form of degenerative disease or indeed any mental or physical disorder such as heart disease, chronic fatigue syndrome, diabetes, epilepsy, anaemia or herpes. The amino acids that are known to be relevant in the fight against cancer - either in a curative or preventative way are:

L-Arginine: This slows tumour growth and helps detoxify and heal the liver. It helps wounds to heal and helps to maintain the immune system. In large doses it may even be curative on its own. One healer, Jimmy Keller, had success with it before his work was rudely interrupted by the US legal authorities.

L-Carnitine: This is a general all round amino acid that enhances the effects of vitamins E and C.

L-Citrulline: This boosts the immune system, protects the liver against ammonia and is an energy booster.

L-Cysteine: This is an antioxidant and a very useful protector against the harmful effects of smoking and alcohol, as well as the effects of radiation.

GABA: Gamma-Aminobutyric Acid. This is good for anxiety, stress and depression. Better than librium or valium, they say.

Glutamine: The most abundantly available amino acid. Evidence shows that it is important for Natural Killer (NK) cells. The more glutamine the more active the NK cells the lower the ability of tumours to grow. Supplementing (0.3 gm/kilo of body weight) can be very beneficial. It is highly recommended for anyone undergoing radiation or chemotherapy as these deplete glutamine reserves. There are anecdotal reports of terminal cancer patients who 'stopped dying' after taking glutamine. It is recommended to take this in combination with another amino acid isoleucine.

Glutathione: This is an extremely important anti-oxidant which protects the body against the ravages of cigarettes, radiation, chemotherapy, heavy metal poisoning and the effects of drugs and alcohol. The best source of the precursors for glutathione is cold processed (or undenatured) whey.

L-Lysine: Important for tissue repair and the production of antibodies, hormones and enzymes. It should be taken before, during and after any operation. This is possibly the most important anti-viral amino acid. It eliminates cold sores and herpes sores very quickly.

L-Ornithine: Important for wound healing

L-Proline: Good for healing. Important for building of cell walls

L-Tryptophan: Mood stabiliser, antidepressant and stress reducer. Good for insomnia. At one time this was banned but it is now available again.

L-Tyrosine: Antidepressant and anxiety reducer.

L-Theanine: Effective against anxiety

They should be taken on an empty stomach. There is no known toxicity: Excess amino acids are burnt off as energy or converted to fat.

Linus Pauling and his successor Matthias Rath claim that high doses of Lysine and Proline along with megadoses of vitamin C are virtually a cancer cure in themselves as these are the building blocks for collagen, the stuff of which cell walls are made. They also block the enzyme that dissolves collagen. They recommend that vitamin C be taken at a level just below bowel tolerance level, and that the same amount of lysine be taken along with about half that level of Proline. A maintenance dose would be vitamin C (6,000mg), Lysine (6,000mg) and Proline (3,000mg) but for treating cancer much higher doses are likely to be necessary—see the section on vitamin C. Testimonials supporting the use of Rath's protocol can be found at www.stopping-cancer-naturally.org/us/testimonials.html.

Lysine and arginine in combination have also been demonstrated as having a beneficial effect on the production of hormones in the thymus gland – which are important for the maintenance of good health.

Cheap source of glutamine and other amino acid products: www.bulknutrition.com

Bee Pollen and Propolis

Beekeepers don't get cancer! Several attempts to find beekeepers who had died of cancer came up virtually empty handed. Only one, in Hawaii, was found to have died of skin cancer. The Russian Georgian peasants who were found to have lived up to 150 years were avid beekeepers.

Bee pollen is one of nature's most complete foods and has long been associated in India, China and even ancient Egypt with healing and energy. A number of animal studies have also shown that it has a strong ability to retard tumour growth. An ounce (28 grams) of bee pollen each day will, according to naturopath Diane Stein, prevent or delay the development of all malignant tumours and will help to reduce the size of existing tumours.

As for propolis, a resin gathered by honeybees from the buds and barks of certain trees and plants, this is known to have antibacterial, antifungal, antiviral, antiinflammatory, and pain-killing properties.

In one study, propolis was found to significantly reduce two cancer markers in the blood.

Beta Glucan

Beta-D-glucans, usually referred to as beta-glucans, comprise a class of non-digestible polysaccharides widely found in nature in such sources as oats, barley, yeast, bacteria, algae and mushrooms.

This is one of those supplements about which some debate is occurring. According to those who like it, Beta-1, 3-D Glucan is a powerful stimulator of the immune system while at the same time being an effective antioxidant and free radical scavenger. Beta Glucan is a safe and non-toxic and shows good effects against cancer. It is best taken with vitamin C as they work synergistically.

While most people agree with these statements, there is disagreement about whether taking this supplement is useful or a waste of money. There is also a lot of dispute about the quality of the products on the market. Some people suggest that the best way of taking it is to eat lots of porridge and/or mushrooms. 10-15,000 grams are required for effective anti-cancer activity.

Immutol is the brand name of a purified beta-glucan product. see www.immutol.com

Brewer's Yeast

Brewer's yeast is inactive yeast that is the by-product of beer making. It is a very rich source of vitamins and minerals, particularly chromium which regulates blood sugar. It has been described as a whole food on a par with chlorella and spirulina. It is also considered by some to be one of nature's cure-alls for everything from diabetes to, well, cancer.

Normally healthy people cannot take much brewer's yeast, as it induces nausea. Curiously though, people with cancers have been found to have a very high tolerance for relatively large quantities of this substance: half a cupful a day or more.

"Supplementation with selenium-enriched brewer's yeast (delivering 200 micrograms of selenium a day) over a period of several years was associated, in one study, with significant reduction in the incidence of lung, colorectal, prostate and total cancer, as well as a reduction in total cancer mortality." Say the author's of information on www.pdrhealth.com.

Interestingly there appears to be a connection between cholesterol levels, inflammation and cancer. A number of anti-cancer approaches are also beneficial against heart disease and arthritis (The Budwig Protocol and Percy Weston's trace mineral product CAA both link their approach to fighting cancer as a way also of fighting heart disease and arthritis.). Brewer's yeast is another substance that has a wide range of beneficial effects including an ability to reduce serum cholesterol. Laboratory tests showed a rise in serum cholesterol was partially or totally prevented when yeast was added to the diet. The rate of reduction in cholesterol levels and cholesterol blockage was directly related to the amount of yeast consumed.

Baker's yeast is not the same and should be avoided. Panaktiv is a liquid form of brewer's yeast available from www.drmetz.de

Co-Enzyme Q10 (CoQ10)

The quinone family of chemical compounds is a very important one for cancer. One of the major chemotherapeutic drugs, Adriamycin, is a quinone. Other quinones are being tested in trials for effects against Alzheimer's and other ailments. Adriamycin is an oxidative quinone whose effects are very different from others, like CoQ10 which are anti-oxidative. Adriamycin is therefore dangerous for people with weak hearts. CoQ10 protects against this effect. Anyone undergoing chemotherapy with Adriamycin should therefore take large amounts of CoQ10.

Co-enzyme Q10 is a quinone which is found almost everywhere in nature - which is why it is called the ubiquitous quinone - ubiquinone for short. But it is present in extremely small quantities - too small to be medically useful. While many quinones have an improved immuno-strengthening effect at very small doses, ubiquinone is not one of these. CoQ10 has an increased effect with larger doses. However, it is known that people with cancer have reduced levels of CoQ10 suggesting that it is used up in fighting the tumour.

A Danish study, published in 1994, found that women with terminal breast cancer did very well when taking 390 mg a day. This amount seemed to be sufficient to prevent further tumour growth and even to cause tumour shrinkage. A group of 32 women with advanced stage breast cancer were given, in addition to the normal treatments of surgery, radiation and chemotherapy, a programme of supplements including 390 mg of CoQ10. Danish cancer specialist, Knud Lockwood said: "I have never before seen spontaneous regression of the type of breast tumours that we were treating in this trial, or comparable regression on any conventional anti-cancer therapy." There are no known toxic effects. Many people take 60-90 mg a day as a general energising tonic.

CoQ10 is best taken as part of what has been called the Stockholm Protocol which included the following supplements (daily amounts): Gamma Linolenic Acid (1.2 grams); Omega 3

Fatty Acids (3.5 grams); Beta Carotene (58 mg or 32,248 IU); Vitamin C (2.8 grams); Vitamin E (2500 IU); Selenium (385 mcg); CoQ10 (390 mg).

In addition high-dose vitamin B complex should be added and the CoQ10 should ideally be taken in an oil base to aid absorbtion–dissolving in olive oil or coconut oil being best.

While the vitamin E level recommended here is very high and should probably be lowered after a few months, the vitamin C level of the Stockholm Protocol has been criticised for being too low, and no one should feel constrained from increasing this by four , five or even more times.

A final note, Life Extension Foundation are marketing a super-absorbable version of CoQ10 – see www.lef.com

Colostrum and Transfer Factor Plus

Colostrum is the pre-milk that new-born babies get from their mother's breast for the first few days they are breast fed. The colostrum available as a nutritional supplement is not sourced from human breasts, however, but from cows.

Colostrum contains many bioactive compounds. A recent study in Sweden focused on alpha-lactalbumin, an immune factor present in colostrum. This was found to cause cancer cells to "commit suicide." Colostrum also contains lactoferrin which is known to prevent or shrink cancers. Conjugated linoleic acid (CLA) and other fats found in colostrum also have anti-carcinogenic properties.

Knowledge of the benefits of bovine colostrum is not new. In India, Ayurvedic doctors have long known about its health benefits and it is so commonly used there that it is delivered by the milkman. As it is a food, there are no toxicity problems.

Some say that the reason colostrum is effective is that it contains transfer factors and that it is much more effective to take a concentrated dose of transfer factors, such as the branded formulation, Transfer Factor Plus.

Transfer factors are tiny molecules found in colostrum which provide information on immunity. If you take these molecules from a person who has recovered from a disease and give them to someone who hasn't, the second person will gain a significant degree of immunity and ability to fight back. Research on these transfer factors has been going on for over 50 years. One study into their potential for cancer patients looked at 20 terminal cancer patients whose average life expectancy was 3.7 months. The patients were given 9 capsules per day of Transfer Factor Plus™ along with a number of other supplements: digestive enzymes, probiotics and vitamins. After eight months, 16 of these individuals were still living and were either in remission, improving or they had stabilized. There was clear evidence also that the immune system had been boosted by over 400 percent, measured in terms of natural killer cell function.

Transfer Factor Plus can be obtained from www.my4life.com

Human breast milk has also been shown to have a strong anti-cancer effect in the laboratory, killing over 40 different kinds of cancer cell in test tube studies. One of the arsenal of compounds that helps achieve this is a protein called alpha-lactalbumin. So if you have a supply of fresh breast milk at hand, do make use of it.

Ellagic Acid

This is a naturally occurring polyphenolic constituent found in 46 different fruits and nuts – in red raspberries in particular but also in strawberry, blueberry and walnuts. It is also, it seems, a highly potent anti-carcinogen which has the ability to inhibit mutations within a cell's DNA. In some studies cancer activity was stopped within 48 hours.

Normal cells have a life cycle which, like all life cycles, involves birth, maturity, old age and death. In the case of cells, when they die they are replaced. The process of natural cell death is known as apoptosis. Cancer cells, however, do not die. Instead they multiply, first dividing into 2 cancer cells, then 4, 8, 16, 32 and so on - and they all continue to live. Ellagic Acid has the effect of causing cancer cells to undergo normal cell death within a matter of days.

There is a lot of excitement about the potential benefits of this chemical, and even the American Cancer Society has not been able to ignore it–though it unhelpfully informs readers that it is not available as a supplement. Nevertheless, they are technically correct – any supplement claiming to contain ellagic acid is a fraud. However, supplements containing ellagitannins will provide the raw materials which are converted to ellagic acid in the body. The raspberry's seeds contain the highest concentrations of ellagitannin.

I would start my internet search at www.ellagic.net and compare this product with others available from other sources. For skin cancer there is Raspex SPF-30 skin gel which is made from meeker raspberries and has a strong ellagitannin content. See www.smdi.org/products.htm

Enzymes (Digestive)

The reason enzymes are important is this. Digestive enzymes are produced by the pancreas. When there is cancer in the body one of the ways the body reacts is to see it as a foreign protein that needs to be digested. Unfortunately, the cancer is an efficient producer of chemicals that destroy these enzymes. This forces the pancreas to work harder to produce more enzymes. The result can quickly be an exhausted pancreas, especially as the pancreas may have been weak in the first place.

To help the pancreas, you should drink green juices, cut back on eating meat, occasionally fast, and supplement your diet with pancreatic enzymes. Pancreatic enzymes should be taken when your system is most alkaline: namely, when you awake, and between 2-3pm in the afternoon.

There are a number of different kinds of proteolytic digestive enzyme: proteases digest proteins, lipases digest fats, and amylases help to digest carbohydrates.

Enzymes not only attack cancer cells directly but also promote immune activity by helping stimulate production of a substance called tumour necrosis factor (TNF) which attacks cancer cells. They also interfere with metastatic activity, so stopping the cancer cells from spreading.

The most important source of proteolytic enzymes is the pancreas. Enzyme formulations often combine pancreatin with papain, a powerful enzyme derived from the papaya, and bromelain, an enzyme derived from the pineapple.

Pancreatic enzymes should play an important part in any overall anti-cancer strategy and should be taken in large quantities. One highly rated enzyme product is made by the German Wobe Mugos company and is marketed as Wobenzyme. Pancreatic enzymes were the cornerstone of Dr William Kelley's anti-cancer program (see page 277) – he cured his own terminal pancreatic cancer with their help. His enzyme formulation can be bought from www.2line.com/drkelleyHOT.html

Dr. Nicholas Gonzalez, who is now the leading proponent of the Kelley approach to cancer treatment, also uses enzymes as a central part of his cancer cure. He is said to favour Pork Pancreas made by www.nutricology.com. Serrapeptase is another enzyme which has strong anti-inflammatory properties which may make it part of a useful package of anti-cancer enzymes.

Fulvic Acid

Not all ancient deposits of vegetation turned into oil or coal. Some simply became what is known as humic deposits. Some of these deposits are very rich in a substance called fulvic acid. It has recently been discovered that fulvic acid is absolutely essential for plant health, and the same is true of animals and man. However, because of modern farming methods, the plants we eat are depleted of this acid. In addition to being necessary for the absorption of minerals and vitamins, fulvic acid has shown extremely powerful anti-viral activity as well as being a potent cancer fighter (it appears to interfere with a cancer tumour's ability to grow). Recent scientific investigations of this complex chemical appears to indicate that it is one of the finest electrolytes known to man; that it assists with human enzyme production and is also a very powerful anti-oxidant and free radical scavenger.

There are a number of products on the market claiming to contain fulvic acid - mainly colloidal mineral mixes. Vital Earth Minerals (www.vitalearth.org/index.htm) market the product with the best reputation, Fulvic Mineral Complex. On this website you will find an article discussing the benefits of fulvic acid.

Glyconutrients

Glyconutrients are the name given to eight essential saccharides (sugars). These are: mannose, glucose, galactose, xylose, N-acetylglucosamine, N-acetylgalactosamine, fucose (not to be confused with fructose), and N-acetylneuraminic acid. These are required to make glycoproteins, which in turn are essential for cellular communication—poor cellular communication leads to poor immune response and vice versa. Medicinal mushrooms and aloe vera are particularly high in these glyconutrients.

It is important to note that glyconutrients need to be taken everyday for extended periods of time to be effective. While there are some expensive glyconutrient supplements available (e.g.. those sold by Mannatech) many people make up their own inexpensive glyconutrient powder by mixing together the following in roughly equal parts: kelp powder, fenugreek powder, whey protein concentrate powder (with added enzymes is best), brewer's yeast, shark (or bovine) cartilage powder, psyllium powder and lecithin powder – add shiitake mushroom powder, cayenne pepper (optional). Buy one pound of each item and mix together thoroughly. Eat one full teaspoon twice a day. Another recommended mix consists simply of one table spoon of apple cider vinegar with one tablespoon of blackstrap molasses. Molasses is the syrup that remains after refined sugar is crystalised and extracted from sugar cane. It is a rich source of minerals and glyconutrients though its high iron content means it is not a perfect source for people with cancer – cancer cells need iron for cell division. Against that, it is high in potassium and is an alkali ash food which is good. Or, of course, you can simply take aloe vera, which is another excellent source all on its own.

Lycopene

Lycopene is a caretenoid that is found in tomatoes and a number of other vegetables/fruit: red guava, red grapefruit, red pepper, watermelon, papaya and sweet potatoes. High lycopene intake is associated with lowered incidences of prostate and colon cancer. Some studies indicate that upping intake of cooked tomatoes is beneficial. In one anecdotal case, a 62-year-old man with advanced prostate cancer experienced regression of his tumor after taking 10 mg of lycopene per day and 300 mg of saw palmetto three times per day.

Melatonin

Until recently the functions of the pineal gland have remained pretty much a mystery. However, melatonin, the pineal gland's chief hormone is now receiving a lot of attention. For one thing it is now known to regulate the circadian rhythm, the body's biological clock. It is used as an antidote to jet-lag and as a supplement that is helpful in reducing anxiety, panic attacks and migraines in addition to being an effective sleeping pill, especially as a safe way to get insomniac children to sleep. It does not have the side effects of other sleeping pills and does not interfere with REM (rapid eye movement) dream states.

Now, new studies are suggesting that it also bolsters the immune system, keeps our cells in a good state of repair, is an powerful anti-oxidant (5 times more powerful than vitamin C), protects against electromagnetic radiation and the toxicity of chemotherapy, slows the growth of tumours and cataracts and keeps heart disease at arm's length. As one cellular biologist, who takes 1 mg every night, said in a Newsweek article "I want to die young as late in life as possible, and I think this hormone could help." (*Newsweek*, Aug 7, 1995)

An Italian study has shown that a nightly 10 mg dose has significantly improved one-year survival rates of metastatic lung cancer.

While no one is suggesting that melatonin on its own is a cure for cancer they are saying it is an important weapon. As we grow older we secrete less and our sleep patterns become disrupted. And sleeplessness leads in the long term to ill health. Research shows that tumours are switched on during the day and switched off at night. The longer the day (i.e., exposure to light), the longer the cancer cells are switched on. Dr. David Blask who has researched the impact of sleep on cancer says: "With constant light, tumors grow seven times faster and soak up incredible amounts of linoleic acid, During the day, the cancer cells are awake and linoleic acid stimulates their growth. But at night cancer cells go to sleep. When we turn on lights at night for a long time, we suppress melatonin and revert back to the daytime condition."

This may explain why nurses who often work the night shift have higher rates of breast and colon cancer.

To be effective, melatonin must be taken at night before going to bed. Most people get good effects from doses of 1-10mg but there is no sign of any toxicity at higher doses and some therapists are using as much as 50mg doses as part of their protocol. No scientist has yet developed a concentration capable of killing a mouse, and human volunteers who took 6 grams (6,000mgs) a day for a month merely reported some stomach discomfort and residual sleepiness. As one researcher noted, "Its nastiest side effect is sleepiness."

Roger Coghill, a scientist who runs his own laboratory in Wales, believes that melatonin is the secret to longer lives – but he also believes that doses in the one gram and more range are not the way to take it. He believes that the best way is to take it in its natural food form: banana, super green drinks, peanuts – or, even better, in the form of Asphalia, his trade name for a food supplement made entirely from Festuca Arundinacea, a meadow grass with the highest known physiological level of plant melatonin in the world. St. John's Wort is another melatonin-rich botanical which aids sleep and is often used as an antidepressant.

However, Dr. Steve Martin, who writes a blog at www.grouppekurosawa.com, makes the point that melatonin is not very bioavailable when taken as a pill. He believes it should be dissolved in milk along with vitamin D3 and taken at night for best results. He suggests 5,000IU of vitamin D3 along with 6mg of melatonin as a breast cancer prevention regime but for those who already have breast cancer, especially estrogen dependent cancer, then much higher amounts of both should be taken.

Other sleep aids: tryptophan, lavender essential oil, St. John's Wort herb, Valerian herb, Miracle Mineral Supplement (sodium chlorite). Two writers to a health group I subscribe to raved about their sleep-promoting protocols. One claimed benefits from a combination of a calcium-magnesium tab with a few tabs of brewer's yeast. The other protocol was 600 mg of tyrosine, 200 mg of tryptophan with zinc and kelp (amounts unspecified). All of these, unlike sleeping pills, promote a deep, restful, natural sleep.

Methyl Jasmonate

This is a chemical found in jasmine oil – and also in grape skins. Indeed it is one of the major odour components of jasmine. Research published in Nature, the scientific journal, (published online 14 August 2003) determined that Methyl Jasmonate was a highly efficient attacker of leukemia, breast and melanoma cancer cells. This chemical needs to be dissolved in distilled water and inhaled through a steam vapour inhaler. [Warning: Do not swallow it, as this is dangerous.] It is recommended that this could be done once a week for a number of months. More frequent inhalations should be avoided at first because there is a danger of overpowering the body with toxic breakdown products. This chemical is considered to be highly effective. It is not yet available from the normal run of supplement suppliers. You will need to get it from a wholesale chemical supplier. It is widely used for food preservation purposes.

Quercetin

Quercetin is a flavonoid which is found in apples, onions, and black tea – and it may be the reason why eating two apples a day has been touted as a natural way to prevent cancer. Quercetin has demonstrated a wide range of health benefits in areas as diverse as asthma and heart disease. In relation to cancer it has also been suggested that it is a potent anti-cancer agent and should be seen, as one Mayo Clinic researcher commented, as a "chemopreventive and/or chemotherapeutic agent for prostate cancer." However, its benefits are not confined to prostate cancer.

For anti-cancer effects a daily intake of a minimum of 1,500 mgs (in divided doses) is necessary, though no negative side effects are associated with intake levels three or four times more than this.

Resveratrol

Resveratrol is an antioxidant found in grape skins – particularly the skin of the red grape - raspberries, mulberries and also peanuts. It functions as an antifungal agent. It has also been found to be a very powerful anti-cancer agent promoting cell death in cancer cells. Laboratory tests have clearly demonstrated that resveratrol may help prevent both heart disease and cancer. Resveratrol is widely available as a nutritional supplement but the question of how much is needed to prevent or attack cancer is not known. When buying resveratrol, check carefully the amount per serving and choose the highest dose you can find. Longevinex is the most highly rated brand at www.longevinex.com–note that this also contains quercetin. A good mix.

Urea/Urine Therapy

Urea is a substance found both in the blood and the urine. High urea levels are associated with good health. While urea itself can be bought cheaply, the best source is in the form of whole urine. That's right. You should drink your own pee! Urine is not dirty, as many people imagine. It is packed full of agents that help combat bacteria, viruses and fungi. Applied to burns and wounds, it speeds up healing. It's free and it's healthy.

We've probably all laughed when we read of an Indian Prime Minister or a Chinese businessman extolling the virtues of drinking their own urine. But there are good reasons to suppose that it is good medicine. Certainly, we shouldn't laugh. Morarji Desai, once Prime Minister of India, lived to the ripe old age of 99 all the while extolling the virtues of a daily glass of his own urine.. Over 200,000 Japanese gargle or drink urine everyday and this therapy is promoted by Japan's Miracle Cup of Life Institute. Urine drinking is also catching on in Europe, particularly in Germany. In India it goes by the name Shivambu therapy.

One proponent of urine drinking is Hong Kong businessman, Lee Hak-shing, who claims to have cured himself of a number of ailments including rheumatism, headaches, bladder stones and skin allergies. A Japanese doctor, Dr. Ryoichi Nakao explains this effect by noting that urine contains interferon, a natural immune substance found in the body.

Auto-Urine Therapy (i.e., drinking one's own urine) is a health modality that has a lot of research behind it, all indicating favourable results for a wide range of health issues. And interest in urine is not confined to China, Japan and India. In America, Dr. Burzynski, who developed the antineoplaston therapy (see p. 271), derives his peptides not from blood but from urine. He says: "Urine is not really waste material, but probably the most complex chemical mixture in the human body, and therefore it can deliver us virtually any information about the body. So from the cybernetic point of view it is just a treasure of information." Blood is not such a complex mixture as it contains fewer chemicals. So urine tests reveal more about the body than blood tests.

The use of chemicals derived from urine, is not new. During the Second World War, British cancer researchers tested a urine derived product that they called H11 and used it on 243 terminal cases. Forty percent of the cases apparently recovered. However, what exactly this product contained is not known, as the research did not receive any support, and the details that have survived are very sketchy.

One of the major constituents of urine is urea. The average adult human excretes about an ounce of urea a day. One Greek doctor, Evangelos Danapoulos, has treated cancers in and around the eye by injecting urea, with, he claims, almost complete success. Urea has no side effects. In animal studies, urea has been injected directly into tumours, particularly melanomas, with the result that they regressed or were eliminated.

While Danapoulos claims it is virtually non-toxic, American researchers suggest that the maximum concentration to be used should be 40 percent.

Urea can also be taken orally, and this has, it is claimed, a strong beneficial effect on the liver and through that to the lungs. One way to make it more effectively distributed to other tissues and organs is to mix the urea with creatine hydrate, a chemical that also has a history of being used to fight cancer, being the supposedly active ingredient of a now much maligned anti-cancer drug known as Krebiozen.

Directions for mixing: 28 grams of urea are dissolved in a quart of water. This quart is divided into seven portions. One portion is drunk every 90 minutes through the waking day. This can be taken with 3.5 grams of creatine hydrate, divided into seven doses of 0.5 grams and eaten with a peanut butter sandwich to mask its unpleasant taste.

Or you can, as many Indians, Chinese, Malays, Japanese, Germans and others do, and drink your own urine. Walter Last, an Australian natural therapist, says this: "I also know personally of several cases of cancer cures exclusively or mainly due to urine therapy; sometimes the addition of urine therapy to a natural cancer program appeared to be responsible for the successful outcome."

Walter Last recommends a urine fast as a great way to heal almost anything. During the fast, the only liquid taken in is one's own urine. All the urine excreted should be drunk. Non-chlorinated water should be added if necessary to bring the total liquid intake to 5 litres.

For those who object to drinking their own urine, there is a company in India that proclaims the virtues of cow's urine and sells a number of products derived from it - see www.cowurine.com

Methylglyoxal

Another constituent of urine is Methylglyoxal ($CH_3-CO-CH=O$ or $C_3H_4O_2$), an organic compound found in many food items. This substance has had an interesting history as a potential cancer treatment – but each time the research has threatened to show the effectiveness of this compound, it has been sidelined.

Dr. William Koch (1885-1967) was one of the first to investigate this area, and he was able to produce a 'reagent' - which he called glyoxilide - that was successful in curing a number of cancer cases—except for those that had previously been treated with radiation. The full story of his attempts to get his treatment accepted is provided at www.williamfkoch.com. His failure to do so made him so furious that he refused to provide any details of his later research. He kept his formula a secret. In short, he went into one of the great sulks of cancer history. Albert Szent-Gyorgy, of vitamin C fame, also appears to have isolated the substance and discovered its anti-cancer effects. However, once again nothing came of this research. More recently, it was investigated by a team of cancer researchers in Calcutta led by Prof. Manju Ray with seemingly extraordinary results.

In 2001, Indian biochemist, Prof. Manju Ray, trialled the drug on 19 patients with 'very advanced stages' of cancer. Of these, all of whom would normally have died within months, only three did in fact die; five had their cancers stabilised, and eleven were effectively cured. Further studies resulted in an overall cure rate of 70 percent in cancer patients who were diagnosed as terminally ill. It is very likely the cure rate would higher if taken at earlier stages.

Even better, methylglyoxal, unlike other chemotherapy drugs, is virtually non-toxic for normal cells. As a cancer drug, it works by starving cancer cells of ATP (adenosine-5-triphosphate). Cancer cells require large amounts of ATP to fuel their growth.

"We have what we think magic bullet against cancer," says Manju Ray. So far, it has been found to work against colon cancer, acute myeloid leukemia, non-Hodgkin's lymphoma, and cancers of ovary, breast, liver, lung, bone, gall bladder, pancreas and oral cavity.

The drug was developed by the Indian Association for the Cultivation of Science (IACS), a Calcutta (Kolkata)-based research organisation. They were funded by the Department of Science and Technology and the Council of Scientific and Industrial Research. For many people, this itself is a major problem, as IACS is not a medical institute, and professional egos have been severely ruffled. This is of course not the first time that the discoveries of biochemistry have been attacked by the medical profession. Vituperative attacks were published in the Indian press, and little has appeared in print since then.

However, Prof. Ray stands by her claims. According to her, chemists have known about the Methylglyoxal molecule for about four decades and its anti-cancer effects in animals have also been studied. "But surprisingly, no one bothered to initiate further research leading to human trials," she said. Her lack of surprise comes from the fact that Methylglyoxal is not patentable. No one is interested in doing research on possible anti-cancer cures that won't make big profits.

Researchers were initially concerned about the possible dangers of Methylglyoxal, but when it is taken in combination with protective agents such as ascorbic acid and vitamins, it had no major toxic effect.

The problem, however, is how to get hold of this drug and what dose levels to take it in. As yet it is not widely available. However, against this picture of a side-effect-free cure all, a less attractive image is appearing.. Dr Vincent Gammill who has used methylglyoxal has this to say: "I don't recommend methylglyoxal for general use. There is too much of a risk of formaldehyde in the manufacturing process, it is easily oxidised, and it can be toxic. It does have its uses and I occasionally use it - maybe 10% of the time. It is not curative, it is expensive." He also warns of a potential for harm to eyes, pancreas and heart. "The incautious use of methylglyoxal would certainly increase the risk of rapid ageing." Enquiries can be made to Dr. Vincent Gammill at the Center for the Study of Natural Oncology (www.natural-oncology.org).

However, a German doctor, Dr. Dieter Reinstorff, has gone back to the Koch research and has prepared a homoeopathic formula that appears to be methylglyoxal based and that he calls SSR Super Quinone. At US$300 a course of 14 vials, this is quite expensive. For more details contact Dr. Dieter Reinstorff, Bruno-Lauenroth Weg 31, 22417 Hamburg, Tel.: 040/ 5 20 25 02, Fax:. 040/5 20 33 10.

Two other Methylglyoxal products that are available and may be useful are Koch's TMT homoeopathic remedies and a methylglyoxal MG Concentrate, which can be bought from www.gethealthyagain.com.

Or it may be that simply drinking one's own urine will provide sufficient quantities to effect a cure.

Two recent books on the benefits of urine therapy for those who wish to follow up on this subject are *The Miracles of Urine Therapy* by Dr. Beatrice Bartnett and *Your Own Perfect Medcine* by Martha Christy.

HERBS & BOTANICALS

Introduction

That plants have medicinal properties is not a subject about which there is any disagreement. The medicinal qualities of many plants are well-known. Hippocrates used to prescribe willow bark for a number of ailments - later the active ingredient was isolated and marketed under the name of aspirin. However, with the rise of science, single-substance drugs became the order of the day, and herbalism to a large extent went underground. It became a woman's area of expertise. Old women's recipes were handed on from mother to daughter.

In eighteenth-century North America, a woman by the name of Mary Johnson came to the attention of the medical authorities. It appeared she was working as a healer and was claiming success in the treatment of cancer. The House of Burgesses of the General Assembly of Virginia appointed a committee to look into the case. Mary Johnson's medicine was a mixture of garden sorrel, celandine, persimmon bark and spring water. The committee took evidence over a period of six or seven years, 1748-54. They listened to the testimony of many witnesses who had taken the remedy and who had been cured. The result? Mrs. Johnson was awarded 100 pounds to aid her work.

This is a rare tale of diligent and generous assessment. The outcome of the investigation would be very different today - for the simple fact is that herbs represent a fundamental challenge to the ruling medical paradigm.

This ruling paradigm argues in a reductionist way as follows: If there is anecdotal evidence that a herb has a specific medicinal property, then it is possible that the plant in question contains a specific chemical that can be called the active ingredient. The plant is then studied to determine what its chemical contents are, and these are tested one at a time until the active ingredient is identified. Then this isolated substance can be tested scientifically to assess its range of action and ideal dosage. It will also, incidentally, be possible then to manufacture the chemical directly in large quantities without having to go through the arduous and expensive process of extraction from plant sources. This illustrates the fact that the ultimate aim of chemical research is to create, on an industrial scale, single chemicals in pure form.

By contrast, Mary Johnson proceeded by mixing a number of herbs together - in what proportions is not known. She was operating according to very different principles. While the scientist is looking for pure unadulterated chemicals, the herbalist is seeking to blend combinations of many different chemicals.

There is no evidence, in relation to the work of healing and curing, that single-substance chemicals are superior to herbs. In fact, there is good reason to believe they may be inferior. Why? For three reasons. First, there is the problem of resistance. Invading organisms such as bacteria and viruses are able to resist pure chemical forms quite effectively. That is why bacteria are increasingly becoming resistant to antibiotics, and it's also why the body is able to resist chemotherapeutic drugs - and if we remember, doctors are now mixing these chemotherapeutic agents. That is, they are starting to mimic the herbalist.

Secondly, the negative side effects of purified molecular forms - which are the basis of all drugs - are rarely present when herbs are used. This is not to say that herbs are always safe. They aren't. But such side effects as there are tend to be muffled by the presence of the surrounding chemicals in the composite herbal structures found in nature. The following two examples demonstrate this point clearly. Smokers take into their bodies a great deal of nicotine every time they light up a cigarette. Yet, if they were to place one drop of pure unadulterated nicotine on their hand, by mistake perhaps in a chemical laboratory, they would have only a few seconds to live. Pure nicotine is one of the most potent poisons known to man. Nicotine in herbal form takes 20 or 30 years to achieve the same result.

Marijuana, to take another example, besides being an illegal drug has clearly demonstrated medicinal qualities. It is known among other things to reduce the effects of nausea. Scientists extracted the active ingredient THC from the marijuana plant. Unfortunately, not only was this less effective than the original herbal marijuana but its side effects were such that half the patients testing it said they preferred to throw up than continue with it.

The third, and perhaps the most important, reason is the fact that the concept of the single active ingredient is almost certainly wrong. It is much more likely, in any herbal substance, that one dominant active chemical is boosted by the presence of others. When separated from these surrounding molecules, it may no longer have the expected effect. The process by which two chemicals contribute to a more pronounced effect is known as synergy. We can even imagine a situation where none of the ingredients of a particular plant have any effect on their own - but when present in an organic whole, they combine to have an effect.

This point about 'organic wholes' is central to the herbalist's credo. In the herb, compounds are interconnected in a coherent structure and have certain qualities both separately and together that are entirely absent from all artificially created chemicals. As we have seen, organic germanium is health giving, while the chemically identical inorganic germanium causes kidney damage.

Some people demonstrate the difference between organic and inorganic forms by using the metaphor of music. If you press the A key on a piano, you will create three kinds of vibrations. One is the vibration that creates the note A, but mixed with this will be overtones that make it clear to any listener that the note A comes from a piano and not a violin or clarinet. In addition, there will be other vibrations that stem from the interaction of the particular musician and the particular instrument. The writer Dean Black, in describing this fact, makes the point that if the music were a herb, then the active element would be the A note - it is the most noticeable property of the sound and it's the only one that can stand alone.

"[However,] None of the three vibrations define the note's entire function, and some of the note's most interesting properties - it's 'piano-ness' and its 'tone quality' - don't exist anywhere except as they somehow emerge like magic when the vibrations blend together." (Dean Black, 1988)

Herbalists believe that the chemical properties of a whole plant operate in much the same way and that we lose these properties when we break the plant up.

However, there is one criticism of herbs that does carry some force. The problem is consistency. Whereas drugs from one batch will always be identical to drugs from another, this is not true of herbs, which contain too many ingredients in variable concentrations. One ounce of ma-huang grown in America may be very different in quality from an ounce of the same herb grown in China. Because of this variability, they argue, it is impossible to adequately test the precise effects any herb might have. Because these objections don't apply to drugs, they say, drugs must be better. Some herbal companies have taken note of this criticism and it is now fairly common to find mention of standardisation (i.e., that what they offer in one batch will not differ from what they offer in another batch produced months later). Nevertheless, this standardisation will apply only to some of the herb's chemical contents, not all.

The conflict of herb versus drug is, in miniature, the war between factory and nature, between West and East, between 'scientific' techno-medicine and holistic healing. How is it that there is no official recognition that herbs play a part in the treatment of cancer? Because it is impossible to prove this effect under the conditions of proof currently laid down - and it would cost US$200-300 million to attempt to do so. No herbal or pharmaceutical company would consider spending that kind of money on an unpatentable medicine. The rules of the scientific game have been designed with this objective in mind.

Warnings *Herbs*

Safety: Once we accept that herbs are a soundly based approach to medical treatment, we need to know which herbs are recommended for the prevention or cure of cancer. Before that a warning is in order. Herbs cannot be presumed to be safe just because they are herbs. Some herbs are poisonous. Pregnant women, in particular, should not take a herb without consulting a professional herbalist. Anyone taking a herb should read up on it first. Not everything that is 'natural' is safe. Remember, Socrates committed suicide by drinking a herbal concoction of what was undoubtedly organic hemlock.

However, it should be remembered that many herbs and other treatments will cause a negative reaction of a temporary sort—known as a healing crisis. As the herbs work on the liver, toxins are released which cause all kinds of negative reaction from headaches to skin eruptions. These healing crises—known as Herxheimer reactions - are usually short-lived and should not last longer than a week or so. Persistence of ill effects after this duration should be taken as a strong indication that whatever herbal preparation you are taking should be discontinued. It is also a good idea to drink lots of water to flush these toxins out of the system as quickly as possible. If a healing crisis seems to be particularly uncomfortable then it makes sense to take a rest from the treatment or a number of days to avoid over-taxing the body.

Pregnancy: There are three conditions in which rapid cell division occurs in the body: cancer, the healing of wounds, and pregnancy. This means that any herb that is effective against cancer is totally contra-indicated for pregnant women.

The Herbs

Some herbalists claim that there are over 3,000 herbs displaying some form of anti-cancer effect. The following list therefore does not pretend to be exhaustive.

Aloe Vera

Aloe vera helps the body fight infections and malignant cells. It is also a detoxifier.

Aloe vera may or may not, on its own, be a cure for cancer, but it has demonstrated a strong ability to enhance the immune system's response to cancer, and it eliminates toxic wastes. This has a revitalising effect on the body. It is also important for immune system defence.

Most products make use of the inner gel, which is heat processed. This destroys many of the benefits. Look out for a whole-leaf, cold-pressed aloe vera product.

Historical side note: One aloe vera extract, called Albarin, given intravenously, was used in a number of Florida clinics in the early 2000s with, apparently, enormous success. There were claims of 90-percent-plus cure rates among terminal stage cancer inmates at a hospice. However, the FDA clamped down on it, and nothing has been heard since. Quack hype or FDA scandal? Who knows?

Bindweed

RECNAC ('cancer' spelled backwards) is a progressive cancer therapy centre in Wichita, Kansas, based at the Center for the Improvement of Human Functioning International, www.brightspot.org.

Bindweed came to the attention of their research team as an anecdotal report from a woman who claimed that an Indian shaman had given her a tincture of Bindweed (*Convolulus arvensis*) with instructions to use the substance daily. She did so and a few months later was found to be cancer free.

Their research showed that bindweed is a powerful anti-angiogenesis factor – about 100 times stronger than shark cartilage. They also found that this effect is even stronger when bindweed is used in conjunction with an immune stimulant combination, Muramyl Polysaccharide-Glycan Complex (MPGC).

Proposed doses are 6 capsules of bindweed (250 mg) plus 6 capsules of MPGC (250mg) a day. These products can be purchased from Aidan, Inc. by telephone at (800) 529-0269. Bindweed is sold as C-Statin and MPGC is sold as ImmKine. Other sources are available on the internet.

Bloodroot

Bloodroot is a herb that has demonstrated very powerful anti-cancer properties. Bloodroot, (*Sanguinaria Canadensis*), is native to the woods of north-central United States and Canada. Its tap root exudes a blood-coloured juice from which its name derives. It was one of the most popular herbal remedies among Plains Indians, who used it internally for sore throats and respiritory ailments and externally for growths on the surface of the body. It is this last property that makes it interesting for people with cancer - especially for those with melanoma or other surface tumours. Quite simply, bloodroot dissolves any form of malignant growth while leaving healthy tissue alone.

There is a long history of bloodroot being used as a herbal salve from the 1750's on promoted by a succession of converts—some of whom were healers while others were bona fide doctors.

Dr. Andrew Weil, author of *Spontaneous Healing*, used some on his dog, who was suffering from a large surface tumour. For three days he smeared a small coat of paste on the tumour. He stopped on the fourth day because he was alarmed to see blood. It seemed that the tumour was separating itself from the flesh around it. He disinfected the wound and kept an eye on developments. Two days later the entire tumour fell off, and the raw flesh around it quickly healed up. "The end result was a perfectly circular, slightly depressed area of skin, with no trace of tumour. The bloodroot had removed it more neatly than one could have done with a scalpel...the dog had shown no signs of discomfort." (Weil, *Spontaneous Healing*, 1995)

An extraordinary set of photographs showing this effect can be seen at www.silvermedicine.org/clay-cansema-silver1.html and also at www.cancerx.org.

Here then is a herb that directly attacks cancers while leaving normal healthy tissue unharmed. It forms a scab over the cancer and expels it from the body. No secondary infections follow. One of America's leading experts on salves used against cancer, Ingrid Naiman, has written: "Bloodroot has been researched and determined to be a potent anticancer agent. Besides the laboratory tests, tens of thousands of people have been treated by lay practitioners as well as medical doctors for at least the last 150 years. Of these, roughly 80 percent experienced remission of malignancy and longer life expectancies than people with similar conditions who chose different treatments."

Bloodroot is easily and quickly absorbed into the body so it is possible that the bloodroot will seek out tumours and eliminate them even though they are not on the surface.

TumorX Salve and Cansema are both products that contain bloodroot. However, the Cansema brand products are no longer available. The manufacturer, Alpha Omega Labs, was put out of business by the FDA, and the proprietor, Greg Caton, imprisoned for supposedly running a 'cancer cure scam'. However, information about Tumor X salve is available at www.cancerX.org. The product can be ordered by phone at (USA) 229-365-7222. They are also available at www.simpledefeat.com. A bloodroot tincture for internal use is available from www.cancersalves.com. Another black salve is sold at www.austinpages.com/yp/balm under the name Balm of Gilead. See also: http://plantcures.com/herbsforcancer.html

As these sources may or may not still be operating by the time you read this, I am including the following instructions for making one's own bloodroot paste.

1/2 cup powdered Blood Root (Sanguinaria Canadensis)
1/2 cup Zinc Chloride, crystals or liquid
1/2 cup common white flour
1 1/2 cup warm water
100ml Chaparral extract or 100gm of powdered Chaparral (Larrea mexicana)

Pre-mix all but the water, thoroughly, before adding to the water. Use a stainless steel double boiler. Put in water, and then stir in the other ingredients. Stir in well using a wooden spoon. Cook for thirty minutes over boiling water, stirring constantly.

Application is much the same as Cansema. Apply a thin layer (2-3mm) of the paste over the affected area and cover for 24 hours. Then remove the covering but do not disturb the lesion at all, do not attempt to pull the cancer out at any time, it should fall out in 10 days or so. Some people with sensitive skin put vaseline around the cancer so that the paste does not irritate the skin.

Boswellia — Indian Frankincense

Boswellia has an anti-angiogenetic effect on cancer, interfering with the tumour's development of a blood supply system. However, it has another effect whose value appears to be particularly directed to men of advancing years who are more and more likely to get prostate cancer. One way to protect against prostate cancer is to inhibit an enzyme known as 5-LOX, which inflames the prostate and which is promoted by a diet that is rich in meat. An extract of Boswellia, known as AKBA, has been shown to be specifically useful in the suppression of 5-LOX. It can be obtained in a product called 5-LOXIN available from www.lef.org

Cannabis

The anti-nausea impact of cannabis and the family of chemicals it contains – the cannabinoids – have already been mentioned. However, the smoking of cannabis has also been found to have direct anti-cancer effects – by inducing apoptosis and by preventing the development of a blood supply to tumours. Cannabinoids have also been shown to have the impact of reducing resistance to chemotherapy drugs, so helping make chemotherapy drugs more effective.

The benefits have been shown in the case of a wide range of cancers – including breast, lung, etc.– but the main benefits might be most readily seen in the case of glioma and other brain cancers for which there are few other options. Cannabinoids are toxic to glioma cells while, at the same time, helping to protect normal brain cells, known as astrocytes, from oxidative stress.

The medicinal use of cannabis is legal in some countries and states, but not all.

Cat's Claw (Uncaria tomentosa) and Samento

Studies have shown that Cat's Claw stimulates the immune system, prevents mutations, stops the spread of cancer cells, inhibits the development of leukemia cells, kills viruses, reduces inflammation and helps cell healing. It was also used as a contraceptive by the local people whose original use led to its discovery. Cancer patients taking it have found that it is helpful in reducing the side effects of chemotherapy and enhancing vitality.

This Peruvian herb is made from the bark of a South American plant. The effective part of the plant is the inner bark. Apparently some Cat's Claw products also contain outer bark, which is ineffective. The herb has a high tannin content that may cause gastric, liver or kidney problems. When taking, avoid milk or other dairy products. *≡ watch*

3-6 grams per day (9 x 350mg capsules in 3 doses, 30-60 min. after a meal).

A very powerful form of Cat's Claw is called Samento; Samento extracts are also available on the internet.

Chaparral

Chaparral is a desert plant covering large areas of southern California and Arizona. It has small brittle leaves and these have been used by the local Indian people to make a health tonic tea. It has an extremely unpleasant and pungent smell and bitter taste.

One dramatic case of a cancer cure using chaparral alone occurred in 1967-8. The patient was a man by the name of Ernest Farr, an 87-year-old man who had had four operations on a malignant melanoma and had been told there was no point to further operations. He drank chaparral tea over a period of four months. The cancer shrank almost entirely away and was still very small nine months later. Clearly something in the chaparral had worked. Scientists investigated and found the chemical substance NDGA. This was already a well-known chemical as it was used to preserve butter in the tropics. It is a very powerful anti-oxidant. It is not known whether it works for all cancers - one test found little activity against breast cancer, while another found it to be effective against gastrointestinal cancer.

However, there is a caution, according to one anecdote, a woman taking chaparral in large quantities suffered severe liver damage. Ernest Farr took 7-8 grams of fresh chaparral leaves and steeped them in a quart of hot water. He drank 2-3 cups a day. Farr lived to the age of 96 when he died of the same melanoma. It appears that his doctor had refused to allow him to continue taking chaparral tea. As with other herbal cancer cures, chaparral needs to be continued after the tumour appears to have disappeared.

Curcumin *yes!*

Curcumin is an extract from the herb turmeric, which is getting very serious attention from cancer researchers. Studies show that curcumin can block cancer-causing enzymes and interfere with the development of new blood supplies; in other words, it is anti-angiogenic. It is also an anti-inflamatory and helps maintain the health of the liver.

Evidence that it is highly beneficial comes from comparing cancer rates in Sri Lanka where the cancer mortality rate per 100,000 is 26.1 for females and 29.3 for males. This compares with US rates or 138.6 for women and 206.0 for men per 100,000. This difference is highly unlikely to be due to genetic or hereditary factors, for two reasons: 1) the population of Sri Lanka is ethnically very varied and 2) the cancer rates of Sri Lankan immigrants to North America and Europe rise considerably within just a generation or two. In Sri Lanka, a typical diet includes large amounts of turmeric. However, for the cancer patient, pure curcumin is required and a dose of 4-5 grams a day is recommended. However, curcumin capsules are useless, as the curcumin needs to be dissolved in fat before being ingested. The best way to take it is to buy curcumin powder, and dissolve it in warm coconut milk or cream and drink it. This has the effect of targeting the dissolved curcumin at the lymphatic system which is where it is needed.

Pregnant women should note this: because it acts as an anti-angiogenesis factor it must be avoided during pregnancy!!

Recent research at the M.D. Anderson Cancer Center in Texas confirms that curcumin is a powerful anti-cancer agent which encourages normal cell death (apoptosis). Curcumin works synergistically with vitamin D (or natural sunlight).

nowadays - 2018 supplement is combined with peperine a black pepper exact supposedly for better absoption

Feverfew

Scientists have found that parthenolide, an extract of the feverfew plant (Tanacetum parthenium), is a highly effective agent against malignant stem cells. The first laboratory investigation found that it was potentially curative in cases of myeloid leukaemia - without harming normal, healthy blood cells. Because the focus of feverfew's activity is against stem cells, such a result indicates that feverfew–also known as batchelor's button–is likely to have an impact on all cancers. Until now, feverfew has been mainly associated with reducing fevers and treating migraines.

More recently, it has been suggested that pathenolide should be taken in combination with a prescription drug Sulindac to inhibit expression of Nuclear factor–kappaB (Nf-κB), a transcription factor essential for cell division. It is activated in response to a number of factors that impose stress on the body: inflammation, viruses, etc.–and, importantly for us, by cancers and carcinogens. Interestingly radiation and chemotherapy also provoke activation of Nf-κB.

One approach to attacking cancer is to prevent cancer cells from dividing – and inhibiting expression of Nf-κB is one way to do this. A simple way of achieving this, according to Stephen Martin, PhD is to combine the feverfew extract parthenolide and the prescription drug, Sulindac – a non-steroidal anti-inflammatory drug also known as Clinoril. Martin recommends mixing the contents of 10 capsules of Nature's Way feverfew herb (which is standardised at 0.7 percent pathenolide) with some form of fat– say coconut milk. Do this twice a day. In addition take a 200mg tab of Sulindac three times a day. This combination will, he claims, have a strong inhibitory effect on cancer cell division. To further enhance the anti-cancer effect, Stephen Martin recommends taking Vitamin E succinate.

next page

Interestingly, the combination of curcumin (4-8 grams/d) and feverfew (4grams/d) both dissolved in some form of cream of coconut milk is also considered to be effective. One user of this regime has dubbed the combination "Curfew" – it's lights out for cancer.

Incidentally, high intracellular levels of vitamin C also appear to inactivate Nf-κB – yet another way in which vitamin C in very high doses appears to work against cancer.

Graviola *also mentioned in Bill Henderson's Book*
especially good for chemo resistant cancer!

Graviola is a South American plant with a wide range of medicinal uses. It has recently come to the fore as a very potent anti-cancer herb. In a 1976 plant screening program by the National Cancer Institute, the leaves and stem of Graviola showed active cytotoxicity against cancer cells, and researchers have been following up on this research ever since. We can assume that their long interest in this plant is itself an implicit validation. But since they are not interested in validating herbs, but rather in the extraction of pure chemicals that can be patented, much of the research on Graviola focuses on a set of phytochemicals called annonaceous acetogenins, which have been shown to have potent antitumour (and pesticidal) properties. Graviola produces these natural compounds in leaf, bark and twig tissues. Suggested dose: 4 capsules (600mg/cap) a day.

N-Tense is a branded formulation that has received a lot of attention in alternative cancer circles. It combines graviola with 7 other herbs, including cat's claw. The ingredients are graviola (50 percent), guacatonga, mullaca, vassourinha, espinheira santa, mutamba, bitter melon, and cat's claw. There are other liquid extracts of graviola on the market. Pawpaw, a cousin of graviola, is considered to be even stronger.

Green Tea

A number of studies have shown that green tea helps protect against a variety of cancers, such as lung, prostate, and breast, but the mechanisms for these effects are not known. It is now suspected that EGCG (epigallocatechin gallate), a powerful antioxidant, may be the reason for its effectiveness. EGCG binds to a protein found on tumour cells and dramatically slows their growth. According to researchers, the concentration of the antioxidant having an anticancer effect was equivalent to that found in the body after drinking only two to three cups of green tea. This is a key component of Matthias Rath's anti-cancer protocol (see p. 281). pg 282

Papaya and Pawpaw

The fruit that Americans know as the pawpaw (*Asiminia triloba*) is not the same fruit as the papaya (*Carica papaya*) – which confusingly is also known in Australia as pawpaw. However, both have an important part to play as anti-cancer therapies.

The Papaya

The papaya is an excellent fruit. It contains more vitamin A than carrots and more vitamin C than oranges. It is particularly noted as the source of the enzyme papain (but only in the unripe fruit and the seeds of the ripe fruit)—which has powerful anti-cancer properties in its own right. Barbara Simonson, author of *Papaya: Healing with the Wonderfruit*, recommends eating and juicing the skin as well. She claims it can cure cancer. "I have a friend, Halima Neumann, who was healed from stomach cancer by drinking the juice of papayas for six months, half a liter each day, and after that eating half-ripe papayas every day."

But this does not exhaust the potential of the papaya. Harald Tietze, an Australian who has actively promoted the health benefits of the papaya, reports that the leaves of the papaya plant have cured a number of cases of cancer.

He recommends that a handful of leaves can be put in a saucepan with boiling water and left to simmer for an hour. The resulting 'tea' can be diluted and drunk throughout the day. One man who read Tietze's advice, mentioned it to a friend: 'I told him to 'stuff a handful of pawpaw leaves into a saucepan and fill with water; boil, simmer for one hour and drink it till it comes out of your ears'. The friend followed this advice and, according to the anecdotal report, five weeks later he 'had no trace of cancer whatsoever'.

Papaya leaves and other products can be obtained from The Kombucha House, which also sells other papaya concentrate products. For further information go to www.kombucha-house.com

The Pawpaw

Let us now turn to the North American pawpaw, the fruit of which looks somewhat like a thick, short banana. This herb too is considered to have powerful biologically active effects against cancer – but in this case it is not the leaves but the bark and twigs. When buying 'pawpaw extract' from a North American herb supplier, it is this product that you will be getting.

Pawpaw extract contains a group of chemicals called acetogenins – which interfere with the production of ATP, a chemical that is necessary for cellular energy. The impact on ATP is more critical for cancer cells than normal cells and results in the reduced growth of blood vessels that nourish cancer cells. Very importantly, it is one of the few herbs that has shown itself to be effective in inhibiting the growth of MDR (multiple drug resistant) cells. *Chemo resistant cancer—!!*

Pawpaw is a cousin of the graviola, guanabana, and soursop trees. However, the acetogenins extracted from pawpaw are reportedly even more active against cancer than those extracted from these other sources.

Pawpaw is also effective against viruses and reduces the side effects of chemo. A number of people have found it useful to combine pawpaw with CanCell (see p. 237). One reported the benefits in this way: "It [pawpaw] stopped pain and bleeding and when later I added Protocel I saw a tremendous lysing. The pawpaw had broken down a huge amount of waste and the Protocel went in and flushed it all out."

↓ toxins coming out of your body
sweating, runny nose, diahrea

dosage next page →

Jerry McLaughlin, professor of pharmacognosy at Purdue University, claims that pawpaw extract, which contains over 40 cancer-fighting compounds, is many times more potent than the leading chemotherapy drug Adriamycin, and yet, at the same time, totally without toxic side effects to normal healthy tissue.

Four capsules of standardized extract of Pawpaw are taken per day, until cancer goes into remission. While taking pawpaw, it is important to avoid at the same time taking megadoses of Vitamins A, C and E; alpha lipoic acid; CoQ10; SOD; and 7-Keto, as these inhibit the effectiveness of the Pawpaw. It is helpful, however, to supplement with concentrated doses of protease (a protein digesting enzyme) and other natural immune enhancing supports such as noni juice, beta glucans, arabinogalactan, colostrum, reishi and maitake mushrooms, and cordyceps.

Warning: some people taking pawpaw have reported that it either caused or exacerbated severe depression. *ooof*

Pau D'Arco — *may be worth looking into* *this is mentioned on Chris work's website .chrisbeatcancer.com*

In 1967, the Brazilian newspaper O'Cruzeiro reported the story of a cancer-stricken girl from Rio who continually prayed for a cure. In a dream or vision, she saw a monk who told her that she would recover if she made a tea brewed with the bark of the pau d'arco tree. The monk returned in a second vision and told her which specific pau d'arco trees she was to use. Whether these visions were true - perhaps a response to a subconscious recognition of the medicinal powers of this tree – or whether they were simply a necessary guise in which to cloak a desire persuasively, the girl was given the tea she required and she recovered.

She was not alone. Many others have claimed their cancers have gone into long-term remission after drinking pau d'arco tea. Anecdotal evidence and folk practice throughout South America appears to justify the claims made for this tree bark. Besides cancer, it is supposedly effective against diabetes, ulcers and rheumatism to name a few - and applied to the skin is good for burns. The inner bark of the tree contains many chemicals that are known to have anti-tumour effects: tannins, quinones and triterpines and others. There are many different varieties of the pau d'arco tree - and each variety seems to have its own range of medicinal characteristics. Its anticancer effects have been demonstrated in a number of animal studies. Pau d'arco - also known as lapacho and taheebo - is available as a bark, in powdered form, and as an alcoholic extract.

Unfortunately, there have been suggestions that a lot of the pau d'arco on the market is of poor quality. A number of studies on the alcoholic extracts commercially available in Europe and North America consider them to be medically useless as they do not appear to contain the active ingredient, lapachol. Others argue that looking for a single active ingredient is wrong: pau d'arco contains at least 12 quinones of which lapachol is only one.

To make a tea add six tablespoons of the bark to four cups of boiling water. The water is kept boiling until it reduces to three cups. This takes about five minutes. The tea is then cooled and then filtered. Three to eight cups a day should be taken, each cup sipped slowly but steadily. The tea not being drunk should be kept refrigerated. Toxicity is low. The symptom to expect from over consumption is a slight skin rash.

The following websites have been suggested as good resources and sources of good quality herb: www.pau-d-arco.com; www.princetea.com; www.herb-care.com

Pycnogenol

Pycnogenol is derived from the bark of the French maritime pine tree (*Pinus maritima*), and is a complex of more than 40 antioxidant compounds. It has been called the most powerful antioxidant discovered by science. However, it is not just an antioxidant but has shown direct and powerful anti-cancer activity. In one anecdotal report by Dr. Lamar Rosquist, a Canadian doctor who is actively promoting pycnogenol, a woman with terminal breast and lung cancer started taking pycnogenol in large quantities (200 mgs x 3 times a day) along with colloidal silver and aloe vera. One month later she was cancer free. It is being taken very seriously and a number of clinical trials are in progress to evaluate its effectiveness.

Salvestrols

These are phytonutrients found in fruits and vegetables—and more so in organic produce – which have only recently been isolated and studied. The results are exciting for people with cancer. The way it works is this: cancer cells contain an enzyme protein called CYP1B1. If we can find a way of triggering this protein it will release chemicals within the cell that will quickly kill it. And this is what salvestrols do. They activate this enzyme. Professor Burke, the co-discoverer of these phytonutrients, likens this protein to a Trojan horse. Unfortunately, the food content of salvestrols is generally too low to provide enough. A concentrated salvestrol extract, called Salvestrol, has been developed. It is cheap and widely available on the internet. It is so cheap that it has been proposed that people of all ages should take it simply as a cancer preventative.

Saw Palmetto

This is the herb for anyone with prostate problems. It is usually considered useful for mild to moderate prostate enlargement. However, in-vitro studies have shown it to have a general anti- cancer effect with prostate cancer cells responding most readily. When purchasing, make sure the strength is 85-95 percent fatty acids and sterols. Take 160 mgs twice daily.

A Note on Prostate Health

In addition to saw palmetto, a number of other herbs are useful in maintaining a healthy prostate gland: pygeum, stinging nettle, isoflavones (genistein and daidzein), rye pollen, phytosterols (e.g., sitosterol), and lycopene. In one reported case, a 62-year-old man with advanced prostate cancer experienced regression of his tumor after taking 10 mg of lycopene per day and 300 mg of saw palmetto three times per day. Researchers attributed this effect more to the lycopene than the saw palmetto.

People with prostate cancer, in addition to the saw palmetto, should take zinc (50-60 mgs daily), because their prostate fluids are low in this mineral. Magnesium has also been shown to be beneficial for the prostate.

Wormwood (Artemisinin)

Wormwood has long been used by herbalists as a bitter herb to improve digestion, to fight worm infestations (as its name suggests) and other parasites and as a useful remedy for liver problems. An extract from wormwood, artemisinin, which was known to the ancient Chinese as a malaria cure, has recently re-emerged as an anti-cancer treatment on its own.

Artemisinin works because it interacts biochemically with iron, a mineral which is needed by cancer cells as it is necessary for cell division, and for that reason usually advised against as a supplement. The surface of a cancer cell has many more iron-attracting receptors than the surface of a normal, healthy cell. When artemisinin comes in contact with the iron a reaction takes place, releasing a burst of free radicals that kills the cell. Although it is normally not advisable to take iron supplements in the case of cancer, when taking artemisinin, the reverse is true, as we wish to flood the cancer cells with iron.

In one study, researchers fed rats a substance known to induce multiple breast tumors. All the rats were then fed a normal diet but half were given a 0.02 percent dose of artemisinin. Over 40 weeks investigators monitored tumor formation in the rats. Ninety-six percent of the rats that did not get artemisinin developed tumors. In those that did receive the substance, only 57 percent developed tumors. In addition, artemisinin-fed rats had smaller and fewer tumors than non-atemisinin-fed rats.

Artemisinin has a good safety record because it has been used extensively against malaria. The problem is that wormwood herb has variable levels of artemisinin—and indeed a particular batch may not have any at all. It is therefore better to take a standardised extract. 1,000-2,000 mg per day per 100 pounds/45 kilos of body weight, divided into 4 doses, is considered appropriate in the case of cancer, but it can be toxic at very high doses, so any negative side effects should indicate that a reduction in dose levels is desired.

In TCM (Traditional Chinese Medicine), wormwood is considered to be a "cooling" herb. If you find yourself tingling (too cool), you might want to reduce the dose. Artemisinin should be taken with food. Using an essential fatty acid (flax oil, cod liver oil, lecithin, or wheat germ oil) will help absorption. Artemisinin is not considered a stand-alone cancer cure, but part of an overall, aggressive, anti-cancer program—including high doses of pancreatic enzymes (on an empty stomach), CoQ10 and a detox program— a source can be found at: www.altcancer.com/artemis.htm

.

Herbal Formulas and Combination Therapies

Alsihum (Alzium)

Alsihum - also called Alzium – was developed by a biblical scholar, Chaim Kass, based on 500-year-old Hebrew and Arabic texts that contained herbal recipes for cures for colds, flus and other ailments. These were tested and found to be effective. They were subsequently tested on cancer patients with some success – In the first study, 2 out of 30 terminal patients had long-term remission. Alsihum is a 100 percent natural herbal compound developed by researchers at CED Tech Health in Jerusalem, Israel. The formula consists of 9 herbs in a base of water and alcohol. The formula includes cone flower, myrrh, skullcap, burdock, saffron and cayenne. For further information and to order, contact info@cedtechhealth.com

Anvirzel

The oleander is an extremely poisonous plant which nevertheless has been widely used in several folk medicines. Its use against cancer has been reported in the Caribbean, North Africa and India. A Turkish doctor, Dr. Huseyin Ozel, developed a herbal cure involving oleander extracts which he trademarked under the name Anvirzel. The roots, leaves and flowers are treated in such a way that the resulting liquid is entirely non-toxic. The product received a US patent in 1992 and a company called Ozelle Pharmaceuticals started work to try and get approval for the drug. It has since been trialled in Ireland with good results. No side effects were reported and it had clear anti-cancer effects along with pain-relief. According to a report on the trial quoted by Moss, 1998: all 46 patients "have shown improvements that have surpassed or defied expectations of conventional treatments."

Other reports indicate that this is a very highly effective anti-cancer treatment for all cancers, and, unlike the oleander plant, completely non-toxic. Anvirzel is administered either orally or by daily injection. It appears to be only available at present from Salud Integral Clinic in Honduras www.saludintegral.hn. For another oleander-based herbal combination see OPC (Page 164).

Carctol

Carctol is a combination of Indian herbs that was formulated by an Ayruvedic doctor, Dr. Nandlal Tiwari of Jaipur. It is available on the internet from www.anticancerherb.com. www.carctolhome.com is another useful website . The product is reported to be completely non-toxic and has been tested in both India (Institute of Medical Sciences) and London. The British newspaper, *The Daily Telegraph*, recently covered the story of Gwen Garner, a woman who had both a primary bladder cancer and a secondary pancreatic cancer. Being told there was nothing more the doctors could do, she went on a course of Carctol. Within 6 months the pancreatic cancer growth had stopped; the original bladder cancer disappeared.

Carctol is supposedly excellent when used during radiotherapy and chemotherapy, preventing patients from becoming neutropenic (i.e., there is no compromise of white cells).

Carctol is a combination of the following herbs:

Blepharis Edulis	200 mg
Piper Cubeba Linn	20 mg
Smilax China Linn	80 mg
Ammani Vesicatoria	20 mg
Hemidesmus Indicus	20 mg
Lepidium Sativum Linn	20 mg
Rheumemodi Wall	20 mg
Tribulus Terrestris	20 mg

Anyone taking Carctol is recommended to maintain a vegetarian diet. At a minimum, patients are advised not to eat "acid foods" like unripe fruits, tomatoes, vinegar or oranges. Carctol works best with a good digestive system.

Normally one capsule is taken four times per day, but a maximum of eight is not unusual. Pre-boiled and cooled water is recommended, not tap water.

The effect is supposed to be slow and steady and normally a six-month period is recommended.

Curaderm (BEC5)

This is a cream which has demonstrated strong healing activity against a number of skin cancers. It was developed by Dr. Bill Cham, an Australian biochemist, and is based on a plant– *Solanum sodamaeum* – which is known in Australia as Devil's apple or Kangaroo apple. It is not a burning salve like bloodroot, but its effectiveness has been demonstrated in a number of studies at reputable London hospitals. The cream is also promoted as beneficial for psoriasis and eczema.

BEC5 can eradicate non-melanoma skin cancers, specifically basal cell carcinoma (BCC) and squamous cell carcinoma (SCC). It is also effective against benign tumours and other skin irregularities, including keratoses, sun spots and age spots.

One important point to note is that it is vital to use the cream before any surgery has taken place. This is because cancerous tissues on the skin are connected to cancerous tissues below the surface. The cream can then eliminate all these cancerous cells one after the other. Surgery may eliminate surface cells without impacting on the cells below the surface. The cream then cannot get access to the deeper lying cells.

It is available from www.curaderm.net and a number of other websites.

Skin Cancer Warning: If you have skin cancer, be very careful what the oncologist rec
One skin cancer medication, Aldara, which contains the chemical imiquimod (IQ), has be
since 1986 to be itself a cause of cancer. "It is so dangerous that the American Cancei
The National Cancer Institute, and others have determined it is a carcinogen, and have μaced it
on their lists of most hazardous chemicals. IQ has even been listed as a laboratory chemical hazard
by the US Occupational Safety Health Agency. Yet, doctors worldwide are prescribing it, willy-nilly,
to "cure" skin cancers" (Elaine Hollingsworth, an Australian skin cancer patient who nearly died
using it, writing in *The Townsend Newsletter*, May 2006) See also her own website:
www.doctorsaredangerous.com

Other creams recommended for skin cancer: PDQ Cream has been recommended by a
person with skin cancer as being beneficial. Look at www.behealed.biz for further details.
Another useful product is Raspex SPF-30 skin gel, which is made from meeker raspberries and
has a strong ellagic acid content. www.smdi.org/products.htm

Danggui Longhui Wan

This is a mixture of Chinese herbs that is used in Chinese medicine, particularly against leukaemia.
The active herb was found to be indigo, which contains indirubin, purified extracts of which have
been shown to be potent inhibitors of cell proliferation (i.e., they help stop the growth of cancer
tumours). Indirubin is a component of a number of herbs, and extracts of these herbs may be found
through a normal internet search. Interestingly, one easily available source of indirubin is available at
no cost whatsoever – in one's own urine.

Eli Jones Syrup

Dr. Eli Jones (1850-1933) was one of the earliest doctors to consider that cancer could be treated by
medical means (i.e., with medicines) rather than by surgery or radiation. His comment: "Four-fifths
of the cancers I have seen in the past forty years had been operated on and the cancer returned
worse than before. Other cases have tried the X-ray, Radium, Escharotics and Hypodermic
treatments, etc., etc., before I saw them, with the same results" (quoted in Moss, 1998).

Dr. Jones formulated a herbal syrup which he called Compound Syrup Scrophularia. It
contains poke root, figwort, may apple and a number of other herbs. This can be obtained from
Dr. Ingrid Naiman, www.cancersalves.com.

Essiac *# Courtney From Chris Wark ~~~website~~
chrisbeatcancer.com drank this along with protocol
Bill Henderson

The official story of Essiac starts in 1922, when a young nurse by the name of Rene Caisse was given
the names of a number of herbs by an old woman who had cured herself of breast cancer by
drinking a tea containing these herbs. This old woman had got the remedy from a native Ojibwa

next pg →

Indian. Some time later, her aunt was diagnosed with terminal stomach cancer and given six months to live. Caisse remembered the herbs and, with the doctor's consent, gave them to her aunt , who went on to live another 21 years. She was given more cases and these also healed. The doctors were so impressed they petitioned the Canadian government in 1926 to give Rene Caisse facilities for research. The result? They tried to arrest her for treating cancer without a medical licence. Fortunately for her she had the support of nine very eminent doctors so they desisted.

She gave the Essiac combination (named by reversing her own name) not only in the form of tea but also - in a modified form - by injection in the site of the cancer. She found this to be quicker and more effective.

In 1938 a Commission of Enquiry conducted an investigation. Unlike Mary Johnson, Rene Caisse did not receive a generous appraisal. It concluded that all of the patients who came to testify on her behalf, none had ever had cancer - despite their X-rays and medical documentation. Despite harassment, she continued to give patients her herbal treatment - without making any charge. In one case she records that her treatment for cancer had the interesting side effect of also curing the patient's diabetes.

There are currently a number of variations of the same basic Essiac formula on the market - Essiac, Tea of Life and Flor-Essence and possibly others - but they all share the same official ingredients, which are Burdock Root, Turkish Rhubarb, Slippery Elm and Sheep Sorrel. Additional ingredients found in commercial Essiac teas are: red clover blossom, kelp, blessed thistle and watercress. The tea can be drunk both as a treatment for cancer or as a preventative health tonic.

Rene Caisse died in 1978 at the age of 91. In 1983, Bruce Hendrick, Chief of the Division of Neurosurgery at the Hospital for Sick Children in Toronto, wrote to the Canadian Minister for Health and Welfare asking her to authorize clinical trials on the effectiveness of Essiac tea. In his letter he said: "I am most impressed with the effectiveness of the treatment and its lack of side effects." Further support for its effectiveness comes from Dr. Charles Brusch, personal physician to President John F. Kennedy, who also claims to have been cured of his cancer using Essiac.

The Canadian Cancer Society nevertheless maintains a cool distance. It considers Essiac to be a questionable or unproven method of cancer treatment. Canadian health laws prohibit it from being marketed as an anti-cancer treatment but they accept that it is not harmful and it is available on prescription - but the prescribing doctor must first get authorization from the Deputy Director of the Health Protection branch. They warn that Essiac may cause some nausea or diarrhoea. They also warn that it is not established that the commercial brands named above are in fact made with the true Essiac recipe. Nevertheless, the manufacturers of Flor-Essence and Tea of Life are able to produce testimonial letters from people who claim to have been cured by the herbal tea. One of the main constituents - Burdock root - has demonstrated anti-tumour activity on its own but, as with all herbal formulas, it is the synergistic effects that are important and which remain largely unexplored.

See what brand Courtney used

Green Sap

This is a secret herbal formulation created by a Uruguayan oncologist that contains a high triterpine content and which claims to have strong anti-cancer activity. It is unsubstantiated by any large scale studies, but they offer a number of case histories of people who have been cured. For further information go to www.gotitas.com. It is non-toxic and it is claimed to be supportive for people undergoing chemotherapy and radiation.

It is certainly true that triterpines, a family of essential oils found in many plants, seem to be one of the most potent ingredients in many herbs and plant extracts associated with long life. And, of course, long life can be seen simply as a life not shortened by cancer. The following are known to contain significant quantities of triterpines: Siberian Ginseng; Licorice root; Gingko leaves; Gotu Kola; and, interestingly, soybeans. These herbs have shown significant anti-tumour activity in studies in the US and Finland. Gingko has also been shown in animal studies to make aggressive cancers significantly less aggressive.

In addition, olives contain oleanolic acid, a triterpine, which is being examined with great interest by the Japanese as a chemopreventive of cancer.

HANSI

HANSI is an acronym for Homeopathic Natural Activator of the Immune System (It works better in Spanish!). Argentinian botanist, Juan Hirschmann, using his knowledge of plants created a number of homoeopathic-concentration cures for a number of diseases. He called his product HANSI. It contains homoeopathic concentrations of ten or so plants including cactus, aloe, arnica and licopodium, along with Lachesis derived from the venom of the bushmaster snake. From his Buenos Aires clinic, he has treated tens of thousands of cancer patients – representing every type of cancer. He claims to have achieved a great deal of success, supported by reviews and testimonials. He markets his products from the Bahamas. There are injectable and oral versions (the injectable versions are apparently more effective). In one study involving 87 terminal-stage pancreatic cancers, 60 were still alive after one year even though the standard prognosis was for death to occur with 3-6 months. It is also claimed that HANSI allows patients to tolerate radiation much better. Promotional material for HANSI quotes a medical researcher, Darryl M. See, M.D. as saying: "Over the past two years I have been involved in screening various herbs and homeopathic preparations for in vitro immune-stimulating effects. Among the 200 or so that I have tested, HANSI proved to be among the most effective in increasing natural killer cell function."

HANSI sells for US$1,300 for a 90 day supply. Critics of HANSI question this cost and ask what raw materials they are using – in undetectable homoeopathic quantities – that could possibly justify that price. For more information contact www.angelfire.com/in3/hansi or email: hansiargentina@hotmail.com

Hoxsey Formula

In 1840, a man by the name of John Hoxsey had a horse with a cancerous growth. Thinking there was nothing he could do he turned the horse loose on a pasture. Amazingly, the cancerous growth soon began to shrink and eventually it fell off. Hoxsey observed the horse and saw that it liked to go to a certain part of the pasture and graze on the plants in that place. If we accept that animals have an instinct for healing plants—and there is a great deal of evidence that they do - then there is nothing strange about this story. Hoxsey collected the plants in that area and experimented with them in various combinations. Eventually, he made a formula that was handed down from father to son until it reached Harry Hoxsey in 1919.

Hoxsey began opening cancer clinics around the USA. He had seventeen when the cancer establishment started to crack down. Morris Fishbein of the American Medical Association offered to take over the treatment. His deal was that Hoxsey would receive nothing for the first 9 years and after that, he would receive 10 percent of the profits. Not surprisingly, Hoxsey said no. Fishbein then arranged through his powerful political connections to have Hoxsey arrested 125 times in 16 months. The charges all dealt with practising medicine without a licence. The cases were all thrown out of court. But eventually, Hoxsey was forced to close down.

In 1963, his chief nurse opened the Bio-medical Center in Tijuana, Mexico, and Hoxsey's herbal treatment is still available there. The current formula includes the following :

Red Clover (Trifolium pratense)
Burdock root (Arctium lappa)
Barberry bark (Berberis vulgaris)
Licorice root (Glycyrrhiza glabra)
Buckthorn bark (Rhammus purshiana)
Prickly Ash (Zanthoxylum americana)
Chaparral (Larrea tridentate- a late addition to the formula)
Stillingia (Stillingia sylvatica)
Cascara amarga (Picramnia antiderma)
Potassium iodide

Patricia Spain, who did a study of the herbs for the US Congress Office of Technology as part of its assessment of alternative cancer therapies, wrote in her report: "More recent literature leaves no doubt that Hoxsey's formula...does indeed contain many plant substances of marked therapeutic activity."

While there are a number of formulas on the market, one that combines the main Hoxsey herbs with other herbs of known efficacy is marketed as Blood Support and is available at www.baselinenutritionals.com

Imupros

This is a concentrated formulation of a number of herbs, vitamins, minerals and other substances. It is used in Holland and Germany as part of a general anti-prostate cancer protocol.

Prof. Ben Pfeifer, Director of Aeskulap Cancer Center, Switzerland has had great success in treating patients with prostate cancer with a combination therapy that includes Prostasol, MGN-3 (Biobran), curcumin complex (3 grams a day) and Imupros. He quotes a success rate of two thirds of his patients showing clear beneficial responses.

Imupros is a combination of vitamin E (tocopherol succinate), vitamin C, cholecalciferol. epigallocatechin gallate (EGCG), calcium carbonate, selenium, genistein, lycopene and zinc.

Imusan

This is another rather expensive but widely used combination of Chinese herbs and mushrooms specifically designed to enhance the immune system. 1 capsule of Imusan (300 mg) contains:

Pyrola Rotundifolia (wintergreen): 30mg
Xian He Cao (Agrimonia Pilosa): 24mg
Yan Hu Shuo (Corydalis Yanhusuo): 24mg
Ganoderma Lucidum (Reishi): 24mg
Shi Suan (Lycoris radiata): 24mg
Mou hui toui (Patrinia hetrophylia): 24mg
Di bu long (Stephania delavayi): 23.7mg
Hua jian jiu teng (Stephania sinica): 23.7mg
Rabdosia Rubescens: 21mg
Cheng-min chou (Cistance deserti cola): 19.5mg
Liang miau zhen (Zanthoxylum nitidum): 15mg
Ginseng: 12mg
Pollen: 12mg
Glycyrrhiza glabra: 3mg

Iscador

This therapy is closely associated with institutions associated with Rudolf Steiner's Anthroposophical movement. It is well-known in Germany.

Iscador is the trade name for a number of preparations made with different types of mistletoe that grow on different kinds of tree and therefore exhibit different properties. These are further combined with homeopathic doses of such metals as silver, copper and mercury. Although condemned by the American Cancer Society, it is approved for use in Germany and Switzerland. The Lukas Clinic in Arlesheim, Switzerland is the major centre where this therapy is carried out.

However, any doctor can procure the capsules. Contact www.lukasklinik.ch

The Iscador is given by subcutaneous injection at a site close to the tumour, starting with low doses and gradually increasing them until the patient reacts by showing a clear objective or subjective improvement in general health, the tumour slows down, or there is a fever reaction. This is seen as a good sign.

Does Iscador work? A lot of evidence suggests it does. One of its most obvious effects is that it increases the size of the thymus gland substantially by nearly 100 percent in some animal studies and the thymus becomes much more active. This is a very significant finding. Iscador works both by attacking the cancer cells directly and by enhancing the immune system.

Not all cancers respond well to Iscador. Leukemia, for example, does not. It works best with carcinomas and melanomas.

Although mistletoe is poisonous, Iscador is relatively non-toxic. It is suggested that it can accompany any other anti-cancer treatment, as no negative interactions with other medications have been reported. However, it should not be taken by people with heart problems, pregnant women and people taking a prescription drug containing a monoamineoxidase (MAO) inhibitor.

It is often combined with a vegetarian diet excluding mushrooms, tomatoes, new potatoes as well as sugar, hard fats and alcohol. In addition, patients following an anthroposophical regime are encouraged to engage in artistic activities including dance as well as having heat baths, oil baths and massage.

In addition to fighting cancer it has the effect of aiding sleep, providing pain relief and stimulating weight gain. Many patients report being reinvigorated. For further details go to www.iscador.com.

Jason Winter's Tea   *I think Chris @ chrisbeatcancer.com drank this*

Sir Jason Winter was a Hollywood stunt man who cured himself of cancer. His tea contains red clover and green tea extract–both of which are known to be beneficial for cancer patients – plus a secret herbal ingredient – about which nothing sensible can be said. It is available from his website at www.sirjasonwinters.com

PC-SPES, PC-HOPE and Prostasol

First a warning. The herbal combination PC-SPES was withdrawn suddenly from the market early in 2002. This product had been aimed at men with prostate cancer (hence the 'PC' bit in the name). However, scientists who were studying it discovered that it also contained small amounts of Xanax (a brand name anti-anxiety drug), DES (an artifical estrogen) and warfarin (rat poison – also used to thin the blood to prevent clotting). The herbal combination, to the extent that it was successful (and it seemed to have been), appears to have worked as a herbal hormone therapy – and warfarin is indeed regularly prescribed to men undergoing regular hormone therapy for prostate problems, as there is a danger of blood clotting as a side effect of the treatment. Other side effects of the orthodox hormone approach are breast development, impotence and loss of sex drive.

There are two warnings to be made in this context. The first warning is that herbal combinations may contain undeclared elements that you would rather not have. The only way of defending yourself against this possibility is to take only combinations recommended by sources of information that you trust (and of course trust can be established only over time). Internet forums are useful for getting a variety of viewpoints and experiences. The second warning is that, although the internet is a wonderful resource, it needs to be approached with care. Information on the internet is not dated. There are still many sites recommending PC-SPES as a worthwhile herbal combination, even though it has been taken off the market.

In fact, the company that took PC-SPES off the market have returned with a new product, PC-HOPE, which has the following declared ingredients: reishi (Ganodema Lucidum), Baikal scullcap (Scutellaria Baicalensis), rabdosia (Rabdosia Rubescens Hara), Dyer's woad (Isatis Indigotica Fortune), mum (Dendranthema Morifolium Tzelev), saw palmetto (Serenoa Repens), San-Qi ginseng (Panax Notoginseng) , and licorice (Glycyrrhiza Glabra L.). These are the same ingredients that PC-SPES had, but there are, they now claim, no hidden extras.

A similar product, and according to the forums a cheaper one, is offered by Dr. Kurt Donsbach. Called Prostasol (previously PC-Plus), it has the same ingredients (more or less).

There are many testimonials in the forums as to the effectiveness of both PC-HOPE and Prostasol in lowering PSA levels speedily and also inhibiting cancer.

Dr. Donsbach admits that Prostasol is loaded with phytoestrogens which will cause breast sensitivity, but he says this can be treated with progesterone cream and curcumin. He makes no mention of other side effects, but it would be worth enquiring. For more information go to www.donsbach.com

Tian Xian

This herbal combination of 30 Chinese herbs is famous throughout China – to the extent that there are many fake versions on the market. It appears to be effective against cancer, as a support for those taking chemotherapy and as a pain reliever. It was formulated by Chinese herbalist Dr. Wang Zhen Guo, who describes its action in this way: "Tian Xian Liquid removes body heat, is a toxin neutral-izer, purifies blood, stops pain, supplements (energy), and regenerates blood." It is available as a liquid, capsules and as suppositories.

Unfortunately it is also very expensive. For further details see www.tian-xian.com. For testimonials go to www.cancer-central.com

Sho-saiko-to

Kampo is the traditional herbal medicine system of Japan. Sho-saiko-to is a kampo herbal formula for the liver. There is growing interest in these herbal formulas and their potential for cancer patients. Most research has focused on its benefits as an adjuvant therapy with chemotherapy and radiation. Studies show clear survival benefits for those taking kampo herbal combinations such as Sho-saiko-to (the largest selling of these preparations). However, given their proven benefits for the liver, many people are taking Sho-saiko-to as part of an overall herbal anti-cancer strategy irrespective of whether or not they are having chemo.

Sho-saiko-to's ingredients are: Bupleurum root (Bupleurum chinense), Pinellia tuber (Pinellia tuberifera), Scutellaria root (Scutellaria baicalensis–also known as Baikal skullcap), Jujube fruit (Zizyphus jujuba), Ginseng root (Panax ginseng), Licorice root (Glycyrrhiza uralensis), and Ginger root (Zingiber officinale).

Recommended dosage: 7.5 grams of the formula.

The Japanese government regulates preparation of these formulations very tightly and their quality is considered to be very high. For more information go to www.honsousa.com

Zyflamend

Inflammation is associated with cancer development and is promoted by an enzyme-protein complex called cycloaxygenase-2 (COX-2). When COX-2 is inhibited, inflammation and pain are reduced.

Zyflamend is a herbal combination that has shown anti-inflammatory impacts (as a COX-2 inhibitor) and additional major anti-cancer effects against prostate cancer cells in the laboratory. In one study it reduced cancer cell proliferation by 78 percent. It contains holy basil (a COX-2 inhibitor), turmeric (contains curcumin), ginger (inhibits both COX-2 and 5-LOX), green tea, rosemary, hu zhang (contains resveratrol), Chinese goldthread and barberry (COX-2 inhibitors), oregano (contains more than 30 known anti-inflammatory compounds), and scutellaria – also known as Baikal Skullcap (a COX-2 inhibitor).

Zyflamend also inhibits activation of NF-kappaB–a transcription factor that is crucial for cell division and therefore incidentally a promoter of cancer. So this is also good news.

It is widely available from internet suppliers.

Botanic Healing Systems
Ayurvedic Medicine

Ayurvedic medicine is a 6,000 year-old system of medicine with a great pedigree and many formal institutional structures: medical schools, hospitals, research facilities and so on. The key difference between Ayurvedic approaches to health and the Western approach has been nicely summarised by Dr. Ron Kennedy: "The Ayurveda holds that we are thoughts which created bodies. In Western medicine we are material (body) which creates thoughts."

The Ayurvedic doctor does not attempt simply to heal the body. He seeks to heal the whole person including the mental part of the person. And because thoughts manifest themselves in the biochemistry of the physical body, such therapies as meditation, yoga, energy medicine and emotional healing, can all have a place in the healing work that is done. One aspect of Ayurvedic medicine is panchakarma, which seeks to achieve a deep cleansing of the physical tissues of the body.

This is a system of medicine that has developed a deep understanding of herbs – and India is the source of many unique herbs. There are a growing number of ayurvedic resources on the internet. One good starting point is www.cancerlinks.com/ayurveda.html

One herbal combination arising out of Ayurvedic medicine, that is considered to have exciting potential as a cancer cure, is Carctol; another is Maharishi Amrit Kalash - an ayurvedic herbal preparation made from extracts of 44 herbs and fruits. There is little evidence as yet, but it appears to have demonstrated some anti-cancer activity and also appears to be helpful in suppressing the side effects of orthodox treatments.

TCM: Traditional Chinese Medicine and Herbs

The Chinese view tumours as the 'uppermost branch' of the disease not its root. They consider cancer to be caused by a wide range of external or internal excesses (i.e., an excessive dose of a cancer causing chemical or an excessive dose of bad emotions). All forms of excess result in the 'chi', the body's living energy, becoming blocked in some way. Some Chinese doctors prefer to treat cancer with herbs alone, while others try to mix Chinese herbs with Western chemotherapy and radiation. In fact, many doctors in China are looking at Chinese herbs in an entirely Western scientific way—looking at them for their anti-cancer effects. The traditional herbalist sees cancers simply as symptoms and uses herbs to bring the body into a state of healthy balance.

Fu-zhen therapy, an immune enhancing herbal regimen, has had very good results when compared with just chemotherapy and radiation. In one study of 76 patients with stage II liver cancer, 46 were treated with Fu-zhen herbs in combination with chemotherapy and radiation. 29 survived one year and ten survived for three years. Only six of the thirty given chemotherapy and radiation alone survived one year. In fact, there are reports of success from using the herbs alone.

The most commonly used Fu-zhen herbs are astragalus, ligustrum, ginseng, codonopsis, atractylodes, ganoderma, actinidia and rabdosia. Actinidia is a root that contains the polysaccharide ACPS-R. In one study, when injected into mice, 90 percent of tumours stopped growing. Another study showed a 50 percent success rate with liver cancers.

Doctors at the Beijing Institute for Cancer Research have found that a herbal tonic usually prescribed for kidney ailments, known variously as Golden Book Tea or Six Flavour Tea had a highly significant effect when combined with chemotherapy against small cell lung cancer (SCLC). It appears that all traditional kidney tonics may have these beneficial effects. Other commonly-used Chinese herbs:

Astragalus: This is a Chinese herb used mainly for patients with heart disease or high blood pressure. It has recently been shown to have a very strong normalising effect on people with damaged immune systems. It is therefore recommended not only as a cancer prevention/cure but also as a herbal support for people undergoing chemotherapy and radiation. Dose: 1-3 400 mg capsules per day.

Tang kuei (Angelica sinensis): This is a highly reputed blood tonic and has had successful results in treating cancer either alone or in combination with other herbs. Women have used it as a douche against cervical cancer.

Juzentaihoto: This is sometimes known as JT-48 or JTT. It is a blood strengthening herb and is reportedly very effective in helping chemotherapy patients recover.

Jiaogulan (Gynostemma pentaphyllum): This is another Chinese herb with a growing reputation and is apparently known as the herb of immortality. Like other herbs it has a wide range of beneficial actions including tumour suppression.

Tripterygium Wilfordii Hook: This is a vine used in TCM for relieving symptoms of rheumatoid arthritis. In Chinese it is known as Lei Gong Teng. (In Cantonese: Lui kong teng.) One of its key active compounds is triptolide, which has been found by scientists at Stanford University School of Medicine to have tumour killing effects. It provokes programmed cell death. Triptolide can be sourced on the internet, but at $65 a milligram it is quite expensive and would need to be taken under close medical supervision. However, the herb itself is not expensive and is considered to be highly effective as an anti-cancer agent.

Kanglaite (KLT): . This has been clinically trialed with very positive outcomes. Mainly used as an adjuvant therapy, alongside chemotherapy and radiation, it nevertheless has cancer retarding and immune system enhancing properties. KLT was developed using an extract of the herb known as coix seed (semen coicis) which is a cooling herb used for supporting the spleen in Chinese medicine. For more information go to www.kanglaite.com. For details of coix seed see: www.tcmtreatment.com

This brief discussion of these few Chinese herbs does not exhaust the subject. There are certainly many other Chinese herbs that will be beneficial.

It should be noted that traditional Chinese herbalists have an attitude to the value of a herb that is totally opposed to the way Western doctors view drugs. For a Western doctor the best kind of drug is one that has a specific effect against a specific ailment. The more generalised a drug's effects, the less it is valued. In fact any drug that claims to be a cure-all will be automatically disregarded as being valueless. In Chinese herbalism the reverse is true. For them, the most inferior herb is the one that acts against a single specific problem. The most valued is the one that has a broad spectrum of effects. Since herbalists seek first and foremost to promote total health and so aid the healing of the individual, this makes sense.

The point can also be made here that most Chinese herb books do not list cancer as a disease that herbs can fight. Instead they list the herbs that are effective in strengthening the immune system. More specific agents may be listed as anti-viral agents.

Chris Teo's Herbal Centre   *I checked out his website - he also recs almost veg diet.*

Chris Teo is a retired Professor of Botany and a dedicated Christian who has, in a very short time, built up a worldwide reputation for his herbal cures for cancer. He is not an orthodox Chinese herbalist, but this seems the best place to discuss his work. Living in Penang, Malaysia, he has not had the problems that many herbalists in the West. If he had attempted to do what he has done in the USA, he would have been pilloried as a quack and a charlatan.

"I am glad that I live in the East. Here, herbal medicine is part of our oriental heritage. So I am not treading on hostile ground when I talk about and practice herbal medicine. Of course there are doctors who are against me and label me a 'quack'. But there are many other doctors who agree with my work and even refer their patients to me."

Teo has formulated 60 herbal combinations for different purposes using herbs that he grows on his own farm or which he imports from China. Malaysia is, we should remember, one of the world's richest herbal terrains. With these herbs he has treated, with a great deal of success, many hundreds of people, many of whom were considered terminal. He has had a great deal of success – though he refuses to put this success in percentage terms – not just in making tumours disappear but in helping people become well and free from pain. He has also formulated herbal regimes for people who are still undergoing radiation or chemotherapy. This is a low-cost service. He does not charge for his consultations only for the herbs.

If you think Malaysia is too far to go for a cancer cure, the writer Bernie Siegel has revealed an interesting fact. Life expectancy for cancer patients undergoing treatment is directly proportional to how far they have to travel, and by implication how much energy they have to put into it. In short, those who travel furthest for their cancer treatments live longest.

For more information look at Chris Teo's website at www.cacare.com. *it doesn't get*

people live years with their cancer on hold - it doesn't get worse - the teas look awful though.

The European Herbal Tradition

We should not forget that Europe too has a strong herbal tradition which is nurtured particularly in the Germanic countries. The following herbs are proposed as being good for cancer by Maria Treben, a renowned Austrian herbalist, and Dr. Vogel, an internationally renowned Swiss herbalist.

Horsetail tea (Equisetum arvense): This is one of the most ancient of cancer cures. The horsetail can also be used in the form of a poultice. Horsetail is rich in silica.

Calendula (aka Marigold): A fresh juice of all the plant - leaves, stem and flower - should be drunk regularly.

Yarrow (aka Milfoil - Achillea millefolium): This is especially recommended for women.

See next page for Liver strengthening herbs - very important for cancer

→

Stinging Nettles: The whole plant is used. It has a great reputation for blood cleansing. Pick them in May and store for the winter.

Butterbur (Petasites officinalis hybridus): This is highly recommended both as a cancer treatment and as a pain reliever. This is the basis of Vogel's herbal product, petaforce.

None of these herbs have negative side effects, and they can be taken in large quantities.

Maria Treben recommends, as a general cancer treatment, a tea made with 2 litres of water, 300 gm of Calendula, 100 gm Yarrow, 100 gm Stinging Nettles.

For leukaemia she recommends a tea consisting of St. John's Wort (15 gm):, Dandelion Roots (15gm); : Speedwell (20 gm);Wormwood (20gm); Bedstraw (25 gm); Yarrow (25 gm); Goat's Beard (25 gm); Elder shoots (30 gm); Calendula (30 gm), Greater Celandine (30 gm); Stinging Nettle (30 gm).

This mixture is mixed dry, and 1 heaped teaspoon is placed in a cup and boiling water is poured in and left for half a minute to two minutes (longer with dried herbs, shorter time with fresh herbs). Make 1 to 2 litres for a day and put in a thermos and sip. One cup is a quarter litre.

Dandelion root alone has some anecdotal support as a cancer cure. A farmer by the name of George Cairns is so convinced of its merits he took out a lengthy ad in the Chicago Northwest Times extolling its merits. According to him, he was on his death bed when the idea of taking dandelion came to him. He picked some fresh roots, took off the leaves and – without washing the soil off – he put the roots out to dry. He suggests putting them in an incubator, under a hot bulb or in the hot sun for 5-6 days or longer. When they can be easily crumbled, the bulbs should be pounded to a fine dust using a mortar and pestle. Half a teaspoon of the resulting powder should be dissolved in water and taken once a day. He attributes a number of cures to this – though admits that it does not appear to be beneficial for skin or brain cancers.

Soil, incidentally, has a long association with health. Eating pesticide-free soil is good for you. A few centuries ago, a sick farmer would get a sod of soil brought into him so that he could breathe in its healthy vapours. More recently scientists have discovered that a common soil bacteria, Mycobacterium vaccae, has an effect on us equal to some brand name anti-depressants. So get out into the garden and get your hasnds dirty. It's good for you.

Liver-Strengthening Herbs:

Poor liver function is considered to be a clear pre-curser to cancer. It is therefore considered important by many herbalists to strengthen or maintain good liver health with such herbs as: Milk thistle, Artichoke, Dandelion, Burdock and Rosemary.

Other Botanic Systems

Aromatherapy

In France, aromatherapy is widely accepted as a clinically effective therapy for a wide range of chronic illnesses. French doctors often apply it as part of a total treatment plan. There are good reasons why aromatherapy might have a useful part to play in a health restoration strategy.

First, it is well established that a large number of oils have an immune system enhancing effect—far too many to be listed here. A number of commercial aromatherapy websites have useful information resources (e.g., www.akobiaromas.com).

Secondly, a number of oils are believed to have a broad anti-carcinogenic effect. The following have been proposed by Robert Tisserand as possibly falling into this category: Cedarwood, Cypress, Eucalyptus, Hyssop, Bergamot and Geranium. Frankincense

There is also evidence that Lavender, Niaouli or Tee-tree oil smeared on the skin before radiation may help prevent burning and scarring of the skin. A bath in these oils before treatment may have beneficial effects internally (3-4 drops in a full bath).

Thirdly, there are those oils that are considered to be beneficial for the liver, rosemary being one. Since the liver has been implicated by many as the source of cancer, these oils may have a general preventative role to play. Rosemary herb has also been considered useful for cancer-protection.

No discussion of aromatherapy oils should ignore what in my house we call 'magic oil'—Lavender oil. Before any kind of medical intervention, lavender oil should be rubbed on or bathed in (4-6 drops in a full bath). After any surgical treatment add lavender oil to the damaged tissue. It is famous for its healing effects when it comes to burns. If I cut myself I pour lavender oil on the cut knowing that the cut will heal quickly and that there will not be any septicaemia. If I have difficulty sleeping I rub some lavender oil under my nose, and then I know I will soon fall asleep. In short, lavender is a great healer and relaxant. My rule is this: When in doubt use lavender. Lavender can be applied without risk directly to the skin.

Apart from their healing potential, there are the psychological benefits of aromatherapy baths and massages that help reduce stress and enhance psychological well-being.

Warning: Many of these essential oils are highly potent and most should not be rubbed directly on the skin in their concentrated form (exceptions are lavender, tea tree, rosemary and peppermint). Putting a few drops in a bath is a very effective way of absorbing the oils – the skin is a highly absorbent organ. Do not exceed 5 drops of any oil - or 15 drops in total - in any bath.

Also, the quality of oils on the market varies widely. As with food there are organic and non-organic oils. It is important to ask for oils of therapeutic quality.

Flower Therapy

It is part of common folklore that some people have green fingers. They appear to have a special intuition for plants and that plants respond to their touch. "All flowers talk to me, and I reply," said the chemist George Washington Carver.

One person who had such an intuition was Edward Bach, a Welsh doctor who gave up his practice to develop a healing system based on flower essences. He extracted flower essences by steeping the flowers in spring water in the sunlight. The purpose of these flower essences is to direct our individual spiritual, emotional, mental and physical development in the direction of health. According to Dr. Bach: "[Disease] is the means adopted by our own souls to point out to us our faults, to prevent our making greater errors, to hinder us from doing more harm, and to bring us back to the path of Truth and Light from which we should never have strayed."

For Dr. Bach, disease does not have a physical cause but, rather, it is the result of a spiritual disharmony within the person. It was his belief that each person has a spiritual dimension which is the Soul. This soul is aware of the individual's life mission, which needs to be given expression in the physical, mental and emotional life of that person. But when a person deviates from the mission, or is blind, deaf and unfeeling to the promptings of the true mission, the result is disease. The worst of all the errors is when Love is not freed, but is instead denied. All virtues without Love become destructive. "Righteousness without love makes us hard. Faith without love makes us fanatical. Power without love makes us brutal. Duty without love makes us peevish. Orderliness without love makes us petty." says an anonymous commentator.

Disharmony results in various negative emotional states. By correcting these states, a state of harmony can be restored. The flower essences work, it is argued, by radiating harmonious energy at frequencies that help to correct distortions in the energy field of the patient. The idea has been developed in Australia and America so it is now possible to choose from a range of over 100 essences. Although I have listed this among the botanical therapies, it has perhaps more in common with the vibrational therapies that I discuss in a later chapter.

One way of choosing which flower essence to use is simply to sniff each of the 38 essences that Edward Bach found and to see which of them the mind and body respond to. Another way is to read the list of emotional states that they are good for dealing with. A number of different 'remedies' can be taken at the same time up to a maximum of six.

For emergencies of any kind, and particularly for anxiety attacks, a ready mixed 'Rescue Remedy' is available. I once recommended this to a highly sceptical scientist who was having a panic attack. I asked him later if it had calmed in down. Yes, he admitted, but it could have been a placebo effect. Does it matter? I replied. If it was just a placebo, maybe he needed to take the Rescue Remedy to trigger it.

For the cancer patient who is self-denying, the following remedies may be useful: Agrimony, Centaury, Chicory, Red Chestnut. For those who are overly strict and rigid, Rock Water. Violet gives feelings of placidity, Gentian dissipates depression. For those feeling depression, desperation or despair any of the following may be helpful: Larch, Pine, Elm, Sweet Chestnut, Star of Bethlehem,

Willow, Oak or Crab Apple. For those undergoing recovery from traumatic events: Walnut and Willow. 3-5 drops are taken four times a day with or without water.

Flower remedies are widely available in health shops. There are ranges based on the flowers of America and Australia as well as the standard Bach Flower Remedies.

Miscellaneous

Kombucha (Mogu)

The kombucha is a fungus that looks like a thick, pale yellow pancake. It has the ability to transform heavily sugared tea into a health drink over a period of a week. Kombucha produces acids similar to those made by the liver. It binds with toxins in the colon and disposes of them through normal elimination. Kombucha discourages cancer and promotes good sleep, energy and helps protect against the side effects of radiation and chemo. This is not a new discovery. On the contrary it has been used as a health support for thousands of years. Getting a kombucha should be easy as kombucha divide every week. The length of time it takes to produce the tea is the same time it takes to split into two plates. It's almost the ultimate in natural pyramid schemes.

To make the tea, float the kombucha in a flat ceramic or glass dish and cover it with a any kind of heavily sugared tea you like (to flavour it). You can add ginger. Leave in a warm place and after 5-7 days pour off the drink and take a glass or two a day for the following week while you brew up another week's supply. For more information contact: The Kombucha Network at www.kombu.de/suche2.htm

It is worth mentioning here that ginger has been shown to kill cancer cells in a laboratory study involving ovarian cancer cells. It killed them in two ways: by causing apoptosis (normal cell death) and also by inducing the cancer cells to eat themselves (known as autophagy). Regular drinks of ginger tea made with fresh or dried ginger could play a useful role as part of a varied anti-cancer regime.

OTHER ANTI-CANCER FORMULATIONS

In this chapter I will be looking at a number of formulations and approaches that have been specifically developed to attack cancer directly. Some of these make use of natural products, while others will appear to be highly unnatural. Nevertheless, they all claim a significant degree of success in treating cancer. Also in this list are drugs that have been found, serendipitously, to have an anti-cancer effect although they are not normally used against cancer.

Active Hexose Correlated Compound (AHCC)

AHCC is made from a combination of hybridized Japanese medicinal mushrooms. There are reports that a number of cancer patients suffering from breast, prostate, and other forms of cancer have experienced dramatic improvement and even full remission after taking AHCC.

Most of the research has been done in Japan where AHCC was developed. In one study of five breast cancer cases given 3 grams of AHCC a day, 2 (40 percent) had gone to complete remission by the end of the 8 month study. It should be noted that participants in these kinds of study have usually been considered terminal. This is an astonishing result.

AHCC is widely available from internet herbal suppliers.

There are a number of other mushroom extract formulations that have shown effectiveness either alone or, more commonly, as supporting therapies for people undergoing chemotherapy. Among these are PSK (This is the Japanese name. It is also known in China as PSP), Ganoderma, MycoSoft and others. There appears to be clear evidence that these formulations make chemotherapy more bearable and at the same time improve survivability rates.

Bentonite Clay

This clay has a strong healing effect and should be plastered over a malignant skin tumour. See photographs at www.silvermedicine.org/clay-cansema-silver1.html

Beta Sitosterol

Beta-sitosterol is a very common phytosterol. It is widely distributed in the plant kingdom and found in such botanicals as saw palmetto, pumpkin seed and pygeum africanum. It is specifically recommended in the case of prostate cancers. Double blind clinical trials have demonstrated that it is highly effective on its own against prostate problems. In various studies, dose levels of 20-130mg per day have completely reversed enlarged prostates. It is also known that beta-sitosterol can reverse colon cancer and lymphocytic leukaemia. It is also a general booster of the immune-system. Athletes are using it to help reduce inflammation caused by intense physical workouts.

CanCell

The story of CanCell is one of the quirkiest in all the annals of alternative cancer cures. The original formula for CanCell was developed in 1936 by James Sheridan, a chemist. He called his discovery 'Entelev'. Later it was taken up and modified by Edward Sopcak in 1984.

It was Sopcak who called his version CanCell. Sopcak and Sheridan shared an interesting and un-American idiosyncrasy. Neither of them wished to profit from their cancer cure and so would give it away free to anyone who asked. This idealistic stance, however, could not last forever. In recent years, a number of products that are 'CanCell-like' are for sale over the internet: Cantron, Protocel, and Entelev are three competing products. (It is also marketed as Sheridan's Formula, Jim's Juice and Crocinic Acid). The formulas of all these products are slightly different and it may be worth trying a second if the first doesn't appear to be having an effect. Cantron is apparently closer to the original formula than some of the others.

There are even competing theories as to why it works. Sheridan, himself, believed it worked by interfering with the respiration of the cancer cell, while in Sopcak's view it interfered with the cancer cell on the level of vibrational energy causing it to self-digest. Neither Sheridan nor Sopcak claimed that their product was a cancer cure-all. On the contrary, they have consistently claimed a 50-55 percent success rate.

Side effects are apparently minimal.

The main problem with CanCell is that it conflicts with a wide range of vitamins, minerals, herbs, etc.—many of which are also recommended against cancer, chief amongst them vitamin C, CoQ10 and flaxseed oil. The full list of things to be avoided can be found at the CanCell home page at www.alternativecancer.us, but the following items top that list: CoQ10, vitamin E, vitamin C, selenium, Essiac, ozone, ellagic acid, IP-6, L-carnitine, blutathione, glutamine, sea silver, lipoic acid, creatine, taurine, acetylcystein, L-cysteine, ginseng, 714-X, hydrogen peroxide, and colloidal silver.

Since, according to testimonies, this is such an effective way of dealing with cancer it is probably worth choosing this option and monitoring effects closely. If it works, good; if not, then move on to something else.

Protocel is now sold simply as a dietary supplement that will rid the body of 'unwanted and unproductive cells' at www.protocel.com. They have two formulas, of which Formula 50 is considered more powerful. Cantron can be obtained at www.cantron.com

one website said use this with Budwig Protocol. A person in the Henderson book used Protocel & had a lot of toxic die off - sweats, diahrea, runny nose

Cansema / TumorX Salve

These powerful anti-cancer products are pastes made from the herb bloodroot (Sanguinaria Canadensis)—see discussion of bloodroot on p. 212.

Carnivora

Carnivora is an extract from the digestive juices of the Venus Flytrap. This plant is very good at digesting animal proteins, and it caught the attention of a German oncologist by the name of

Helmut Keller. Dr. Keller has tested out carnivora on both animals and humans at his clinic in Germany - with good results. Carnivora contains a powerful chemical, plumbagin, which has demonstrated clear anti-viral and anti-cancer properties in independent tests. It does this by promoting the cellular production of hydrogen peroxide. It is also a powerful healer - yet it is virtually harmless, so much so that Russians have suggested it can be used as a food preservative. Self-administered venus flytrap juice is not advised, as it contains other chemicals that can cause unpleasant side effects. Keller's carnivora has been purified and is non-toxic.

All research on carnivora has been done with injectible extracts. Capsules are available on the internet but their effectiveness is unknown. The drug can be obtained from the Carnivora Research Co., www.carnivora.com

Cesium Therapy (aka High pH Therapy)

This is becoming an increasingly popular approach to the treatment of cancer. It was first promoted in the 1970s and 1980s by Dr. Keith Brewer — and is therefore also referred to as Dr. Brewer's high pH therapy. Brewer noted that cesium, one of the basic chemical elements, was one of the few chemicals that could enter cancer cells — indeed it was readily sucked up by cancer cells — and this uptake was further enhanced by Vitamins A and C, as well as zinc and selenium salts. Inside the body it has the effect of making the cells more alkaline.

When the quantity of cesium taken up was sufficient to raise the cell pH to 8 (a very alkaline state) the cancer cells stopped dividing and soon died. In animal and human tests it has been found that large tumour masses start to shrink over a period of a few weeks. "Also," Brewer reported, "all pains and effects associated with cancer disappeared within 12 to 36 hours; the more chemotherapy and morphine the patient had taken, the longer the withdrawal period."

The basic argument of cesium therapy is the same as for the alkaline pH diet. Cancer cells arise out of an acidic tissue environment and are cured by the simple expedient of returning the cells and their environment to a highly alkaline state.

Take 3-9 grams a day of CsCl [Cesium Chloride] or Cs2CO3 [Cesium Carbonate] along with vitamin C (4-30 grams), and any zinc and selenium salt such as zinc citrate (60-100 mgs) or selenium (200-800mcg). These have a dramatic effect on the uptake of the cesium salt by the cancer cell. The cesium should always be taken with food. The presence of cesium salts in the body fluids helps also to neutralize the acidic and toxic material leaking from the tumor mass and this reduces the risks of toxaemia. This is an important point as some otherwise successful regimes kill the cancer but also kill the patient with the toxic wastes that are suddenly released into the body.

However, a major drawback of cesium therapy is that it can easily cause heart problems since it uses up tissue potassium rapidly. For this reason potassium supplementation is absolutely vital. One person who took cesium with apparently successful results reported that he took the following additional supplements: Potassium (3 grams or more), magnesium (1 gram), CoQ10 (400mg), Pancreatin (10 grams), Neprinol–a combination of nattokinase and serrapeptase enzymes (20 caps), Taurine (1 gram).

These supplements must be continued for at least three months after use of cesium has been discontinued as it stays in the body depleting potassium levels for that length of time.

Potassium is the problem as cesium is known to deplete the body's supplies (and we need 2-4 grams a day) but taking too much potassium can also be problematic.

Side effects of cesium can include tingling around the lips, diarrhoea, constant sweating and other side effects that relate to the die off of cancer cells. It also has a tendency to increase the uric acid levels of the blood which can have a harmful impact on the kidney so uric acid levels need to be monitored carefully. It is best to consult with a sympathetic doctor so that regular tests can be done to ensure all is well while on this regime. One solution is to take the pharmaceutical drug Xyloprim (allopurinol) both before and at the same time as cesium is being taken so that excessively high values of uric acid do not develop.

Cesium can also be taken through the skin. One suggestion is to dampen the skin with DMSO and then spray the cesium on. Use areas of skin close to the tumour or soft areas (i.e., under the arm) where absorption can be maximised. Alternatively dissolve the cesium in the DMSO before putting on the skin.

It sounds as if this should be the eureka cancer cure. Unfortunately, clinics working with advanced cancer patients report that only about 50 percent appear to benefit (though this is exciting in its own right). It has been suggested that the benefits of cesium chloride, or alternatively, ionic cesium, can be enhanced by a low-carbohydrate diet.

Cesium chloride and ionic cesium can be bought from a number of suppliers such as www.rainbowminerals.net and www.cesium-chloride.com.

An alternative way of raising the pH is to take modified liquid silicon. This is marketed as MLS-02. This product has a ph of 14 in its concentreated form but in a 2 percent solution the pH drops to 11. Other chemicals with this pH level would be highly toxic but MLS-02 is claimed to be completely benign and can be used topically on the skin or ingested. For further information go to www.arrowheadhealthworks.com/mLs02.htm.

Finally, it should be said that the increased alkalinity of the body in persons on a long-term treatment with cesium seems to retard the aging process. Dr. Keith Brewer himself started taking CsCl at the age of 87 and at the age of 92 pronounced himself to be fitter, healthier and much more vigorous than five years previously.

There is a cesium therapy discussion group at the yahoo health groups site. Go to http://health.groups.yahoo.com/group/cesiumtherapy

Cimetidine

In 1979, *The Lancet* carried a letter from two doctors at Nebraska University describing the curious fact that two of their cancer patients had both had spontaneous remissions while taking the non-prescription drug Cimetidine, also known as Tagamet, commonly used to treat heart burn. One had squamous cell carcinoma and the other large cell lung cancer. In August 1982, three other doctors reported in *The Lancet* that a patient with stage 4 malignant melanoma had started taking 1,000 mg of Cimetidine and had had an almost instantaneous recovery, with tumours disappearing within a few weeks [Thornes R D, Lynch G, Sheehan M V. Cimetidine and coumarin therapy of melanoma. *Lancet* 1982; ii: 328] Over the years there have been a number of similar anecdotes with a wide range of cancers. This would appear to be a no-brainer. It's relatively safe though it does have the potential to interact with other drugs and in males there is the possibility of breast enlargement. Against that it could be remarkably effective. For a fuller discussion follow this link: www.second-opinions.co.uk/cimetidine.html

Colloidal Silver

Colloidal silver is a powerful antibiotic and anti-viral agent and so is a useful preventative against almost any kind of infection. It disables the enzyme that one-celled bacteria, viruses and fungi need for their oxygen metabolism while in no way harming normal cells.

It is also possible that colloidal silver might have a beneficial effect on cancerous tissues, forcing the cancer cells to return to their undifferentiated state. An orthopaedic surgeon Robert O. Becker found that a low current (high currents promote cancer growth) passed between two pure silver electrodes had the side effect, in one of his patients that he was treating, of curing his cancer.

Whether or not colloidal silver has the same effect has not absolutely been demonstrated. Indeed the problem would be to ensure that the colloidal silver reached the site of the tumour.

There are two main issues relating to the use of silver. The first is whether colloidal silver a solution containing microscopically small particles of silver – or ionic silver, a solution of silver ions, is best. One head to head test came out firmly on the side of ionic silver. However, most solutions are likely to contain both colloidal and ionic silver.

The other question is that of side effects. Silver is generally recognised to be wholly non-toxic. However, the intake of silver salts can lead to a cosmetic condition called argyria, in which the skin becomes silvery grey in colour. It must be stressed that there is absolutely no evidence that the intake of pure colloidal or ionic silver will result in argyria.

In any case, argyria can be treated both by lasers and/or with a self-administered vitamin and mineral chelation therapy (for details see: www.eytonsearth.org/forum/about7.html).

Many people make their own colloidal silver using simple and fairly inexpensive equipment which can be bought on the internet. However, machines that use thin strips of silver wire should be avoided - silver rods are best. Store bought colloidal silver solution can be very variable in quality. It may be better to buy a colloidal silver concentrate and dilute it with distilled water. In this way you have control over the concentration required. For more information about colloidal silver makers go to the Transformation Technologies at www.braintuner.com.

The question of delivery of colloidal silver within the body is usually assumed to be by ingestion. However, if the problem relates to infected lungs then delivering the colloidal silver via a nebulizer – a device used mainly by asthmatics that converts liquid medicine into an aerosol mist – may be preferred. However, if the lung condition is serious make sure you have qualified medical personnel at hand as the impact may be very quick and the immediate response of the body may be negative.

Dichloroacetate (DCA)

In January 2007, an article in New Scientist magazine alerted the world to what may be a cheap, out of patent, cure for cancer. In Lab tests conducted at the University of Alberta, the drug, DCA, which has been used for many years to treat a number of rare metabolic disorders, was found to kill cancer cells in vitro and also in animal studies.

In cancer cells, the mitochondria, which in normal healthy cells are the energy factories, have been switched off. The cancer cell, instead, gets its energy through an inefficient process of glycolysis which requires large amounts of glucose. The mitochondria also control the process of apoptosis (normal programmed cell death). DCA appears to reawaken the mitochondria – and this in turn switches on apoptosis – causing the cancer cells to die. The drug is taken orally in water and is fairly safe though there are some uncomfortable side effects including pain or numbness. Nevertheless, it does appear to be a true cure for cancer. However, I am not holding my breath against the day it will be a standard treatment.

For Leukaemia, Steve Martin (whose grouppekurasawa website I have mentioned a few times) recommends a daily intake of the following combination: DCA (12 mgs per kilo of body weight), caffeine (600 mgs), sodium selenite 1 gram (5 x 200mg), and Vitamin B1 (2-4 grams). This is a stand alone formula and must not, he says, be accompanied by any anti-oxidant supplements.

Digitalis

Digitalis is a well known extract from the foxglove and is used for certain heart conditions. A number of cancer researchers have discovered that it also has a very potent anti-cancer effect for a wide variety of cancers. It appears to work by inducing apoptosis (natural cell death).

Digitalis is currently available in two forms—one of which has no anti-cancer effect. Digitoxin (from Digitalis purpurea) is effective; the similarly named, and now more commonly used, Digoxin (from Digitalis lanata) has no anti-cancer effect.

In 1974, Dr. Bjorn Stenkvist of University Hospital, Uppsala, Sweden, started a long-term study on digitalis. He discovered that of the 44 patients (all of whom had breast cancer) who were on digitalis there was only one recurrence after five years compared with almost 25 percent of the control group who did not take digitalis (21 patients out of a group of 88). The Digitalis had reduced recurrence of cancer by 90 percent. Twenty two years later Stenkvist revisited his patients and discovered that of his digitalis group only six percent had died from breast cancer compared with almost fifty percent of the control group. Details of this and other research supporting the use of Digitoxin can be found at www.second-opinions.co.uk/heart_drugs.html. As Dr. Wayne Martin has commented, "Digitalis is the right drug being used to treat the wrong disease."

Dipyridamole and Anticoagulant Drugs

A cancer that doesn't spread to other sites does not kill the host. If we can impede metastasis to other sites then we have a good way of attacking cancer. The drugs that I will now discuss, which are currently used for various heart conditions, all appear to have the additional effect of impeding metastasis.

Dipyridamole is a drug widely-used in treating patients who have survived an episode of coronary thrombosis. It has very few if any side effects. In *The Lancet* (March 23, 1985, p. 693), E.H. Rhodes et al. of St. Hilaire and Kingman Hospital in Surrey, reported that for the previous 11 years they had been maintaining 30 Grade III and IV melanoma patients on dipyridamole (300 mg a day). The five-year survival rate for the whole group was 77 percent. None of the level III patients had died. Compare this with an expected five-year survival for level IV melanoma of 32 percent.

Dipyridamole works by preventing free floating cancer cells from attaching themselves to the sides of blood vessels at distant sites.

Anticoagulant drugs, which are normally used to dissolve blood clots in patients who have had or who are in danger of having a heart attack, also appear to have an ability to interfere with metastatic developments.

Barry Groves explains the mode of action:: "It was demonstrated as long ago as 1903 that distant metastases from cancer cells circulating in the bloodstream couldn't end up just anywhere; that for a distant tumour to form, it needed a thrombus (clot) at the site of the metastasis to be… In 1958 Professor O'Meara of Trinity College, Dublin, showed that dividing cancer cells were surrounded by fibrils which gave off clotting factors causing the deposition of fibrin." This fibrin has the dual effect of allowing the cancer cells to form a clot at a distant site and at the same time to protect the colony of cancer cells from attack. Any chemical that attacks this fibrin will impact on the ability of the cancer to spread. Drugs that are used for this purpose are warfarin, heparin and streptokinase.

Support for this theory was found in a retroactive study of 1,500 patients (Michaels L. Cancer incidence and mortality in patients having anticoagulant therapy. *Lancet* 1964; ii: 832-5). This study found that the patients who had been on long-term anticoagulant therapy had only one eighth of the expected number of cancer deaths.

In one anecdotal report, a woman who had a widely metastasised endometrial cancer suffered a heart attack and was given streptokinase. An unexpected result was that her cancer went into immediate remission, though for how long is not recorded except that it lasted for several months. For further details of the anti-cancer effects of these drugs go to www.second-opinions.co.uk

DMSO and MSM *may be worth looking into – under guidance of health professional*

Dimethyl sulphoxide (DMSO) is an organic sulphur compound. It is a clear, colourless and largely odorless liquid that has demonstrated clear anti-tumour qualities. Over 6,000 articles in scientific

journals establish a very solid claim for it to be recognised as an anti-cancer weapon. V
freely when treating cancer in animals. It is available on the internet from www.dmso.c
www.dmso.org (two distinct companies).

DMSO can be taken by intravenous injection, orally, or it can be rubbed on. It is absorbed
very rapidly through the skin and this is a very efficient way of getting it to the intended site. Patients
who wish to undergo radiation and chemotherapy should take DMSO as it also reduces both the
pain and the side effects caused by these treatments.

DMSO has a wide range of biological activities. One reason given for this is that it creates
very powerful bonds with water molecules. This allows it to penetrate membranes and to pass from
one organ or tissue to another with great ease.   It has a wider range of biochemical actions than any
other known chemical agent. One Chilean study showed that DMSO in conjunction with low doses
of a chemotherapeutic drug was able to obtain remissions in 44 out of 65 cancer patients. This
result was even more amazing because these patients had all previously had chemotherapy without
success. Twenty-six of the cases involved women with metastatic breast cancer. Twenty-three
obtained remission. Whether the remission was permanent is not known. It is also not known what
effect DMSO on its own, without the chemotherapy, would have had.

DMSO, in a 12.5 percent solution, shows long-term growth inhibitory action on cancer
tumours in laboratory settings.

One dramatic case of a DMSO implicated cancer cure (mentioned in Richard Walters book,
Options) occurred in 1970, when the mother   of 3-year-old Clyde Robert Lindsey of Pasadena,
Texas took her son to see Dr. Eli Tucker of Houston. Clyde had a very deadly cancer known as
Letterer-Siwe disease. The cancer had spread throughout his body and orthodox doctors considered
the case to be hopeless. Dr. Tucker gave the boy a dilute mixture of DMSO mixed with
haematoxylon, a chemical normally used as a dye to trace the location of pathological animal cells.
The haematoxylon-DMSO combination therefore had a special affinity for tumour cells. Inside the
cells the haematoxylon oxidises and this has the effect of causing the cancer cells toto die. Five drops
of this substance in a glass of distilled water every morning from then till now has completely
eliminated all signs of Clyde's cancer and he is, by all accounts, alive today.

It is believed by some that DMSO works by re-establishing aerobic metabolic processes in
the anaerobic cancer cell. This in effect forces the cancer cell to revert to a healthy state. And healthy
cells undergo apoptosis, healthy programmed cell death.. A full description of this process can be
found at David Gregg's site at www.krysalis.net/cancer.htm. (This is an extremely detailed but clear
analysis of a number of anti-cancer approaches by a biochemist. Highly recommended!)

Are there any side effects to taking DMSO? A garlicky taste in the mouth and bad smell on
the breath. Some people suffer from headaches, dizziness and mild nausea. A localised skin rash or
burning feeling can occur on the skin

Warning: DMSO is an extremely powerful solvent. It will dissolve anything, including latex
gloves and plastic. Obviously no one wants anything poisonous to be dissolved and taken into the
body so all jewelry should be taken off and the skin's surface should be cleaned thoroughly before
DMSO is used (According to some, 99.99 percent pharmaceutical grade DMSO is advised. This can

245

next pg

be easily tested as pure DMSO will crystalise at 68°F - in the main part of the fridge for example. If it doesn't crystalise in the fridge it is not pure). DMSO should never come in contact with plastic – only glass and a high quality stainless steel spoon. A dose level of 1-2 teaspoons a day should be sufficient. DMSO is also effective against brain tumours. It has been suggested that a good way of getting cesium chloride into the body is to dissolve it first in DMSO.

MSM supplements are made from DMSO and are thought to have many of DMSO's advantages without negative smell or toxicity. MSM appears to inhibit pain and improve blood flow. It is important for collagen, needed for cell walls and helps the body maintain a good pH level. And there is evidence that it slows the growth of cancer tumours, and may even turn malignant tumours into benign tumours. Some people have combined DMSO and MSM to good effect. MSM is widely and cheaply available and is used as a treatment for arthritis.

Epicor

This is a fermented yeast product that was discovered to have a powerful beneficial impact on the immune system. Used in the process of making animal feed products, it was noted that people working with this product had substantially fewer days off work than workers in other areas of the company. It is now being used by athletes whose immune systems are negatively affected by their low levels of body fat to help them stay unaffected by the colds and flus that are common in top level athletics.

Haelan 951

Haelan is a fermented soy drink which appears to have powerful effects on cancer. One credible witness is Ross Pelton Ph.D. (pharmacist, clinical nutritionist and author of *How to Prevent Breast Cancer*) who was the administrator at an alternative cancer clinic, Hospital Santa Monica. He used Haelan to treat a group of six cancer patients who were suffering the symptoms of cachexia common to late-stage terminal cancer patients. These patients were not expected to live long, in some cases only days.

The six patients drank an eight-ounce bottle per day, and within two days four of them were out of their beds and walking, and within a week they all were. Pelton says Haelan works because of its "high concentration of anti-cancer agents, [and] phenomenal concentration of nutrients, phytochemicals and protein."

In another case, a Texan by the name of Sherman Sanders claims that Haelan enabled him to cure himself of terminal stage liver cancer (cholangiocarcinoma) and to undergo chemotherapy with little discomfort.

A bottle a day is the recommended dose.

A cheaper and, according to some, better-tasting alternative to Haelan is Soy Essence (www.jarrow.com/products/fermentedsoy.htm).

Hydrazine Sulphate

[handwritten: also in Henderson book use with health professional.]

How does cancer kill people? Mainly through causing extreme weight loss and debilitation. This is a process known to doctors as cachexia. Dr. Joseph Gold decided that one way to approach the cancer question was to interfere with this cachexic process. If he could do this then cancer tumours might grow but they wouldn't generally speaking kill the person who had them. Cancer might then be seen in the same way as diabetes: a disease which– if it couldn't be cured - could at least be controlled. At the time Gold was writing, no one knew what caused cachexia.

Gold investigated this question and came to the conclusion that cancer imposes a waste recycling system on the liver and kidneys. The process works like this: cancer uses glucose as its fuel. The waste product that emerges is lactic acid which is excreted into the blood system and is taken up by the liver and kidneys. The lactic acid is then reconverted back into glucose by a process that requires a great deal of energy. The more glucose that is created the more fuel the cancer has to feed on and the more waste products that return to the liver for reconversion. This process depletes the body and energises the cancer. When the body cannot keep up the result is cachexia.

Gold looked for a drug that would interfere with this process. He found it: hydrazine sulphate (or more commonly 'sulfate'). His experiments showed that hydrazine sulphate did indeed have an effect on the cancer energising process by deactivating a key enzyme in the liver. He also found that it had very few side effects. That is to say it was not a very toxic substance in its own right.

His first human guinea pig was a woman who was expected to die within a matter of days from Hodgkin's disease. She was completely bed-ridden and not having eaten much for some time was 'paper thin'. Administration of the drug resulted in very quick improvement. Within a week she was shopping, within five weeks she was pottering about her garden. Dr. Dean Burke, a leading scientist at the U.S. National Cancer Institute who took the side of the alternative approaches to cancer and who attacked the focus on chemotherapy, once declared: "(hydrazine sulphate is) the most remarkable anti-cancer agent I have come across in my forty-five years of experience of cancer." *[handwritten: 8·1973]*

That was in August 1973. So, why isn't everyone now taking hydrazine sulphate? Because it eventually wound up on the American Cancer Society's list of unproven therapies. This was despite the evidence that Gold put forward to support the value of hydrazine sulphate.

Gold claimed that out of 84 patients with advanced stage cancer treated by other doctors with hydrazine sulphate, 70 percent showed subjective improvements (i.e., lessened pain, improved appetite) and that 17 percent had had objective improvements (tumour regression, disappearance of cancer related disorders). These are very good figures given that all the patients were considered terminal and the success rate should therefore have been close to zero percent.

Russian scientists at the N.N.Petrov Research Institute of Oncology in St. Petersburg have replicated these results. In 1974, they used hydrazine sulfate on 48 patients who were considered terminal. They found that almost 60 percent felt subjectively much better, indeed euphoric! Their appetites improved and the pain lessened or disappeared. Over half of these had clear signs of

[handwritten: next pg]

tumour control. In March 1979 another Russian study followed 225 patients. They found that 65 percent had an anti-cachexia response and 44 percent had an anti-tumor response.

Subsequent studies show that it works against every kind of tumour at every stage.

In 1985, Tim Hansen, an eleven year old boy with three inoperable brain tumours was given one week to live. A few weeks later he was put on hydrazine sulphate. When last recorded, he was still taking the hydrazine sulphate as the tumours were still in evidence ten years later - but he was still alive and the tumours had not grown.

Gold's own history of his research and the obstacles that have been put in his way by the National Cancer Institute is published at www.hydrazinesulfate.org.

Gold's recommended dosage for adults weighing over 100 lb is 60 milligrams per day for the first three days, then 60 milligrams twice a day for the next three days, and 60 milligrams three times a day thereafter. This treatment must continue for as long as there is evidence of a tumour in the body. No dose higher than 60 milligrams is to be tried as this can cause nerve damage. For patients weighing under 100 lb the dosage should be halved. Doses should be taken about 2 hours before next meal (i.e., on a very empty stomach).

There are, however, a number of cautions that need to be taken on board by anyone taking this route.

One minor side effect that appears to affect a very small percentage of patients undergoing hydrazine sulfate therapy - and is associated only with high doses for lengthy periods - is a slight pain or temporary numbness in the patient's extremities. This condition is, however, quickly controlled by reducing the dosage.

A much more important concern is that hydrazine sulphate is a monoamine oxidase inhibitor (MAOI) and the following should not be used during hydrazine therapy: Tranquillisers or sedatives in doses greater than 100 mg per day (especially benzodiazepines and phenothiazines) should be avoided, also antihistamines, alcohol and other agents that depress the central nervous system such as morphine. Also vitamin B6 should not be taken. Foods high in tyramine must also be avoided. These tend to be aged and fermented products such as most cheeses, cured meats or fish, sour cream and yoghurt, tofu and tempeh, bouillon cubes, sauerkraut, pickles and yeast extracts. Also restricted are broad beans, avocados, bananas, raisins, figs, dates and dried fruit in general as well as overripe fruit.

The result of mixing tyramin containing foods with hydrazine sulphate can be severes headaches and high blood pressure.

Dr. Gold, developer of Hydrazine Sulphate, specifically warns: "Central nervous system depressants — such as barbiturates, tranquilizers and alcohol — are incompatible with MAO inhibitors and use of the two together could result in extremely dangerous effects." One other reported problem is that it has a tendency to lower blood sugar levels. This needs to be monitored. See the website www.hydrazinesulfate.org for further information. Hydrazine sulphate is cheap and available on the internet.

Immunocal/Undetnatured Whey (Glutathione)

Glutathione is a small protein which is noted for its ability to detoxify the body, binding to such toxins as heavy metals, solvents, and pesticides in a way that allows them to be easily excreted. Glutathione is also an important antioxidant. In relation to cancer, it has been shown to inhibit cancer growth. In general, higher glutathione levels are associated with good health.

Immunocal is the brand name of a product that boosts glutathione levels in the body. Undenatured whey isolate products are also highly recommended as a way of boosting normal cellular glutathione levels while at the same time depleting glutathione levels in cancer cells. Recommended dose is 30-60 grams a day.

IP6 (IP-6)

IP6 is a chemical called Inositol hexaphosphate, which is found naturally in high fibre foods such as beans, brown rice and wheat bran. A number of animal studies, but as yet no human studies, indicate that it is extremely effective against a wide range of cancers. It appears to work against all cancer cells by normalising them—turning them back into normal cells. Interestingly, it has been found to work against every kind of cancer cell studied in animals—and there is no known toxicity.

According to Dr. Abdul Kalam Shamsuddin, Professor of Pathology at the University of Maryland School of Medicine in Baltimore, who developed IP-6, someone with cancer should be taking 4800-7200 mg of IP6 and 1200-1800 mg of Inositol. One reputable brand is Cell Forte. It is available in powder form from www.totaldiscountvitamins.com, and Dr. Shamsuddin recommends two scoops in the morning and two in the evening.

Interestingly, IP-6 has a very broad range of health supporting effects. It boosts the immune system, helps lower cholesterol, prevents kidney stones as well as the complications of diabetes and sickle cell anaemia, and reduces the risk of cardiovascular disease, including heart attack and stroke.

Iridodial

This is an extract of a family of substances found in ants which has very powerful DNA repairing capabilities. Iridodials operate as natural genetic repair kits and they have been shown to have a powerful effect on cancer tumours causing regression even in cancers such as lung cancer that are generally resistant to treatment. Apparently, iridodials are needed by ants that live in areas of strong geomagnetic radiation. There are a number of suppliers on the internet.

Dr. Hans Nieper, the well-known German alternative doctor, considered iridodials to be potentially the most exciting anti-cancer chemicals worth researching at the end of the last century. A liquid extract is available from www.Arrowheadhealthworks.com.

249

Laetrile

Laetrile is the litmus test of all litmus tests. If you find a book on cancer and you wish to know where on the intellectual spectrum the writer is sitting, the quickest and easiest way is to look up 'laetrile' in the index and read what he has to say on the subject. If the writer is against it then the writer is most likely writing from an orthodox position (though some natural therapists are also anti-laetrilists). If, on the other hand, the writer writes with great approval of this substance, then they are talking from an alternative view point. That's all you need to know to make your decision. What you do then is up to you.

Laetrile is the name given by one of its early promoters, Ernest Krebs, to a substance found in concentrated form in apricot kernels and almonds. Also known as amygdalin, nitriloside and vitamin B17, it is found in varying quantities in up to two and a half thousand other plants, many, indeed the vast majority, of which are edible.

In the early seventies, Dr. Harold Manner of the Biology Department at Loyola University, Chicago conducted a study on a strain of mice genetically engineered to produce females that develop spontaneous mammary tumours. Using a combination of enzymes, Vitamin A and laetrile he reported in his book, *The Death of Cancer*:

"After 6-8 days an ulceration appeared at the tumour site. Within the ulceration was a pus like fluid. An examination of this fluid revealed dead malignant cells.. The tumour gradually underwent complete regression in 75 of the experimental animals. This represented 89.3 percent of the total group." (quoted in Moss, 1982)

Further tests on 550 mice, comparing enzymes, vitamin A and laetrile alone and in combinations of two, and in combination of all three together showed that the enzymes alone or in combination with either laetrile or vitamin A produced regression in 52-54 percent of the mice. Laetrile on its own had no visible effect. But when all three were in combination, there was total regression in 36 out of 50 cases (i.e., 76 percent).

So laetrile needs to be taken with vitamin A and enzymes to be really effective.

Pure laetrile, however, has very recently been taken off the shelves in Britain and it has been illegal in much of the USA for decades. Opponents of laetrile argue that it is potentially toxic and can lead to cyanide poisoning. However, this can happen only if pure laetrile is taken orally - because any cyanide that is released does so as a result of the action of the digestive enzymes - and is in any case a largely theoretical fear - very few if any actual deaths have been nailed emphatically to laetrile's door. In the late 1970s an estimated 50,000-100,000 cancer patients were taking over 1 million grams a month (in total – not individually!). Only two or possibly three deaths from an accidental overdose of this substance have been reported – and even these cases are contentious (i.e., there is the distinct possibility that no one has died of laetrile poisoning). Based on these facts, laetrile does not seem to be particulary dangerous or toxic.

Indeed, laetrile-rich foods can be eaten more or less with impunity: bitter almonds and apricots - particularly apricot kernel oil - are eaten in large quantities in the Hunza valley in northern Pakistan. Until modern diets started to impact on their way of life, cancer was unknown.

Anecdotal evidence from a number of doctors supports the use of laetrile therapy. Leon Chaitow, in his book *An End to Cancer?* (1983), quotes the Dutch doctor, H. Moolenburgh: "I have been treating cancer patients for twenty-fice years and introduced laetrile four years ago (i.e., in 1973). That was a turning point. For the first time I saw people who stayed alive in the late stages of cancer, against all expectations." And again: "...a lot of patients with hopeless cancer feel better, have less pain and live longer than I would have expected. And some cases live on and on and on, which could not be expected at all. I did not see that sort of patient before laetrile."

How does laetrile work? There have been two theories. The first is that it is a vitamin and that its deficiency has led to the vitamin-deficiency disease of cancer. For that reason it is sometimes called Vitamin B17. However, it is the second theory that carries most respectability.

According to this theory, laetrile is a parcel that contains poisons. When the parcel is unwrapped the poisons are released. Normal cells do not have the power to unwrap the parcel. Only cancer cells have that power. Laetrile is a substance that can be separated (by certain enzymes, in the presence of water) into glucose, benzaldehyde and hydrocyanic acid. The last two substances are each, individually, a poison but together they work synergistically (i.e., they are more powerful together, in combination, than they are separately). The enzyme that unwraps this package is beta-glucoronidase. This enzyme appears in great quantities in and around cancer cells - but not normal cells.

Laetrile apparently works best on slow-growing cancers in the early stages of malignancy. Late-stage malignancies need to be slowed down. One way of achieving this is through copper replacement therapy - copper is a vital mineral that is eliminated by cancer cells. Copper supplements help to slow down the respiration rate of the cancer cell and this improves the chances of laetrile working.

Proponents of laetrile therapy insist that tumour regression is only one possible result of laetrile therapy. Pain relief and improved subjective feelings of well-being also result. This well-being is the result of the benzaldehyde, which is a known pain-killer.

The question of tumour regression is sometimes brought up as evidence that laetrile is ineffective. Laetrile, it appears, does not make tumours grow smaller. Certainly, at first sight, it seems to make sense that if laetrile does not cause tumours to grow smaller then this is a clear sign that it is an ineffective anticancer agent. This raises an important question about the nature of cancer and tumours.

Laetrilists argue that tumour size is not in fact a good indicator of anti-cancer activity. Their reasoning is as follows. A tumour does not just consist of malignant cells. It also contains a large proportion of normal cells. Chemotherapy attacks all cells so it is not unusual to see significant short-term tumour regression with chemotherapeutic drugs: they kill the malignant and the normal cells together. However, the long-term result may be, in fact, to make the tumour even more aggressive by increasing the proportion of malignant cells. Laetrile, on the other hand, does not affect the normal cells - only the malignant ones. Therefore the tumour will not decrease very much in size. It will simply have been made unmalignant. The body of the cancer may remain, but without the engine.

Laetrilists are almost universal in saying that laetrile therapy must be accompanied by dietary measures - a raw vegetable diet is generally recommended. In fact, such a diet will contain a large amount of dietary laetrile. Indeed, one of the things that makes the laetrile controversy so bizarre is that laetrile is a very common component of food. Between 1,200 and 2,500 plants contain laetrile: most cereals and fruits and many vegetables. Such ubiquity must have a purpose, and surely is evidence of its safety when taken nutritionally. However, laetrile remains isolated in an intellectual no-go area by the medical establishment.

A diet that contains good quantities of the following would be high in laetrile: chick peas, bean sprouts, nuts, mung beans, blackberries, raspberries and the seeds of apples, apricots, cherries, plums and pears. However, bitter almonds are the easiest source: 50-60 a day are recommended.

Laetrile can be injected or taken orally. Treatment generally consists of one to two grams taken orally every day with meals (not more than one gram at any time). Some doctors supplement this with intravenous injections ranging from 3 grams a week to 9 grams a day (for a short period of a few weeks only).

Those who still need to be convinced of laetrile's safety can take heart from an experiment with mice undertaken at a leading US cancer research centre (Sloan-Kettering). For thirty months, mice were injected daily with 2 grams per kilogram of laetrile (equivalent to giving a human a quarter of a pound a day). At the end of the period, these mice were healthier and exhibited better well-being than the control group who did not get any laetrile.

How this experiment and other laetrile supporting research got suppressed takes up a fascinating chapter in Ralph Moss's book *The Cancer Industry*, the best book on the history of cancer and orthodox medicine in the 20th century.

Laetrile is also known as amygdalin or vitamin B-17 by those who advocate its use. Note that it deteriorates very fast and so only fresh laetrile should be used. Many people prefer simply to eat whole apricot kernels. However, larger doses can be taken intravenously – if you can find a doctor who will do this. This is a therapy that is available at some Mexican clinics.

Laetrile is widely available on the internet. One reputable source is www.cytopharma.com. Also look at www.laetrile.info. It has also been suggested that laetrile should be taken with zinc and vitamin C to be properly effective.

Low-Dose Naltrexone (LDN)

Naltrexone (branded under the name: Revia) is an FDA-approved drug originally designed to help wean addicts off heroin. However, in 1985, Bernard Bihari, M.D., a New York City doctor, discovered that very low doses of this drug had a very powerful stimulating effect on the immune system. In addition to stabilizing AIDS, he found that this treatment also had a powerful, beneficial impact on many cancers including cancers such as neuroblastoma, multiple myeloma, and pancreatic cancer, which are normally considered incurable.

Interestingly, this treatment has the effect not of curing cancer but, in many cases where all other treatments have failed, of stopping it in its tracks. This is not 100 percent assured but seems to be a very high frequency effect. However, the LDN needs to be taken permanently as the cancer will start growing again when the LDN is discontinued.

It is safe, cheap and has no side effects (apart from possible sleeplessness in the first week or two of starting) For further details go to www.lowdosenaltrexone.org or www.ldn4cancer.com. It is also effective for a wide range of auto-immune diseases. However, there is a caution. Naltrexone is also known as Antibuse – for those with long memories this was a drug developed to help alcoholics and heroin addicts kick their habit. Normally, if you drink or abuse opiate drugs while taking Naltrexone you will feel ill. However, I am assured that the levels involved here with LDN therapy do not interfere with the enjoyment of alcohol – though one self-described connoiseur of wine says she simply, for no obvious reason, doesn't need to drink as much as she once did.

For those who have a problem obtaining LDN – for the reason that the normal dose is in 50mg tablets while the therapeutic dose is 1.75-4.5 mg (taken once a day at bedtime) – prescriptions can be sent to one of a number of pharmacies in the USA that specialize in LDN. For those without a computer one is Irmat Pharmacy in New York (tel: 1-(212) 685-0500 or 1-(800) 975-2809). A list of other pharmacies is provided on the above websites. Do not take the slow release form.

However, it is much cheaper and easier to dissolve a 50 mg tablet in 50 ml of distilled water and use a dropper to get the amount required (4ml of water will contain 4 mg of LDN).

Lymphotonic PF2

This is a formulation based on a plant extract from calendula, isolated by a top-level Russian team headed by Prof. Doctor Eugenii Severin, President of the Russian Research Center of Molecular Diagnostics & Therapy, Moscow.

One 72-year-old patient with prostate cancer that had metastasized to the bone had a complete remission after using lymphotonic PF2, according to one of the personal testimonials supporting this product. This and a number of other case reports can be found at www.goodbyecancer.com where you can also order the tonic. It is also claimed to be effective in helping reduce the side effects of radiation and chemotherapy.

On a critical note, none of the case reports follow the patients beyond noting their complete remission at the end of a few months of treatment, which took place more than a few years ago. How many had relapses? What other studies have been done since then? I have asked the company for further details but none were provided. This may be a case where the buyer should be cautious.

Alternatively, you can take this as support for the anti-cancer effects of calendula herb.

MGN-3 (BioBran, Noxylane)

This supplement was developed by Dr. Mamdooh Ghoneum, an Egyptian immunologist at Charles Drew University of Medicine and Science, Los Angeles. (I have not been able to find any information as to why it is called MGN-3, but I guess that the first two letters are Dr. Ghoneum's initials). Dr. Ghoneum has said that MGN-3 is, "the most powerful immune complex I have ever tested."

This supplement appears to have a marked effect in increasing natural killer cell activity as well as natural interferon and tumour necrosis factors. It is a potent immune system booster. MGN-3 can also be used to lessen the toxic side effects of conventional cancer treatment.

MGN-3 is made from the outer shell of rice bran which has been enzymatically treated with extracts from three different medicinal mushrooms: Shiitake, Kawaratake and Suehirotake. In Japan, these mushroom extracts have become the leading prescription treatments for cancer.

Articles on MGN-3 quote the story of a 58-year old multiple myeloma patient diagnosed in 1990. He underwent several months of chemotherapy following his diagnosis. Although his condition seemed to stabilize, his blood still showed markers for multiple myeloma eight months after chemotherapy. He then began taking MGN-3, and in less than 6 months, follow-up lab work showed no indication of cancer. In 1998, eight years after his initial diagnosis, he was still alive and cancer-free. He is the first patient known to have survived multiple myeloma, according to Dr. Ghoneum. *Everyone's Guide to Cancer Therapy* certainly concurs that surviving multiple myeloma is not common: "Almost all patients with multiple myeloma who do respond to chemotherapy will eventually relapse if they do not die of some other disease in the meantime."

However, the benefits of MGN-3 are not restricted to any particular cancer, nor to cancer alone. Dr. Ghoneum believes it is of immense benefit for a wide range of conditions - particularly for AIDS. Unlike other forms of cancer treatment, MGN-3 is a totally harmless substance and has no known side effects.

How much should one take? Normal capsule dose is 250mg. To maintain normal good health 2 capsules a day are recommended but for people with cancer the dose should be 12 capsules a day – 1,000 mgs with each meal for the first 2 weeks, reducing to 1,000 mgs a day thereafter. MGN-3 has been shown to be safe to use for long periods of time.

At the time of writing, the US distributor of MGN-3 was having difficulties with the FDA. However, this product is widely available from its Japanese source under the BioBran name. It is also available under the name Noxylane.

Microhydrin (Active H)

Microhydrin (also marketed in Europe as Active H) is a formulated chemical known technically as Flanagan Hydrogen Enhanced Silica. Patrick Flanagan, its creator, who is credited with over 300 inventions, says his inspiration was the fact that people living in northern Pakistan, who are renowned for their longevity and robust good health, benefit from drinking the glacier melt water that comes off the Himalayas. This water, loaded with hydrogen ions, is a powerful health product in its own right. Standard tap water, by comparison, robs the body of hydrogen ions and this results in disease. Microhydrin was developed specifically to provide a ready source of hydrogen ions. It is a mineral composed of silica, potassium and magnesium that has been saturated with hydrogen in such a way that, when consumed, it floods the body with electrons in the form of hydrogen ions. Albert Szent-Gyorgy, discoverer of vitamin C, called electrons 'the fuel of life'.

Microhydrin has shown a number of very powerful effects.

1. It makes the body more alkaline.

2. It is very effective at neutralising free radicals.

3. It assists the oxygenation of cells

4. It helps remove toxic wastes from cells.

5. It increases the electrical conductivity of the body's fluids.

Microhydrin's antioxidant properties have been used by athletes for its ability to increase substantially the oxygen levels of cells. It has been used by mountaineers to climb Everest without oxygen tanks. Anything that increases oxygen levels in cells is good for health and bad for cancer.

A new very much more powerful formula, Microhydrin Plus, is also available. Another product, Hydrogen Boost, appears to be the same but much cheaper.

Oncotox

Oncotox is a propriatory formulation that is well-known among anti-cancer therapists. Formulated by Dr. Donsbach, a well-known alternative cancer therapist who works at the Hospital Santa Monica in Tijuana, Oncotox is a liquid concentrate of five known anti-cancer agents: resveratrol, IP6, lactoferrin, arginine and curcumin. It can be bought from www.donsbach.com/cancer.htm

Phycotene

Phycotene is a complex of 17 different carotenoids and micro-nutrients extracted from Spirulina and Dunaliella algae. It was developed by Dr. Christopher and in research conducted at Harvard university on hamsters, it demonstrated powerful anti-cancer effects - so powerful that one of the researchers, Dr. Joel Schwartz, believes it to be a 100 percent cure for oral cancers in hamsters. No human studies have been done. It is also available as a cream. Source: www.rbclifesciences.com.

Poly-MVA

I've read people on line have used this as a part of their cancer program

Poly-MVA (the initials stand for Minerals, Vitamins and Amino acids) is a patented formulation consisting of the element Paladium which has been complexed with alpha lipoic acid and a number of other vitamins and minerals. It is claimed that this substance is a powerful re-energiser of cells, immune stimulant, chelator of heavy metals, detoxifier, and helps maintain alkaline pH levels. There are a number of convincing testimonials relating the benefits of Poly-MVA for a wide range of cancers, both on its own or as part of a parcel of alternative therapies. There is a big buzz

next page →

about this product and the only problem with Poly-MVA is the price. It is fairly expensive. For further information go to www.polymva.org

Seanol

Seanol is the registered trade name for an extract of marine algae that acts as a powerful anti-oxidant and anti-inflammatory agent. In animal studies, it has shown marked benefits for circulatory problems from blood pressure and arthritis to sexual dysfunction. It is also showing huge potential cancer benefits – it slows down tumour cell division. Testimonials support claims that it is a natural energy booster and that it clears brain-fog. It is sold under the trade name of Fibronol and fibroboost. See www.fibronol.com and www.lifesvigor.com/78100.html

Shark (and Bovine) Cartilage

It is not quite true that sharks don't get cancer - but it is almost true. Cancer is, it appears, very rare in sharks, skates, rays and other members of the elasmobranch family - which includes the dogfish. Why is this the case? According to Dr. William Lane, who has almost single-handedly pushed shark cartilage as a cancer cure, the answer lies in the fact that sharks do not have bones. Instead their skeleton is composed of cartilage which has no blood vessels or nerves. The cartilage contains a substance that inhibits the development of blood cells. Cancer tumours cannot grow without a network of blood vessels to nourish them. The development of a blood supply is known as angiogenesis. In normal adults the blood network is already well developed. Angiogenesis therefore occurs in adults for specific purposes - ovulation and pregnancy, healing of wounds and fractures - and the development of cancer tumours.

Others argue that if shark cartilage works it does so for other reasons. So the question is does it work? One well known experiment conducted in Cuba but followed by the documentary programme 60 Minutes had the following results. Of the original 29 terminally ill cancer patients, 9 died of their cancer within the first 17 weeks of the start of the trial and a further six died of other causes. 14 (48 percent) were alive and cancer free three years later. The protocol they were on was 60 grams/day for the first 16 weeks and then 20g/day thereafter. Apparently, taking 60 grams orally is not easy and some prefer to take it as a suppository.

Claims are also made for the anti-cancer effects of Bovine cartilage. Though why bovine cartilage is supposed to work it is hard to say – cows, after all, do get cancer.

The Chinese have been eating shark cartilage for centuries in the form of shark's fin soup. No Chinese wedding is complete without the shark's fin soup served half-way through the banquet. It is considered to be a rejuvenator and aphrodisiac. One billion Chinese can't be wrong - or can they? An unfortunate side effect of China's growing prosperity is therefore the likely extinction of the shark. In fact this potential impact on shark populations has provoked a great deal of anger against those promoting shark cartilage. However, for what appears to be a more powerful anti-angiogenesis agent, see bindweed (p. 227).

Shark Liver Oil and Squalamine

Squalamine is the first known example of a class of compounds called aminosterols, steroids chemically linked to an amino acid. It is found in   high concentrations in the livers of dogfish and sharks. It has shown   significant anti-cancer activity and is currently being studied at Johns Hopkins School of Medicine. Squalamine can be taken as a capsule. It remains unscathed through the digestive tract and appears to be able to cross the blood brain barrier, making it potentially effective against brain tumours. It works as an anti-angiogensis agent as well as being an immune system booster. Unfortunately, mercury pollution appears to be a problem with shark liver oil, and squalamine products and some investigation may be required to obtain a pure product.

BIOLOGICAL THERAPIES

Introduction

Our bodies have enormous powers of self-healing. The following therapies work by activating the body's own immune system.

Some of these need to be done, or certainly are best done, in a clinical setting, while others, such as homeopathy, can really be done only under the supervision of a trained and experienced professional. Some of these therapies will require you to make use of the services of an alternative clinic – in Mexico or Germany or elsewhere.

Here then are a number of therapies that have potential against cancer.

Coley's Toxins

One highly successful method of curing cancer has remained more or less sidelined for over a century. In 1888, Dr. William Coley discovered accidentally that a man had undergone what seemed like a spontaneous remission from cancer after suffering from a particular bacterial infection. Coley followed this lead and developed a number of toxins that he tested out on other patients, often successfully. His toxins were the by products of two bacteria: Streptococcus pyogenes and Serratia marcescens.

The toxins cause a transient but marked fever accompanied by chills and tremblings. Thus, Coley's toxins is a form of Fever Therapy (see below). A survey of 1,000 of Coley's cases showed a 45-50 percent five-year survival rate. The best results were with giant cell bone tumours where the five year success rate was 80 percent percent plus.

Amazingly, they were then put on the list of unproven treatments by the American Cancer Society, which, as we have seen, seeks to denigrate any non-drug-based therapy.

After decades in the wilderness, it seems Coley's toxins are once again being offered as a treatment by a number of clinics: www.sdiegoclinic.com, www.hufeland-klinik.de, CHIPSA.com, and Issels.com.

For instructions on how to make your own Coley's Toxins go to www.second-opinions.co.uk/coleys_instructions.html

Fever Therapy

One ancient Greek doctor said: "Give me the power to produce fever and I'll cure all disease."

Fever, of course, is not a disease itself but a sign. It is a symptom that the body is fighting off some disease. It is generally a very effective defence. Many invading bodies die when the body's temperature rises. Fevers should therefore be encouraged and not artificially cooled down. Fever therapy is simply the harnessing of this knowledge for the purposes of inducing high fever under clinical conditions. As we have seen, hyperthermia is a subject about which both alternative and orthodox doctors agree—fever is good for you.

An active fever can be induced by the injection of Coley's toxins, the drug Vaccincurin, or Pyrifer. A passive fever can be induced by placing the patient inside a cylinder and subjected to ultra-short waves. Modern medicine has developed other ways of interfering with the thermostats in the brain. They can even raise the temperature of selected portions of the body without affecting other parts. The object is to bring the patient to a state where his body tememperature is 105-108 degrees Fahrenheit for 60-90 minutes. This is the temprature at which cancer cells, but not normal cells, are damaged. During this treatment the body loses potassium and so a potassium-rich diet must be maintained: lots of bananas, rice and potatoes. Healthy cells are not damaged until temperatures rise to 109.5 degrees. Sometimes heat can be applied to a solid tumour through a heat probe placed inside the tumour.

This therapy can even be done at home. The patient can sit in a very hot bath and then lie in bed surrounded by blankets and hot water bottles for five or six hours at a time. For a detailed description of this process you should go to www.curezone.com/Schulze/handbook/hyperthermia.asp.

Passive fever treatments are usually done three times a week for as long as it takes. Fever can even be produced by hypnotic suggestion. Alternatively, one might stand with an onion under each armpit in the hot sun, as one early doctor instructed his patients.

Since fever is the body's mechanism for fighting off disease, it directly promotes the body's own defence mechanisms. Detoxifying enzymes and white blood cells are released into the system in higher concentrations.

Some doctors use this therapy in conjunction with chemotherapy - allowing them to lower doses by a third or a half.

It is not only cancer that responds to fever treatments. One doctor is supposed to have cured two epileptics by having them stand barely dressed for an hour in mid-winter. Then put into a hot bed to let them sweat it out. Syphilis was also cured by fever therapy before the discovery of penicillin. The means by which the cure was effected was to infect the syphilitic patient with malaria. The result? Regular and persistent fevers that took the body's temperature to 104 F or 105 F degrees for the necessary duration. Then the malaria could be cured with quinine. For this line of reasoning Professor Julius Wagner von Jauregg won the Nobel Prize in 1927.

Homoeopathy

Everyone's Guide to Cancer Treatment, 1994 edition, says this of homoeopathy: "Around 1850 homeopathy became popular. This was based on its Law of Similia, which states that disease results from suppressed itch ("Psora"). Over 3,000 drugs, each a highly distilled organic or inorganic substance, were used for cures."

This rather bizarre description does three things very effectively. It says first of all that this is a weird and wonderful delusionary system of treatment; secondly, it gives the distinct impression that it is based on some arcane and difficult system of belief and thirdly the use of the past tense strongly suggests that it no longer exists.

All of this is rather unfair to practising homoeopaths because homoeopathy as a system of treatment is alive and well.

Suspicion of homeopathy runs very deep among the orthodox scientific and medical communities. In 1986, the British Medical Association published a report entitled *Alternative Therapy*. In this report, the authors stated their commitment to scientific method in these words: "scientific method lays...emphasis on observation, measurement and reproducibility". They then went on to say: " It is simply not possible, for example, for orthodox scientists to accept that a medicine so dilute that it may contain not so much as one molecule of the remedy in a given dose can have any pharmacological action."

We can note here that the kind of medicine being described is homoeopathy and that it is being rejected not on the scientific grounds of observation, measurement or reproducibility but on the ideological grounds that they can't understand it - indeed they go on to state that homoeopathy is not 'consistent with natural laws as we now understand them.' There is no suggestion that the problem may be with their understanding of natural laws.

A proper scientific approach based on observation, measurement and reproducibility would approach the question differently. In my view, a true scientist would say: "I don't understand how this works but let's observe and measure and see whether it does in fact have reproducible results." In 1997, *The Lancet* published the results of a meta-analysis of 186 well controlled studies into homeopathy and the results appeared to demonstrate that homeopathy was significantly more effective than a placebo response. However, alongside the study were two commentaries that criticized the results on the grounds that it conflicted with our understanding of reality. As one writer noted: "...to put it starkly, there is no place in our current scientific theories for any possible mechanism by which homeopathy might work" (Dylan Evans, *Placebo*, p.149) – and yet, according to *What Doctors Don't Tell Us* (newsletter 25th May 2006), " In the past 24 years there have been 180 controlled, and 118 randomized, trials into homeopathy, which were analysed by four separate meta-analyses. In each case, the researchers concluded that the benefits of homeopathy went far beyond that which could be explained purely by the placebo effect."

But homoeopathy does in fact have a very clear theory - one which is also shared in certain circumstances by orthodox medicine - and one for which there is scientific support.

Homoeopathy was developed by Samuel Hahnemann as a result of his studies into the effects of quinine. Hahnemann discovered that quinine, in a normally healthy person, creates the same symptoms as malaria. Since it was also a very effective cure for malaria, Hahnemann came to the view that symptoms did not arise from the disease - instead they arose from the body's attempts to fight the disease. So, by exaggerating the symptoms, the disease can be more successfully fought off. Applied to other areas this perception has interesting corollaries. A cough should not be suppressed, rather it should be encouraged. After all the cough arises because the body is seeking to expel something. We should help it, otherwise whatever is causing the irritation will remain in the body. Similarly, a fever should be promoted rather than cooled, the heat of the body is fighting the infection so we should encourage it to stay hot and so help it defeat the infection sooner. This is a perfectly legitimate - and indeed commonly accepted - point of view even among some orthodox doctors.

So, Hahnemann followed this logic through to its inevitable conclusion and suggested that we should use drugs that promote the same symptoms as the disease - this is the real explanation of his Laws of Similars. This is a perfectly simple and reasonable theory and it goes against no laws of nature. Hahnemann made the following observation, "Most medicines have more than one action: the first a direct action, which gradually changes into the second (which I call indirect secondary action). The latter is generally a state exactly the opposite of the former."

We have discovered this effect in chemotherapy. It is the effect known as resistance. A drug attacks the flawed action of the body (i.e., the disease which is embedded in the cells of the body). The cells have a natural tendency to resist this action so they amplify the original effect. Eventually the drug's effects are neutralised. The doctor sees the drug no longer has an effect and withdraws it and the result is that the problem is much worse. Sometimes of course the drug is able to so overcome the cells' flawed action so that a cure is effected. The problem is in those cases where the drug is not effective. Its effects ultimately are to worsen the problem. Hahnemann therefore had the idea of reversing the process. If you reverse the action by amplifying the effect, the cells will resist this by diminishing the cause - and so working towards a cure. When the drug is removed the cells are working in the direction of health.

What causes problems for most people, however, is Hahnemann's discovery that dilute doses of drugs work better than strong doses. Now there is nothing in homoeopathic theory that predicts this effect. It is the result of an observation. Why it is true is not truly known.

Hahnemann, because of his suspiciousness of drugs, wished to use very dilute forms of drugs. He wished to interfere with the body's own healing power as little as possible. It therefore made sense to experiment and see how far he could dilute the drugs before they lost effectiveness. To his surprise, even though he diluted them to a level where, theoretically, they should contain not even one molecule of the original substance - a point known as Avogadro's limit - they were still effective.

Even Hahnemann had no explanation for it except to say it was a spiritual principle. Yet, there is interesting evidence that supports Hahnemann's observation. Researchers using nuclear magnetic resonance techniques can distinguish between homoeopathic dilutions and pure water. Other researchers have shown that homoeopathic dilutions rotate light passed through it in a different way than pure water. But these experimental results are still contentious.

But can homoeopathy help in the fight against cancer? Enid Segall, Secretary-General of the British Homeopathic Association, argues that it has.

"Homoeopathy is very supportive to patients with cancer... Certainly, there are people I talk to regularly who have been cured of cancer with the help of homoeopathy..."

Homoeopathy is a whole-person approach to treatment. It deals with the disease process rather than the disease product. This distinction remains, as we have seen, the great dividing line between alternative/complementary approaches and the orthodox approach. Homoeopaths ask how it is the cancer formed and what in the body's physical ecology is supporting the cancer's growth. In this, they are in agreement with naturopaths and, indeed, with almost every other practitioner of non-orthodox healing. This approach to cancer is largely ignored by the orthodox medical profession who are almost entirely focused on elimination of the disease product, in this case the tumour but have little interest in why the tumour developed in the first place.

Most homoeopaths recognise that removal of the end product - the cancerous tumour - may be a useful adjunct to their treatment. However, toxic chemotherapy is not one of the forms of treatment that they approve of.

Homoeopathic treatment is generally proposed as an adjuvant therapy (i.e., one that supports other, preferably natural, therapies). Indeed, homoeopaths are very cautious about their role in cancer treatment. There seems to be some resistance to the idea that homoeopathy alone would be effective in curing cancer, although they would not deny it was possible. But this generally defensive attitude to homoeopathy is a modern phenomenon. One hundred years ago, J. Compton Burnett M.D. wrote a short book entitled *Curability of Tumours by Medicines*. Here he gives a number of examples of cancer cases that he cured entirely by homoeopathic means.

Here is one case of breast cancer he describes successfully treating:

"(Jessie S) came on May 24th 1888 and informed me that two years previously a lump came in her left breast, which lump persists in growing, and pains. In the left mamma there was a tumour in its outer lower fourth, about the size of a lady's fist.... In three months,... the tumour was gone and thus far has not returned. Thuja 30, Acid nit. 30 and Sabina 30 were used in infrequent dose, and each given during one month by itself alone and in order named...I ought to have added to the foregoing narrative that I forbade salt and milk, other than in very moderate quantities and recommended a partial exclusion of meat from the patient's dietary as also the ovary irritating condiment known as pepper. Pepper, salt and milk are bad in cases of mammary tumours from ovarian or uterine irritation, and many of these tumours are of such origin."

Salt and milk have been widely implicated as nutritional no-nos, but pepper? Modern science comes to Dr. Compton Burnett's support. In 1980, researchers found that mice exposed to black pepper developed significantly more tumours - mainly liver, lung and skin. 77 percent of the pepper treated mice developed tumours compared with only 11 percent of the controls.

Here is another case quoted by Dr. Compton Burnett.

"On November 17th, 1887, I was requested to see a gentleman resident in London who was said to have a very large tumour in the abdomen and no efforts to cure it had been spared....There seemed no chance of a cure and an operation had been declared to be impossible....... the final outcome of all the deliberations was that it was cancer, or at any rate a tumour connected with the spleen which was or had become malignant in its nature, and that the result must necessarily be fatal...I think any practical physician or surgeon will concede that a more hopeless case to cure by medicines is hardly to be found...

"My own plan in difficult cases that seem so hopeless is to lay firmly hold of some point that may serve as a reasonable therapeutic starting point whence to carry out a cure. As a start there is here the traumatic element in the case that is positive, and my own favourite and well-tried anti-traumatic is Bellis Perrenis... Bellis Perrenis as an anti-traumatic and also Ceanothus Americanus as splenic, presented themselves to my mind, but which? Candidly confess, I thought the good man doomed but determined to try and save him, and not knowing which of my two remedies was the more likely to do something quickly, (for the case was urgent - patient's friends had already taken a last look at him as they thought) I gave the two in alternation, and much did I subsequently regret this double shot, for the use of two medicines at one time teaches next to nothing. Bellis o and Caenothus 1X were given in five drop doses every four hours in alternation....The result of this medication was that after a while patient could turn over in bed, then he could get in and out of bed by himself and in 17 days from beginning the medicine..[the] patient came to my West End rooms in a cab with his wife. [Dr. Burnett then describes various changes in the case and changes of medication] He did not need any subsequent treatment and he came to say goodbye on June 24th 1888. He had lost the tumour and the enlargement and induration of the lymphatic in the left side, and he was rapidly gaining flesh and strength...The cure was complete and permanent, which I know, patient turns up in my rooms every three months for his own and my satisfaction. Such a case is an oasis in the desert of a physician's hard life."

These anecdotal cases are quite sufficient to establish a sensible claim that homoeopathy on its own can be effective in treating tumours, even at a very late stage in development.

But Burnett agrees that it is vital for the homeopathic doctor treating cases of cancer to have the full range of othodox medical training to help the diagnosis of the ailments.

We don't, of course, know how many cancer cases Burnett failed to cure but he certainly felt that his success rate was better than anyone else's - and certainly justified greater attention being given to this medicinal   approach to cancer treatment.

Laurie Monteleone, a contemporary American homeopath, explains that there are three approaches that a modern day homeopath might take when treating a cancer patient. The first is to target the tumour by selecting remedies that match the symptom picture of the tumour and these remedies may even be injected at the site of the tumour. Another approach the homeopath might take is to use remedies that improve the effectiveness of the channels of elimination: kidneys, lymph, etc., so helping to detoxify the body. Finally, there is the classical approach which is to consider the whole constitution of the patient and prescribe remedies that strengthen the patient's mental, emotional, and physical state so allowing self-healing to occur.

One anti-cancer therapy that we may soon be hearing a lot more of is the use of homoeopathic nosodes. A nosode, here, is a remedy created directly from diseased tissue – which is then diluted in the same way that other homoeopathic remedies are. (Homoeopathic nosodes have been prepared against nearly every epidemic and endemic disease on the planet. (So forget the flu shot and get a flu nosode.) In the case of cancer, the nosodes are made from the blood of cancer patients who have recovered from cancer or who are in a state of remission. This blood is assumed to contain as yet unidentified immune substances whose healing power can be transmitted to other cancer patients.

The best known example of a cancer-fighting homoeopathic nosode is Carcinosin, created from breast cancer tissue. However, while it has clearly demonstrated to have anti-cancer activity in animal studies, it has not been as effective as had been hoped as a stand alone cancer cure. That does not mean, however, that it is not a useful weapon to be used along with other anti-cancer therapies.

More recently a new nosode, considered to be more potent than Carcinosin, is CarcinPLUS™. This was made from the blood of a woman who had cured herself of cancer using only natural supplements and spiritual healing. (The supplements she used to cure herself were: Proteolytic enzymes–Pancreatin 56,000 USP-units/300mg, Papain 492 FIP-unit/180 mg, Bromelain 675 FIP-unit/135 mg, Trypsin 2,160 FIP-unit/72 mg, Chymotrypsin 900 FIP-unit/3 mg, Rutosid 3 H2O(Rutin) 150 mg; Quercetin–134 mg; Turmeric– 800 mg; Coenzyme Q-10–300 mg; Folic Acid– 800 mg as L-5 methyl-tetrahydrofolate and Omega-3 fatty acids–1500 mg EPA/DHA.)

CarcinPLUS™ is available only by prescription. For more information go to www.homeopathyworks.com and www.phisinc.com

For anyone interested in reading more about homoeopathy, Dale Moss's article in the *Townsend Letter for Doctors and Patients*, June 2004 is worth reading (www.tldp.com).

Moss describes the work of Dr. Ramakrishnan, born into a family of homoeopathic practitioners who nevertheless had to watch two siblings die of cancer as neither responded to any of the homeopathic treatments they were given.

Dr. Ramakrishnan dedicated his life to developing a homeopathic cure for cancer. He described his work in his book that he co-wrote with Catherine Coulter, *A Homoeopathic Approach to Cancer*.

Ramakrishnan's first breakthrough was to abandon the classical approach. As Moss notes, "Classical homeopaths are taught that continued repetition of a single remedy, particularly at high potency, is unwise, because too frequent dosing might worsen symptoms being treated or induce undesirable new ones characteristic of the remedy."

However, Dr. Ramakrishnan took a very different approach, treating cancer as an acute emergency rather than a chronic disease. He chose therefore to give high potency remedies on a daily basis in multiple doses. An aggressive approach to an aggressive disease. Further, he gave his patients daily doses of one remedy for a week and then a second remedy for the following week. The first would be an organ specific remedy and the second a nosode such as Carcinosin. Using what he called his 'plussing method' He dissolved three pellets of each remedy in two small bottles each containing 11 teaspoons of distilled or spring water. The patient takes a teaspoonful of the solution every 15 minutes ten times a day over a 2 hour 15 minute period. Between doses, he shakes or stirs the solution slightly. At the end of the day's dosing, one spoonful of solution remains, which becomes the basis of the next day's dose after the patient refills the bottle with water. This process goes on for one week. The next week, the patient switches to the second bottle. This therapy must be followed for eighteen months or two years until the patient is stable and cancer-free.

Does it work? Dr. Ramakrishnan claims a cure rate for lung cancer of 58 percent; for oral cavity cancer 90 percent; for breast cancer (and prostate cancer) 80 percent; ovarian cancer 69 percent; and cervical cancer 68 percent. For leukemia and Hodgkin's lymphoma, his claimed cure rates are 54 percent and 77 percent, and for brain lesions his cure rate is 70 percent. These are extraordinary figures compared with what orthodox doctors achieve. Sceptics, however, have queried the reliability of these figures.

Dr. Ramakrishnan practices primarily in India, where homeopathy is widely available and respected, so patients will generally seek his treatment in the first place rather than when all else has failed. As Moss says: "Having an intact immune system greatly improves chances of successful treatment."

Dr. Ramakrishnan reports: "I now know which cases will do well and which will not. If I take a case at Stage II, I can be pretty sure of curing it. If the patient is at Stage I and the tumor is removed, then the patient follows with homeopathic treatment, he should do well for a long time, with no shocks or surprises in the case." Cancers at stages III and IV are more difficult to cure but Dr. Ramakrishnan has cured many seemingly hopelessly advanced malignancies.

Finally, Dr. Prasanta Bannerji, a homoeopathic doctor who works in Calcutta has found the combination of two widely available homoeopathic remedies have the ability to reverse glioma, a brain cancer, and is probably beneficial for many other cancers. This was demonstrated in a study led by Professor S. Pathak, Department of Molecular Genetics, at M.D. Anderson Cancer Center. In the abstract of results he states: "Fifteen patients diagnosed with intracranial tumors were treated with Ruta 6 and $Ca3(PO4)2$. Of these 15 patients, 6 of the 7 glioma patients showed complete regression of tumors."

This is the protocol they used:
1) Ruta 6c, in pills No.40, 2 pills a dose, two doses daily, morning and evening.
2) Calcarea Phos 3X, in tablets, 2 tablets a dose, two doses daily, noon and night.

The pills/tablets can be taken on tongue just suck it or chew it. If Ruta 6c liquid is taken, it will be Ok to take 1 dose = 2 drops in a spoonful of water.

For further information contact Dr. Prasanta Banerji at PBH Research Foundation, 10/3/1 Elgin Road, Calcutta - 700 020, India, Tel: +91 33 22472845, Fax: +91 33 22477275 pbhrf@vsnl.com

This is a protocol that appears to be remarkably powerful and of which further studies will be done. To keep abreast of discussions you can go to http://health.groups.yahoo.com/group/Ruta6

Ruta 6 and Cal Phos can be obtained from any online homoeopathic store. One easy to use site is www.abchomeopathy.com–the forums are particularly interesting and many other homoeopathic combinations are discussed.

Live Cell Therapy

In the 1930s a Swiss doctor, Paul Niehans, discovered that it was possible to cure people suffering from a number of conditions using intra-muscular injections containing a saline solution with a suspension of glandular cells. He became famous for offering this treatment as a rejuvenating therapy to film stars and others who could afford it.

One of his associates, Dr. Wolfram W. Kuhnau, adapted the technique and brought it to Mexico where it is offered by the Centre for Holistic Life Extension, www.extendlife.com. Kuhnau has since died but his work is being carried on by Dr. Luis Velazquez.

In this therapy, the foetal cells of the blue shark are injected into the cancer patient. The idea is that the stem cells will detect which area of the body is depleted of healthy cells and will work to

nem. There appears to be little danger in the procedure, which is not a stand alone cancer
 rtainly, cellular rejuvenation by means of live cell therapy has long established itself as a
via herapy.

However, anyone undergoing such treatments should be aware that German studies have linked the therapy with a number of fatal or otherwise serious allergic reactions. Dr. Kuhnau, however, insisted that his therapy was totally safe – and no evidence to the contrary has come to light. Cancer patients receive only three injections, once a week, then two others at three months and six months. Dr. Kuhnau is reported to have treated over 20,000 patients with this therapy over 40 years without any toxic effects greater than some fatigue.

One word of caution: It seams that the biggest therapy scams relate to rejuvenation, weight loss and other cosmetic issues. This is an area where the buyer needs to be particularly aware. A number of websites offer 'cellular therapy' or something similar in pill form. These are unlikely to be effective in themselves and are certainly not effective in relation to cancer.

Oxygen Therapy — rebounder, hyper baric chamber trampolene

"Remember, where cells get enough oxygen, cancer will not, cannot occur." Otto Warburg, 1966

We have already discussed the relevance of oxygen in relation to cancer. Cancers often, if not always, are generated by tissue conditions of low oxygenation. Also they tend to thrive in these conditions. Consequently, it has been proposed that cancer tumours can be effectively prevented and treated by increasing the oxygen levels of the blood and tissues.

The problem is exacerbated by poor food, poor eating practices - fast eating, overeating - lack of exercise, bad breathing techniques, rigid postures (caused by muscular tightness which in turn is the result of stress) - all of which worsen the problem. It is argued that good mental attitudes and meditation work partly because they lead to more relaxed and deeper breathing. The result is that the oxygen content of ill people is very much less than that of well people.

A number of ways of achieving higher oxygen levels in the body have been used - apparently with the sort of success that validates the theory.

Haematogenic Oxidation Therapy (HOT) (aka Ultraviolet Blood Irradiation [UVBI])

This is one variation. It is a simple and painless method of treatment. A quantity of blood, 100-200 mls, is taken from the patient and oxygen is then bubbled through it. The blood is then irradiated with ultraviolet rays for five to ten minutes then left to settle for an hour before being returned to the patient by drip. This is a form of ozone therapy. According to Issels, who used this therapy,

"[The blood] is: sterilized, normalized, regenerated and reactivated. Defense cells regain their aggressive capacity. Returned to the host, these cells can once more attack microbes and cancer-promoting viruses which are characterised by an anaerobic metabolism - making them unable to survive in the actively oxidised environment that HOT creates."

This treatment is generally done on a weekly basis for two to three months or for as long as it takes to achieve the desired result.

A similar treatment, called Recirculatory Haemo Perfusion, is available in Malaysia. See www.ozonehospital.com

Ozone is a very powerful form of sterilising and cleansing agent. The tap water in most continental European towns and cities is ozonated rather than chlorinated. Most German public swimming pools are also ozonated rather than chlorinated. Ozone is a strong anti-carcinogen while chlorine can under certain circumstances promote cancer. Ozone is a far more powerful agent than oxygen probably because it is highly unstable and releases a lot of energy as it transforms into ordinary oxygen molecules. In 1980, *Science* reported a study into the effects of ozonated air on cancer cells. The growth of the cancer cells was inhibited by 90 percent. Ozone has also been implicated in dramatic success stories against AIDS.

Ozone can be injected directly into the muscle, or it can be taken in simply by drinking ozonated water. Some patients have an ozone shower. This involves wrapping themselves naked in a plastic bag or jump suit and blowing in ozone from an ozone generator. It is also common to have humidified ozone applied either vaginally or through the rectum in short 30 second to one minute bursts. This allows a very rich ozone concentration to be absorbed by the blood in a painless non-invasive way.

While, in America, ozone is labelled by the FDA as a toxic gas, in Germany, ozone therapy is very common. Is it dangerous? According to author Ed McCabe, in one year, 644 German therapists reported using ozone therapy on 384,775 patients, a total of 5.5 million ozone treatments, and the incidence of negative side effects was 0.0007 percent.

Some people have claimed tumour-suppressing effects from simply drinking ozonated water. An ozonating machine costs about $175-$300 or more. There are a number of models on the market. It is a simple matter to pass ozone through water for a few minutes immediately before drinking it. A very useful site giving the whole Ozone story is http://www.geocities.com/ojoronen/OZ.htm

Hydrogen Peroxide

Another form of hyper-oxygenation therapy is through the use of hydrogen peroxide. Intravenous H_2O_2 was first used during the 1918 influenza outbreak. It then became widely used for a wide variety of viral and bacterial illnesses, with good results. In fact it was the preferred form of treatment until antibiotics arrived on the scene. The body itself manufactures hydrogen peroxide as a first line of defence against toxins and other invaders.

Hydrogen peroxide can be taken in many ways. Doctors prefer to give it in the form of an intravenous drip, and this is probably the best way when chronic illness is being treated. However, it can be taken at home in other ways. But it is important to note that hydrogen peroxide, in strengths greater than 3 percent, is dangerous. It can normally be bought in strengths of 3 percent or 6 percent from any chemist shop. Food grade hydrogen peroxide is 35 percent. This is the purest form and many advocates of hydrogen peroxide therapy urge users to use food grade H_2O_2 for internal use.

But it must be diluted! Undiluted H2O2 is extremely dangerous. A drop of food grade H2O2 on the skin will cause a white burn mark. Warning: Anyone with children should not have it around the house!

Hydrogen peroxide can be taken orally, it can be added to a bath, it can be rubbed on the skin or it can be gargled as a mouthwash.

Suggested quantities are as follows:

For oral use - either for drinking or mouthwash:

35 percent food grade: increasing daily from 1 drop to 25 drops in a glass of water. However, it appears that not many people can tolerate 25 drops in a glass of water.

6 percent solution: half a teaspoon to two teaspoons in an eight-ounce glass of water.

3 percent solution: should be mixed one part to five parts of water and then drunk slowly increasing from 1 to 5 ounces a day. This regime can be increased to 5 oz three times a day for a week at a time. This all depends on whether it is being taken for curative or maintence reasons. A maintenance programme of five ounces a day, two days a week, is recommended.

It should be noted that not everyone agrees that it should be taken orally. There are arguments about its effects on stomach acidity and bacteria. There is also the question of whether it can be properly absorbed into the bloodstream in this way or whether it is broken down to oxygen and water in the stomach.

Everyone says that hydrogen peroxide should not be persisted with if it is uncomfortable.

Dr. Donsbach of the Hospital Santa Monica argues that a preferable way of getting the peroxide effect without the discomfort is to take the same quantity of magnesium peroxide (magnesium dioxide) instead.

H2O2 should be taken on an empty stomach and at least an hour should separate its use and intake of vitamin C as they negate each other.

For use in baths: half a cup of food grade 35 percent or a pint of 3 percent can be added to half a bath of water. Soak for twenty minutes and it is claimed you will feel feel rejuvenated. To give an indication of how powerful the skin is as an absorbing organ, a 200 pound person can absorb up to four pounds of water from a twenty minute soak in a bath.

Counter-indications: Hydrogen peroxide should not be taken by anyone who has had a transplanted organ. Rejection of the organ may result.

There are also a number of fairly inexpensive oxygen-enhancing products on the market — the following two products combine dissolved oxygen, trace elements and other ingredients: Cellfood and Oxygen Elements Plus. Both of these are available on the internet and come with many testimonials as to their benefits. They combine two approaches – increasing oxygen levels of the body's tissue and the provision of trace minerals – both of which appear to be highly beneficial for   people with cancer.

Pharmaceutical Drugs and Oxygen

Synta Pharmaceuticals Corp. is currently researching a drug that they call STA-4783 which is designed to overload cancer cells with oxygen containing chemicals. It is apparently having some success in extending patient lives with minimal side effects. It is likely that other similar drugs will also come to market and it may be worth enquiring about this approach when discussing therapies with an oncologist.

Stabilised Oxygen & Sodium Chlorite

Serendipity is the word we use when we meet something entirely unexpectedly. You will remember that increasing oxygen to tissues is one way of impeding or even reversing cancer. One product that claims to deliver oxygen to the body is stabilised oxygen – which is, in fact a very dilute solution of sodium chlorite (not sodium chloride which is table salt). Now it is contentious whether or not this product actually does deliver oxygen in a way that is usable by the body. However, that does not mean that stabilised oxygen is useless. In fact it could, if utilised in the correct way, be one of the most powerful anti-cancer weapons in our arsenal.

What happens is that when you mix a few drops of sodium chlorite with vinegar or lemon juice, it releases chlorine dioxide — and, according to a 1999 statement by the American Society of Analytical Chemists, chlorine dioxide is the most powerful pathogen killer known to man!

Jim Humble, a mining engineer, discovered the powerful healing effects of stabilized oxygen while working in Guyana. He has since developed a more concentrated solution – which he calls, perhaps a little unwisely, Miracle Mineral Supplement. His story can be found at www.miraclemineral.org/part1.php.   This is an interesting read. The first half of the book is free, the second costs a few dollars (and you must read both parts because there are cautions that you need to know about – especially in relation to the dangers associated with the rapid unblocking of arteries). What emerges is that this substance is not only fast acting against malarial parasites and viruses – it also appears, in some cases at least,   to help eliminate cancer. What its mode of action is is not clearly understood. It may be that it attacks a viral or fungal cause of cancer or it may be that it reacts explosively in contact with cancerous cells, while remaining completely safe to normal cells.

Miracle Mineral Supplement is inexpensive and available from www.globallight.net . Humble recommends starting with a few drops and then slowly increasing by one drop a day until there is a feeling of nausea. This dose level should then be maintained until the nausea (a Herxheimer reaction caused by the body being temporarily overcome by toxins released by the healing or curative process) is no longer felt. It is then possible to continue increasing the dose.

Virus Therapy

It is known that certain viruses have an anti-cancer effect. People have been cured of their cancers after natural infection with measles and also with viral fowl plague, also known as Newcastle disease. In humans the only known side effect of Newcastle disease is 'pinkeye'. An Hungarian-America doctor Csatary has studied this type of therapy with herpes and influenza viruses with exciting results. Influenza viruses have shown a strong protective effect against a cancer-like disease in experiments with chickens. Since Newcastle disease has the best effects, a live virus vaccine, called the MTH-68 vaccine, has been developed. There are reports of clinical trials in Hungary, but I have not read of any results. Side effects are not, it seems, a concern. Most patients note subjective improvements in pain relief but clear results have not yet been released.

The common mumps virus has also shown anticancer effects in Japanese research. It has been particularly helpful in reducing oedema (swelling of lymphatic system - a common result of radiation), cancerous bleeding and pain. Tumour regression was also noted.

CANCER PIONEERS AND OUTCASTS

Introduction

It comes as a surprise to anyone researching the range of approaches to cancer just how many approaches have been developed – and we should note that many of these have been developed by scientists working within the fold of orthodox cancer research. Unfortunately, as soon as their ideas conflict with the interests of the major pharmaceutical companies, when they refuse to be bought out or relinquish control of their therapy, they find obstacles being put in their way. If they persist, then they are vilified and their work repudiated. They are called quacks or charlatans. Their research is misrepresented. If they work in America, then the FDA comes knocking on the door.

There are clear signs that the interests of the big pharmaceutical companies are being expressed in legislation and repressive legal action both in Europe and the U.S. – and it is very difficult to get any critical analysis of cancer research by the media. Nor do the so called quality press discuss the general failure of orthodox cancer treatments or give impartial consideration of alternative approaches. Our so-called 'free press' would appear to be firmly on the side of big money.

That then is the background to many of these alternative therapies that have been black-balled. Some of these approaches are patented and proprietary therapies that are quite expensive to access, and the success rates are difficult to determine. Others involve combinations of herbs, supplements, enzymes or other freely available products.

Taken together, the work of the men and women described below make us understand something of the dynamic of the world of cancer..

And, lastly, it must be clear to any impartial witness that the men and women whose work is discussed below are extraordinarily stubborn and well-intentioned and that the label 'charlatan', with all its associations of deliberate fraud, is totally misplaced in this context.

Beljanski

Professor Mirko Beljanski was born in Yugoslavia in 1923. He emigrated to France and became a research biologist at the renowned Pasteur Institute where he worked for almost 30 years on DNA and RNA biology. However, he was eventually forced to leave when his innovative ideas drastically conflicted with those of the Institute's director.

After leaving the Pasteur Institute, though under-funded, he continued his research and continued to publish scientific papers, most of which were in French. But his problems didn't end there. The Ministry of Health took him to court for practising medicine illegally. His lab was raided, equipment destroyed and documents seized. The court put a legal gag on him, forbidding him to speak about his products in public. This became public knowledge and caused a big scandal and there were street protests. But in the end nothing came of these protests and Beljanski was effectively side-lined. Beljanski, himself, died in 1998 after years of persecution for his innovative ideas.

One of Dr. Beljanski's key discoveries was that a part of the structure of DNA in cancer cells differs from normal DNA in that it contains some permanently open loops which have been d by carcinogenic substances interfering with the hydrogen bonding between the two strands oi ui.e double helix.

Once these permanently separated sections have formed they allow more carcinogenic substances to come between the two strands of the double helix and the result is to lead the DNA in the direction of uncontrollable replication, resulting in the rapid and uncontrollable growth of cancer cells.

Continuing his work he created his patented Oncotest that allowed him to ascertain whether or not a given chemical was cancerous or not. It also allowed him to work backwards and find substances that helped to strengthen the hydrogen bonds. He formulated a number of products based on certain herbs. Working with some sympathetic doctors he was able to show that his approach did result in cures. The website dedicated to his work www.beljanski.com contains a number of very persuasive testimonials for many different cancers, including brain cancers which are notoriously difficult to cure.

His formulated products are sold exclusively by a New York-based company, Natural Source www.natural-source.com

Two of the products have an anti-cancer effect and two are designed to support patients undergoing chemotherapy and radiation. The two anti-cancer products are called PAO V and ROVOL V. The first contains an extract from the herb Pao Pereira and the second from the herb Rauwolfia vomitoria. These are entirely non-toxic in normal doses to ordinary cells.

PAO V seems to be useful for all forms of cancer including brain cancers while ROVOL V seems best in hormone related cancers but not for brain cancers as the extracted molecule is too large to cross the blood brain barrier.

Interestingly, Beljanski believed that low doses of chemotherapy and radiation are necessary to break open the cancer cells to allow both PAO V and ROVOL V to gain access to the DNA, while high doses of vitamin C, iron, ferritin and vitamin B12 and possibly other natural substances interfere with PAO V. Iron of course is a no-no where cancer is concerned as cancer cells need it in large amounts for cell division.

Burton's Immuno-Augmentative Therapy

Lawrence Burton was not a medical doctor, his doctorate work was in experimental zoology. His specialisation was the relationship between the immune mechanism responses and cancer first in invertebrates, then in laboratory animals and finally, he took the perilous step, in humans. He graduated in 1955 and for the next eighteen years his life was that of any ordinary highly successful scientist. He published in the right places and had a solid job, eventually becoming the senior investigator and senior oncologist in the cancer research unit of the pathology department of St. Vincent's Hospital in New York - a post he held until 1973. It is significant that his cancer research was based in a pathology unit. He was working with real tumours not cell lines, with real patients not laboratory rats.

Burton's work led to the development of a serum that would, he argued, inhibit the growth of cancer tumours. This serum was derived from certain proteins found in blood: a tumour antibody, a tumour complement that activated the antibody, an antibody blocking protein and 'de-blocker' that neutralises the blocker. Burton, with an associate Frank Friedman, isolated these blood fractions. His theory was that when these four elements were in a balanced ratio in the blood, cancer cells would be routinely destroyed. His serum therefore was a way of bringing about this balance and so putting cancers into remission. He called this method of dealing with cancer 'Immuno-augmentative therapy'.

The way it works is that the patient's blood is analysed everyday for the ratio of these four proteins. A personalised serum is then made up to correct any deficiencies in the balance.

Burton's work came to the attention of Pat McGrady, who was an editor working for the American Cancer Society. McGrady later reported seeing Burton inject some mice with his tumour inhibiting factor. "They injected the mice and the lumps went down before your eyes - something I never believed possible." This demonstration was repeated in 1966 before a group of science writers. The result was a story in the *Los Angeles Times* under the headline: "15 minute cancer cure for mice. Humans next". Oncologists present at the seminar claimed that Burton and Friedman were tricksters.

That's when the problems began. Eventually Friedman gave up in disgust and Burton was forced abroad. Despite political interference, the Bahamian government allowed him to set up a clinic in Freeport.

There patients who could afford it made their way to be treated. There were frequent demands from establishment medical bodies for him to conduct clinical trials on his own - a request he spurned for the obvious ethical reason that, when dealing with the terminally ill, this is tantamount to murder.

In 1985 his clinic was summarily closed down. The NCI and other bodies had persuaded the Bahamian government that Burton's serum products were a source of hepatitis B and of AIDS. The evidence supporting this was of very dubious quality. None of Burton's 2,700 plus patients treated with hundreds of thousands of serum injections ever got AIDS. Many people are known to have caught AIDS and hepatitis B from blood transfusions but no blood transfusion service has ever been closed down. Impartial experts pointed out, also, that the serum had been put through the wrong test, a test that produces a large number of false positives.

As for hepatitis, only one of Burton's patients came down with this disease. Contrast this with the fact that, in 1976, in the USA blood transfusions caused 30,000 cases of hepatitis of which 3,000 were fatal. Even before the advent of AIDS, blood transfusions were not a good thing but the general public have not been kept fully informed of the dangers. According to Dr. John Wallace, "Blood should be regarded as a dangerous drug. There are now more than twenty viruses known to be transmissible by transfusion."

A sign reportedly seen in Dr. Burton's waiting room more or less sums it up: "Just because you're paranoid doesn't mean they aren't out to get you."

Outraged patients lobbied Congress and the result was that Congress ordered a study of alternative cancer therapies - a point that, in future years, may be seen as the year the tide turned in America in favour of non-orthodox medicine.

Dr. Burton was allowed to reopen his clinic, which continues the work, even though Burton himself died of heart disease in 1993 aged 67.

And does it work? One patient, Curry Hutchinson, diagnosed as having metastasized malignant melanoma of the lung, told the authors of a *Penthouse* article: "When I came here I was in a wheelchair. My mother had to care for me constantly. Two months later she was able to go home. I'm walking, jogging, swimming - alive...My improvements are unbelievable... Burton's critics claim there's no proof his therapy works. I disagree. I'm proof."

The Center offers a number of other experimental therapies using a number of vaccines. Its website www.immunemedicine.com is admirably clear and straightforward about the costs involved.

Burzynski's Antineoplastons

Dr. Stanislaw Burzynski is both a doctor and a biochemist who works in Houston, Texas. His discovery is that a group of peptides and amino acid derivatives occurring naturally in our bodies have the effect of inhibiting the growth of cancer cells. Burzynski calls these peptides anti-neoplastons.

In Burzynski's view there is a biochemical defence system which allows defective cells to be corrected through biochemical means. Antineoplastons are at the heart of this defence system. Blood samples from cancer patients show that they have only 2-3 percent of the amount typically found in a healthy person.

Burzynski's method simply requires the injection of antineoplastons into the blood stream. The result is tumour shrinkage and even remission. Often this occurs in a matter of a few weeks. Burzynski has been treating patients since 1977. He does not claim to be able to cure all cancers in all patients - but there is strong evidence that many are cured. In one study of 20 patients with astrocytoma, a highly malignant brain cancer, mostly in an advanced stage, four went into early remission, two showed partial remission, and ten showed stabilisation (i.e., tumour regression of less than 50 percent). Some of these subsequently went on to complete remission.

For a long time, Burzynski was considered to be a quack and a charlatan by the FDA and the American Cancer Society but despite decades of extremely unfriendly attention, including the invasion of his clinic and seizure of patient records, he remains very much in business. He has played the system well and is now running over 20 FDA-controlled clinical trials at his clinic.

Burzynski is phlegmatic and considers all this harassment to be normal: "Most medical breakthroughs have happened because there was some lack of suppression by the supervisors of people doing some innovative work."

Burzynski's website is coy about the cost of his treatment. For further information go to: www.cancermed.com. However, a website has been set up by ex-patients, and this contains many persuasive testimonials. See www.burzynskipatientgroup.org

The Hulda Clark Cure

The Clark cure, put forward by Hulda Regehr Clark, is very radical. Indeed, if she is right, the entire cancer research industry can switch off its lights and go home. It is her view that cancer is caused by a parasite - the human intestinal fluke. This causes no major problems in the gut where it normally resides but by some means as yet unknown - but associated with the presence of propyl alcohol - it can move to other organs where it starts creating problems. The problem it creates, if it gets to the liver, is cancer. Her test for cancer is to test for the presence of the marker Ortho-phospho-tyrosine (OPT).

"All cancer patients (100 percent) have both propyl alcohol and the intestinal fluke in their livers. The solvent propyl alcohol is responsible for letting the fluke establish itself in the liver. In order to get cancer, you must have both the parasite and propyl alcohol in your body."

Just as the cause is simple, so is the cure that she proposes: black walnut tincture, wormwood, and cloves. The first two kill adult and developmental stages of over 100 parasites. The cloves kill the eggs. They are to be taken as follows:

1. Black walnut tincture: This should be taken in a glass of water four times a day. Start the first day with one drop each time and increase the dose by one drop a day until on day 20 you are taking 20 drops in water four times a day. Then reduce to 20 drops once a day for 3 months - and then reduced to 30 drops once a day, two days a week. It should be taken on an empty stomach (viz., half an hour before a meal).

2. Wormwood: this herb is made from the leaves of the Artemisia shrub. It is also available from herbalists as part of a combination of herbs. It should be taken once a day before the evening meal increasing daily from one capsule to fourteen. Then maintain this level twice a week forever. As we have seen, studies have shown that wormwood on its own has demonstrated anti-tumour effects.

3. Cloves: obtain whole cloves and grind them up. Cloves that have already been ground do not work. Fill capsules (preferably, size 00 but any vitamin capsules will do) with the ground cloves and take three times a day before meals building up from one capsule a time to three capsules a time. Continue until day 10 and then reduce to 3 capsules once a day for three months - and then just twice a week forever.

Dr. Hulda Clark is a Canadian physiologist (not a medical doctor) who published details of her cure with 100 case studies in her book: *The Cure for All Cancers*. She believes that many, if not most, ailments, from asthma and AIDS to heart disease and schizophrenia, are the result of parasitical infection, and the formula she gives above is one that she believes will rid the body of many of these. She accepts that other formulas will also work. But, in her view, the parasite is only half the problem, the other half is the propyl alcohol. Most people can process this effectively, and so it causes no problem whatsoever. But people developing cancer have an impaired ability to do this. For this, she blames the presence in the liver of aflatoxin B. This is a known carcinogenic substance found in mouldy food.

One way to deal with the problem, she argues, is to eliminate propyl alcohol from the system. Unfortunately it is a common ingredient used in the food and cosmetics industries. Check the items in your bathroom and you will find most contain one of the following ingredients: propanol, isopropyl alcohol, isopropanol and so on. Even if not listed, she claims that propyl alcohol is so commonly used for cleaning industrial equipment that it will very likely be present in minute quantities in a wide range of modern retail goods - but for those people with an impaired ability to break it down, even these quantities are sufficient to cause cancer. She particularly fingers hair and cosmetics products, sugar, carbonated soft drinks and even bottled water, fruit drinks. and vitamin supplements. She makes an exception for vitamin C as this helps the liver to break down propyl alcohol by directly attacking the aflatoxin.

Her four point plan for regaining health is simple but extreme: remove every unnatural chemical substance from your mouth, from your diet, from your body and from your home.

Clark has become very famous and is probably number one on the FDA's ten most wanted list. And there are grave doubts about her facts. Scientists point out that there is no evidence at all that the human intestinal fluke is present in epidemic quantities in the USA; quite the reverse. They dispute the validity of her test for the presence of cancer and point out that very few if any of her claimed cures are in any way validated independently.

My own view is that Clark has definitely not satisfactorily proven her case, but it may be that she is on to something – and as we have noted, wormwood has demonstrated anti-cancer activity. I would invoke the risk-benefit analysis and argue that since the herbal part of her cure is cheap and not harmful we can happily do this – but only as an add-on to a more substantially supported therapeutic regime.

Dr. Govallo and VG-1000

Valentin I. Govallo, M.D., PhD, Director of the Laboratory of Immunology in Moscow and author of 290 scientific articles and 20 books, including *The Immunology of Pregnancy and Cancer* (1993), is clearly no charlatan. His credentials are scientifically impeccable. But the results of his labour, a substance that is almost wholly non-toxic–it causes some slight fever and chills when first injected – and which cures over 75 percent of late-stage cancer–has been totally ignored by the leading medical journals in America. And the whole world is influenced by what the leading American medical journals choose to publish.

Govallo's perception is that the biochemical way in which cancer develops in the body and protects itself from the body's immune system seems to bear a striking resemblance to how an embryo protects itself from being attacked as a foreign object during pregnancy. Govallo had the brilliant idea of using a placental extract to immunize the patient against the foetus-like cancer. This is the basis of his anti-cancer vaccine which he has called VG-1000.

According to Govallo, in human trials, he has achieved a whopping 77.1 percent five-year survival rate–remember, these were all so-called terminal cases, no longer responsive to surgery, radiation or chemotherapy. Unfortunately, Govallo admits that "it is not exactly clear how the placental extract effect works."

And equally unfortunately, no one in the American cancer establishment is interested in following up on this. Joseph M. Miller, M.D., who has written the only review of the treatment to date, wrote: "If the results are accurate, this innovative approach could be one of the greater discoveries of the twentieth century."

VG-1000 is a non-toxic, organic product that doesn't so much attack the cancer cell as simply turn it off. VG-1000 appears to be most beneficial in treating carcinomas and melanomas, and it is also indicated for some sarcomas and in leukemia. Patients who have been subjected to chemotherapy or radiation tend to respond more slowly to VG-1000 as they have a depressed immune system. However, patients who have had neither radiation nor chemotherapy respond well. VG-1000 treatment is available at The Immuno-Augmentative Clinic in Freeport, Grand Bahamas and also CHIPSA - Center for Integrative Medicine in Tijuana, Mexico (www.CHIPSA.com).

In Europe, VG-1000 can be obtained from Autobiologics BV and from the affiliated organization, The Placenta Research Foundation. Director William H. van Ewijk, M.D. (MA) Ph.D., Autobiologics BV will make VG-1000 available to qualified doctors only. For more information contact Autobiologics BV, JOL 24-19, 8243 GN Lelystad, The Netherlands. Tel. +31 (0) 320 247 326 Fax. + 31 (0) 320 247 327. autobiologicsplacenta@wxs.nl

Dr. Joseph Issels

Dr. Joseph Issels, working in Bavaria, and basing his approach on Gerson's work, established what he called a whole-body therapy to deal with the whole-body problem of cancer. The therapy is in fact a combination therapy including ozone/oxygen treatments, diet, fever therapy and even low-dose chemotherapy and radiation.

For Issels the body has four interrelated defence systems. First, there are the lymphocytes and antibodies that are normally considered to be the entire immune system. Secondly, there are the eliminating and detoxifying organs: liver, kidneys, skin and intestine. Thirdly, there are the friendly bacteria in the epithelial tissues of the body and lastly there is the connective tissue where organic salts are stored and toxins are digested or bound chemically to make them inert. He also made a big point of insisting that infected teeth and tonsils should be removed - including all teeth filled with mercury amalgam and teeth whose pulp has been removed through root canal treatment. He believes that these impair the immune system.

External observers have calculated that 17 percent of his patients go on to long-term remission. Since most of them were diagnosed as terminal when they arrived at his clinic, this is an excellent result. The Issels Clinic currently claims an amazing overall 87 percent success rate with early-stage cancers of all kinds.

But Issels was not left free to pursue his own therapies. He was blacklisted by the American Cancer Society in 1958. In 1960 he was arrested on charges of fraud and imprisoned without bail in a cell block containing only convicted murderers. This attempt to intimidate him eventually failed. After five years of court case after court case He was finally acquitted of all charges. But in the meantime his clinic was forced to close.

In 1970, a documentary about his work was made by the BBC but the scheduled release of the programme was first cancelled under pressure from the British medical establishment then, in a response to criticism over censorship, eventually rescheduled. A re-edited version was aired. Nevertheless, great interest was aroused by the programme, so much so that the medical establishment moved more firmly to discredit Issels. They sent a five man team to Issels' Clinic. They arrived in January 1971 to do their study. Two of the team were outspoken opponents of Issels, and only two of them could speak German. They spent three and a half days at the clinic. On their return they rushed out a report that concluded his treatment was ineffective. One critic of the report had this to say: "The sum of the team's arguments that Dr. Issels cures are not really cures boils down to this - 'we cannot accept the cures because cancer is incurable'...I hope readers will not have missed the logical imperfection in the team's reasoning."

The loss of business and the constant weight of pressure - nuisance calls, refusals by medical journals to accept advertisements, internal criticism from his own staff, tampering with postal deliveries of medicines - eventually forced Issels to close his clinic in 1973.

Issels work is being continued at the Hufeland Klinik, Bismarckstrasse, Bad Mergentheim, Germany, Phone: (49) 7931 8185 and at the Issels Clinic in Tijuana Tel: 888-447-7357 from the USA and Canada, 001-480-585-6804 from Europe/Asia. Email: informationcenter@issels.com. www.issels.com

William Kelley

Kelley is the odd one out in this company in that he wasn't a doctor, cancer researcher or a naturopath. In fact he was a dentist from a small town in Texas who in the early 1960s discovered that he had terminal stage pancreatic cancer. People generally don't survive long after receiving such a diagnosis. Kelley lived another 40 years.

He cured himself by a combination of diet, detoxification and, most important of all, the taking of pancreatic enzymes. According to Kelley, all cancers are really only a single disease caused by a deficiency of proteolytic, protein digesting enzymes (i.e., pancreatic enzymes–particularly trypsin and chymotrypsin).

In his theory, cancer arises when three events coincide. First there is the presence on an ectopic germ cell, secondly there are female sex hormones, and thirdly there is a deficiency of active pancreatic enzymes. In this theory, the cancer develops in the same way that an embryo develops. This is known as the trophoblast theory and it has a long and distinguished history. But back to Kelley. In his view, cancer progresses because there is a lack of cancer-digesting enzymes in the body. The solution, therefore, is to get pancreatic enzymes to the place where the tumour is growing, in a concentration that is sufficient to stop the cancer's growth, but not too high as that would cause the tumour to break down too rapidly and that in turn would release toxins into the body faster than the body can cope with. What is required is a slow regular decrease in the tumour's growth. In addition, he recommended physical manipulation of the body (chiropractic, osteopathy and so on) and prayer.

An interesting side note on the possibility that cancer might be curable by chiropractic: Hanna Kroeger, now more famous as the founder of a respected herbal brand, claimed to be able to stop Leukemia in less than one week by making an adjustment to the tail bone. She apparently did this on hundreds of people. This may sound mad but we should remember that bonesetting has a long history and was associated with curing disease, not simply mending bones. Chiropractic has managed to develop as a profession in the last 120 years despite enormous pressure from established medicine – it must have something going for it. For more information go to www.kroegerherb.com and buy her short book: *Free Your Body of Tumors and Cysts*.

Returning to Kelley's dietary regime, this was at first simple but then became extremely complex, based on a theory of metabolic types.

It would be nice to say that he grew old to be a wise healer. Sadly this was not the case. He did not have the personal resources finally to withstand the witch hunt that was launched against him, and he ended his days as a clinically paranoid racist. He became convinced that the world's supply of pancreatin – the main element of his cancer programme had been deliberately contaminated with a deadly bacteria by the US government. Dr. Nicholas Gonzalez, who first came across Kelley's work when he was a medical student, studied the records of those who had followed the Kelley programme and found that of his first 139 patients, representing people with all types of cancer, and all of whom had come to Kelley as a last resort for whom no further conventional treatment could be offered, 93 percent were effectively cured.

Dr. Gonzalez has taken this work forward and adapted it. He is now the leading proponent of the Kelley approach. He recommends up to 45 grams of pancreatic enzyme a day taken in a number of equal doses. He offers at his clinic a rather expensive therapy, but, as Kelley himself said, there is only one person who can treat a person's cancer, and that is the person who has the cancer.

For further information contact www.dr-gonzalez.com and/ or www.drkelley.com. Pancreatic enzymes are discussed on page 201

Dr. Catherine Kousmine's Combination Therapy

Catherine Kousmine (1904 -1992) was a Swiss-trained doctor of Russian origins who from a very early age felt strongly that dividing the body into specific areas of expertise was the wrong way to focus on the question of health. She therefore became a GP in order to work with whole body solutions.

Early on in her career two distressing failures to treat children who had cancer lead her to conduct her own small-scale animal research at home. She found that through dietary means she could protect animals that she subsequently injected with tumour extracts. She would inject them and they would reject the cancerous growths that were created. Despite enormous professional pressures and public criticism, she persisted in using her methods with those patients who took responsibility for their own treatment. She publicised her work in a number of books that have been translated from the French into Italian and German, but, interestingly, never into English. Her success rate? While no statistics are provided, and the picture is obscured by the fact that many if not most of her patients had already undergone surgery and radiation before coming to her, nevertheless, according to one doctor, 'Survival rates are much higher than what could be expected.'

In her view cancer was caused by a number of factors, one of which was stress, which she believed had a measurable impact on the micro-organisms in the body. Another cause is a diet which is deficient in vitamins, minerals and trace elements. In her view surgery and radiation might be acceptable as a means of getting rid of the existing tumour but they would not result in a cure for the cancer if the terrain in which the cancer had developed remained unchanged. And changing the terrain is not something that surgery or radiation can address.

Kousmine eventually established a system of curing cancer that rested on what she called the five pillars.

1. Diet: Raw fruits and vegetables, whole cereals, the Budwig Protocol (flaxseed oil and cottage cheese [to which Kousmine added: the juice of a whole lemon, a mashed ripe banana or honey, and whatever fruits are in season])–no meat.

2. Intestinal Health: She recommended regular fasts and enemas. A clean colon was, for her, of vital importance. She suggested daily enemas.

3. Promoting a positive alkali/acid balance: To achieve tissue pH to 7.5, she recommended the use of potassium and magnesium citrate.

4. Use of supplements: The supplements she advised were: Vitamins B (no B12), E, C (high doses), selenium, zinc, polyunsaturated fatty acids (capsules of evening primrose oil and fish liver oil), and magnesium salts.

5. Use of some low-level chemotherapy: She recommended Endoxan (2x100mg pills a week).

Central to her therapy is the health of the liver. This can be promoted by means of relaxation, moderate sport, exercise, fresh air, sunbathing, sleep, a good diet of raw fruits and vegetables and good intake of vitamins. Liver health is compromised by stress (worries), lack of sleep, fatigue; poor diet, constipation, chronic and recurrent infections, too much alcohol, smoking and too many drugs, even simple pain killers such as ibuprofen, heavy foods (fats, eggs, chocolate, milk and any food treated with chemicals).

Kousimine was an important figure in Continental Europe and it is surprising that her ideas have not received a wider audience in the English-speaking world, where she remains virtually unknown. For further information (in French) see www.kousmine.com

Gaston Naessens and 714-X

Gaston Naessens was born in Roubaix, France in 1924 but has done most of his work as a pioneering scientist in Canada. Among his inventions was an extremely powerful light microscope – he called it a somatoscope - which used ultraviolet and laser technology and which was capable of very powerful magnification - up to 30,000X - and which, unlike any other microscope before (with the exception of that developed by Rife) enabled the viewer to examine living tissue. Unfortunately for Naessens the electron microscope, which is capable of even higher levels of magnification, was developed soon after. Nevertheless his invention remains the most powerful microscope capable of looking at fresh, living and moving, unstained blood and tissues. Naessens too believed that disease was caused by a microbe that was capable of changing size and at a certain time in its life cycle was a bacteria and at another was a fungus.

His contribution to cancer was the development of 714-X which is now available at a number of centres, is inexpensive and by all accounts very effective. However, it took years of pressure and persecution for practicing medicine illegally before it became available.
714-X? It sounds like a new jet fighter but is in fact a derivative of camphor, with an extra nitrogen molecule attached, combined with organic salts (according to one source, 714X contains "a mixture of camphor, ammonium chloride and nitrate, sodium chloride, ethanol, and water"). This substance was developed by Naessens on the theory that cancer cells require high levels of nitrogen. In order to protect themselves from the immune system the cancer cells release a substance which he calls co-cancerogenic K factor, or CKF for short. 714-X neutralises this factor. This prevents the cancer cells from being able to hide from the immune system. The result is that the cancer tumour is gradually eliminated from the body by the body's own natural defence system.

714-X is administered by injection into the lymphatic system, usually in the groin area. A course of daily injections for 21 days is followed by a 3 day rest and then another 21-day cycle is begun. This continues for as long as necessary but for cancer patients this usually means 7-12 cycles. AIDS patients are also benefiting from this treatment.

One patient, a Mr Ganong, receiving this treatment found that his tumour shrank so much after two months that his surgeon decided to operate. When he went in, he found the tumour: "had been changed into an apparently non-threatening jelly-like mass he'd never seen the likes of before" according to his son (quoted in Walters, 1993). Another patient diagnosed with metastatic prostate cancer in 1977 was still cancer free in 1989 after using 714-X

Other doctors using this substance report very impressive results. Although it is administered through injections, the entire course is relatively inexpensive.

Information on doctors using this treatment and/or treatment with 714-X is available from the following organisations:

1. Centre d'Orthobiologie Somatidienne de l'Estrie (C.O.S.E.), 5270 Fontaine, Rock Forest, Quebec J1N 3B6, Canada, Phone: (819) 564 7883

2. Canadian Institute of Alternative Medicine, 715 Bloor Street West, Toronto, Ontario M6G 1L5, Canada, Phone: (416) 530-0473

Dr. Hans Nieper

Hans Nieper, 1928-1998, was a German doctor who achieved a great reputation as a natural healer. Being German meant that he was able to carry on his cancer work untroubled by the American medical establishment. At one time, he found himself in the interesting situation of treating Ronald Reagan's cancer while at the same time being persecuted by the FDA.

Nieper has sometimes been dismissed as a dreamer and not a serious scientist. Nevertheless there has been little investigation of his contention that mineral orotates, a kind of salt, are effective in transporting minerals such as potassium and magnesium into cells – particularly cancer cells – and that this helps to maintain cellular health. In his view, the taking of magnesium orotate would have the effect of reducing the recurrence of cancer by four fifths. "The rate of new cancerous diseases with long-term magnesium orotate therapy is perhaps less than 20 percent of the frequency otherwise expected, at least for the first 10 years of the observation period."

He was an early promoter of bromelain, the pineapple enzyme, as a way of dissolving the protective shield around cancer tumours that protects them. He also promoted the use of iridodials (see p. 248).

Dr. Matthias Rath

Dr. Rath is the new star of the alternative medical universe. He worked for some years with Linus Pauling and since Pauling's death has taken on his mantle as the world's leading exponent for vitamin C. He is a research scientist.

Rath's answer to cancer seems very simple. According to him, all metabolic disease involves a collagen dissolving process. Collagen, if you remember, is the substance from which all cell walls are formed. The key building blocks for healthy collagen production are a plentiful supply of vitamin C, L-Lysine and L-Proline. These also block the enzymes that do the work of dissolving the collagen and maintaining proper cellular health. Take these three supplements, increasing steadily until you are taking as high a dose as can be tolerated – and the cancer's growth will be checked, even reversed.

A final component of his protocol for cancer is a substance that is found in green tea, a polyphenol catechin known as epigallocatechin gallate (EGCG)– this is available in pure form only for the purposes of laboratory based cancer research but it is a significant component of green tea extract.

A full explanation of his cellular medicine and cancer is available at his website as a free e-booklet. See www.health-foundation.org

If Rath's answer to cancer is considered to be too simple a programme, we might respond by asking: why shouldn't the answer to cancer be simple? The answer to scurvy was simple (take vitamin C); the answer to beri-beri was simple (take vitamin B1). Both of these were metabolic diseases that had complex symptoms that led eventually to death. Both were easily and quickly cured once the answer was discovered. Why should cancer not be the same?

Dr. Wassil Nowicky and Ukrain

Dr. Nowicky is another very stubborn research scientist, based in Vienna, who has persisted in the face of great opposition to develop, test and promote his answer to cancer: Ukrain, named after his native country. For the last twenty or more years he has been in the absurd position of being firmly backed by the Austrian Ministry of Science and blocked at every turn by the Austrian Ministry of Health.

Ukrain is a patented formula which combines a potent herb – greater celandine – with a chemotherapeutic drug called thiotepa (thiophosphoric triaziridine). It has been well studied – mainly in Germany, Belarus and Ukraine - and in Ralph Moss's words: "What makes Ukrain so unusual is that this forced marriage of herb and drug yields a compound that is lacking in toxicity in normal cells. Yet it seems to have a strong affinity for killing cancer cells." It is delivered by intramuscular injection.

The US National Cancer Institute tested it on 60 different cancer cell lines, and it was 100 percent effective against all. Unfortunately, it has not been quite so successful in real cancer cases though results are still extremely impressive. Dr. Wassil Nowicky, its developer, himself claims that in cases of terminal stage cancer it can be 30 percent successful, and 90 percent successful in early stage cancers.

So why isn't it being widely used in the cancer hospitals of the world? That is a question that the medical authorities should be asked – and indeed should be asking themselves. Details of research and a record of the obstacles that have been put in the way of Dr. Nowicky can be found at his website at www.ukrin.com.

Ukrain is a medium to long-term treatment which has been shown to be very effective against all kinds of cancer. It has even cured cases of terminal-stage melanoma. It is administered by a doctor ideally in a clinical setting supervised by a doctor—however, patients can buy it directly.

Curiously, or perhaps not so curiously, the American Cancer Society has shown no interest in this therapy.

Ukrain is available only from the clinic of its inventor, Dr. J. Wassil Nowicky, and is produced by his company JW Nowicky Pharmaceuticals. Imitation products are apparently available on the internet but should be avoided. According to Nowicky, the alkaloids in the milk of greater celandine vary in quality depending on what time of the year they are harvested. Only he knows when to collect the herb. For further information contact Dr. Wassil Nowicky at nowicky@ukrin.com

Alternative Cancer Clinics

While some cancer clinics offering non-orthodox therapies appear to be able to operate in the USA, Germany, France, England and elsewhere, very often they find themselves blocked or harassed. This is particularly true of the USA. The result has been that a number of clinics have gone off-shore – mostly to the town of Tijuana, Mexico – a town conveniently located just across the US-Mexican border close to San Diego. Often there will be a presence of sorts in the USA. For example Dr. Vincent Gammill has offices in Solana Beach, near San Diego, California, registered as the Center for the Study of Natural Oncology (www.natural-oncology.org), where, as he says: "Primarily we just research and problem solve." However, he is associated with the San Diego Clinic in Tijuana (www.sdiegoclinic.com). I mention this, as Dr. Gammill is very approachable and has a lot of fans. However, there are many other clinics, many of which also have their supporters. There are far too many to list here, but anyone looking for one will find lists of clinics at the following internet links:

www.cancure.org/directory_mexican_clinics.htm
www.cancure.org/directory_clinics_outsidepercent20US.htm
www.cancertutor.com/Other/Clinics.html
www.cancercure.ws/clinics.htm
www.annieappleseedproject.org/gerclinstor.html

ENERGY MEDICINE

Introduction

We have become so used to thinking of medicine in terms of pills, capsules, tonics, injections and so on that it may come as something of a shock (to make a rather obvious pun) to learn that there is a growing interest in the use of magnetism, electricity, colour spectrum radiation and other forms of more subtle vibrational energy as tools for healing – specifically for cancer.

While some of these ideas may be uncomfortably new-agey, others are grounded in good old electrical engineering and electromagnetic science. It is a highly controversial area and has a long way to go before it gains popular, let alone professional, acceptance.

Let's start at the beginning. It is generally accepted that 'radiation', which is another way of saying energy of various frequencies from an external source, can positively or negatively affect the body. Radiation may manifest different wave patterns – sine, saw-tooth and square waves. These have different biological effects with the more normal sine wave radiation being the least effective for medical purposes – possibly because it is too smooth. These vibrations vary in force from extremely weak subtle energies, such as the energies that emanate from a lump of crystal salt, to powerful penetrative energies such as X-rays. Light too is a form of energy. Any specific energy differs from another specific energy in one way only – its wavelength.

The second fact we need to understand is that everything, every single thing on the planet (and in the universe), has a unique vibrational signature that defines it.

Then there are the magnetic fields. Whenever there is a difference of polarity between two points we have a flow of energy and when we have such a flow one of the results is an electromagnetic (EM) field. Given that every atom contains positively charged protons and negatively charged electrons, we see that even single molecules must emanate an EM field. The same is true at the cellular level and beyond. The body itself has an electrical-magnetic field, which is the combined field of every single living cell in the body. Also, of course the world as a whole has a magnetic field..

In this chapter we are going to explore how energy has been used in healing..

Early Pioneers
Nicola Tesla and the Tesla Coil

Probably the first successful attempt to build a healing machine was by Nicola Tesla. Tesla was born in Smijlan, Croatia in 1856 and immigrated to the United States in 1884. He worked for a time as Thomas Edison's assistant but then, after falling out with his boss, he became Edison's greatest rival.

Tesla was a true genius—many of whose inventions have subsequently been attributed to others. Perhaps the most important of his intellectual bequests was the fact that he invented AC electricity. To him also we owe neon lights, speedometers for cars and even the world's first hydro-electric plant located at Niagara Falls.

But our interest in Tesla here is the fact that he developed a machine – the so-called Tesla Coil which produces energy waves which he insisted had the effect of energizing him and helping him to work long hours without getting tired. He persuaded his friend Mark Twain to experience it, and he too enjoyed the benefits - until apparently he found himself afflicted with a sudden bout of diarrhoea.

The Tesla coil produces pulsed EM fields that radiate broadband, wide spectrum energy. As with the Rife machine (see below), a little goes a long way. He found that an hour in front of the machine was too long.

He was not alone in thinking he had invented something useful. This was a time when the controlling bodies of American science had not built up their political muscle to the extent they have today. Doctors and inventors felt free to experiment and to comment honestly on what they saw. On September 6, 1932, at a seminar presented by the American Congress of Physical Therapy, held in New York, a Dr. Gustave Kolischer announced: "Tesla's high-frequency electrical currents are bringing about highly beneficial results in dealing with cancer, surpassing anything that could be acomplished with ordinary surgery."

There are a number of websites that show illustrations of various electrical apparatuses that go by the name of Tesla Coils. One designed for classroom use can be bought from www.sciplus.com. A good general information resource is www.amasci.com/tesla/tesla.html. The following warning, however, should be noted: Tesla coils and other high voltage devices may present a lethal electrical shock hazard! Do not touch them while they are in operation.

A number of other pieces of equipment that are claimed to be developments from Tesla's work and which are available for health purposes are offered by the following website: www.myholistichealthshop.com. These include a high-frequency violet ray and a 'molecular enhancer' – www.altered-states.net is another interesting site that sells a wide range of devices.

Since Tesla, there has been a strong tradition of developing electromagnetic devices including Lakhovsky's Multiple Wave Oscillator, The Rife Generator, the Tesla Photon Machine, the Pappas Pulsed Magnetic Induction Device, the Light Beam Generator and the V.I.B.E. (Vibrational Integration Bio-phonic Energizer).

Lakhovsky's Multi-Wave Oscillator (MWO)

Georges Lakhovsky was a Russian émigré scientist living in France in the years immediately after the first world war. He knew of Tesla's work and developed these ideas going on to publish an article entitled 'Curing Cancer with Ultra Radio Frequencies' in 1925.

Lakhovsky invented the Multi-Wave Oscillator (MWO) which produced a wide range of waves from very low to very high radiowaves with lots of "extremely short harmonics." The MWO consists of two antennae with a number of concentric rings - the high voltage discharges move from one ring to the next and in the process create complex multiple wavelength electrostatic fields. Anyone using the MWO sits between these circular antennae while the high voltage, multiple frequency electrostatic fields are received and absorbed by the tissues. A very interesting website that contains a translation of Lakhovsky's article is www.altered-states.net

His explanation for why it worked was that "The cell with very weak vibrations, placed in the field of multiple vibrations, finds its own frequency and starts again to os_...ate normally through the phenomenon of resonance."

The MWO produces a broad range of high frequency pulsed signals that radiate energy into patient via two resonators: one resonator acting as a transmitter and the other as a receiver. The patient sits on a wooden stool in between the two resonators and is exposed to these energies for about 15 minutes. These energies increase the resonance of healthy cells and create disequilibrium in disease organisms.

Bob Beck (about whom more below) popularised this machine in the States in the 1960s and has published designs. These are available on the web. However, attempts to market the machine in the USA have met with severe FDA disapproval. However, I did find one US site of interest at www.zephyrtechnology.com.

Another convert to the MWO, Ralph Bergstresser, decided that the best way to resist FDA pressure was to seek protection for medical freedom under the freedom for religion laws. He founded a church that worshipped the machine. For a couple of years, he and his followers were able to go to church, sit around the MWO - which was placed on an altar with resonator antennas glowing - and receive the 'blessed waves' from the Sacred Oscillator. However, he was eventually thrown in jail. But he emerged a year or so later undeterred and continued to manufacture and sell the machines along with other electromagnetic devices (see www.purpleharmonyplates.com).

The Rife Square-Wave Frequency Generator — *might be worth looking into*

Round about the same time that Lakhovsky was working in France, a San Diego inventor by the name of Royal Raymond Rife was inventing perhaps the most famous of all the healing machines: the Rife Ultrasound Frequency Generator.

Before inventing the Rife Generator, he built an extraordinarily powerful light microscope with a magnification of 60,000X which made it possible to study living bacteria and viruses – unlike the standard microscopes then and now that required tissue to be dead before it can be viewed.

As a result of watching living bacteria he saw something very interesting - the bacteria could change their forms from bacillus to a fungus to a virus. In all he identified four forms, one of which - the monococcoid - he found in 90 percent of cancer patients. Another form - the BX form - was he claimed the form in which it caused cancer. Any of the forms could change into a BX form within 36 hours.

The idea that relatively harmless bacteria can change into cancer-causing viruses is utterly rejected by most scientists - but Rife is not alone in his belief. We have already seen that Gaston Naessens, who himself, independently, developed a similar microscope, saw similar events unfolding through the lens and, as a result, developed his anti-cancer substance 714-X .

Having discovered these microbes, Rife experimented by passing energy frequencies through the microbes. He found that each microbe had a frequency that would cause it to resonate and then explode (just as a champagne glass explodes when a sound of the right pitch hits it).

Rife then built a generator that emitted radiation of various frequencies that destroyed the microbe that he had identified as the one that causes cancer – which he called the BX virus. It was tested at the University of Southern California in the early 1930s. Rife reported the results: "16 cases were treated at the clinic for many types of malignancy. After 3 months, 14 of these so-called hopeless cases were signed off as clinically cured."

The patients were treated every 3 days - this was found to be more effective than daily treatment, the reason being that the lymphatic system had to deal with the toxicity created by the dead particles of the BX virus. In fact all the patients in the study eventually recovered. The machine had a 100 percent cure rate in cases of terminal cancer. If there are cures for cancer this is certainly one of them..

There is no doubt about the authenticity of the research - nor of the high quality of the scientists who participated in the study: it included a university president, a director of a major medical school, Northwestern Medical School, and other eminent doctors. The study was run under the auspices of the American Medical Association of Los Angeles, personally facilitated by the President, Dr. Milbank Johnson. So what happened?

The story is that Morris Fishbein, who (despite a complete lack of medical qualifications) headed the American Medical Association, was also a front man for the pharmaceutical industry. Through his efforts pressure was exerted on everyone involved to distance themselves from the machine. Some key supporters were bought off with large grants to allow them to retire in peace - and silence. Others, it is claimed, were killed. At least two unnatural deaths occurred among key supporters of Rife. One was poisoned and another was burnt to death when his laboratory burnt down. Equipment was stolen or tampered with. The manufacturers of the equipment were forced by various means into bankruptcy. It was, by all accounts, a mean and nasty war.

However, some doctors continued to use the machine. In 1940, Dr. Arthur Yale reported the results he had obtained using Rife's generator. He reported on four cases that would have been fatal within 90 days. One was a 53-year-old man with a grapefruit sized tumour in the rectum. Within a week, the pain had gone and within sixty days the entire tumour had disappeared. Pain relief, it should be noted, is a possible sign that the cancerous stage of cachexia has ceased.

The AMA reacted to all of this work by threatening doctors who used the machine with loss of license and even jail terms. Rife himself was taken to court. A laboratory that was investigating Rife's claims was burnt to the ground in 1939, killing the key researcher. Rife continued his work despite this pressure. However, harassment continued. One of his partners, Jim Crane, was sent to jail for 3 years in 1961. He was not allowed to defend himself with evidence showing the machine's effectiveness.

As for the machine, there appears to be absolutely no doubt that it worked then and works now. The underlying principle is that every living organism has an internal vibratory frequency - and that life without this frequency signature is impossible. If this frequency is altered or if the power of the frequency is amplified then the organism can be destroyed. So the objective of the Rife generator is to tune into the natural resonance of disease causing microbes and then to increase the intensity of the frequency until they disintegrate.

The Rife generator then is a machine that is capable of producing frequencies and directing these frequencies through the body. Note that Rife used square-wave frequencies, not the normal smooth sine-wave form. Usually, the machine is used to send frequencies throughout the whole body - but it is also possible to direct the waves to specific parts of the body.

Proponents of the Rife frequency generator say that any illness -- from athlete's foot to yellow fever -- can be treated effectively using this machine. Usually, patients will sit for a period of time not exceeding 40 minutes, with their hands holding metal cylinders and their bare feet resting on metal plates. The left hand and left foot are hooked to the same output; similarly the right hand and right foot. The patient then receives a sequence of specified frequencies ranging from 1 to 10,000 Hz. The intensity of these frequencies is individually modulated so that the patient will feel the pulse in the hand and wrist.

A number of machines purporting to be Rife Generators are on the market. You can also buy software that claims to convert your own computer into a Rife generator. One issue with these machines is whether analogue is better than digital (almost certainly yes – because, with digital outputs there is always a gap between one frequency and the next and microbes will be under evolutionary pressure to occupy these gaps. With analogue machines there are no such gaps).

Another issue that buyers need to consider is whether to have a machine that goes through a pre-set programme of frequencies – or whether to take a machine that is programmable to specific frequencies specified for the particular disease.

It seems at first sight that a programmable machine capable of targeting specific disease would be best. Most of these machines will come with a protocol of which frequencies should be used for which health condition. The problem is that there is no general agreement as to which frequencies are specific to cancer. Also of course, once again, the pressures of evolution will mean that microbes will eventually change frequencies. One researcher, Gary Wade, has solved this problem by creating a machine that has a 45-minute programme that covers all ultrasound frequencies within the relevant range. Gary Wade will make a machine specifically upon request (current cost US$1,560). He can be contacted at: Transformation Technologies , 4110 Lyceum Ave. LA, CA. 90066 Toll Free 1-877-287-0912 (310) 823-7016 Fax (310)823-5028 E-Mail vristo@earthlink.net

There are many other machines on the market with prices starting at around US$1,500. See www.staytuned.ws for example.

People undergoing therapy with this machine must make sure they drink plenty of water before and after using the machine - and they should expect to feel tired afterwards.

Also, it should be noted that the generator produces ultrasound frequencies which tend to dissolve blood clots. Therefore, the unit should not be used within several weeks after major or minor surgery, nor on anyone who has phlebitis, who has had a stroke or who is pregnant. For more information also see: www.rifetechnology.com

Prioré

The next important figure in the history of healing machines was an Italian who settled in France and who invented a machine that appeared to cure not only cancer but parasite infections. It did this not by directly attacking the tumour or the parasite but by stimulating the host's cells to eliminate the source of disease. This was witnessed over the years by a number of eminent scientists.

In 1953, Antoine Prioré began treating human patients whose cancers had been judged hopeless – and many were cured. His medical colleague maintained a huge file of these cases, but the file later was mysteriously lost. But Prioré faced enormous hurdles in his attempt to get recognition for his work. Given the fact that he was a simple electrical repairman living in Bordeaux and had no academic status at all, this was an uphill task and he was to die in the early 1980s a broken man.

Part of the problem was that he was utilizing concepts that had at that time no theoretical framework. There is nothing a scientist hates more than something that works but which appears to be meaningless gobbledy-gook according to the current theory. It appears that Prioré found a method of using a fixed magnetic field in combination with electromagnetic radiation.

It may be relevant that his initial inspiration came from seeing that a piece of fruit that had fallen near a machine that gave out electromagnetic radiation did not go rotten for a long time.

Everyone who worked with him at various institutions was convinced that he was able to cure cancer, first in animals and then in humans. And it must be the case that his first equipment must have been cheap to make and portable. Over the years his dream was to make bigger and stronger machines but sadly these never materialized.

There are organizations in France seeking to replicate his work. Sadly, little is known about the exact specifications but it is surmised that Prioré is unlikely to have used a finely tuned machine. It is likely to have produced frequencies across a broad range and the strength of the magnetic field also does not appear to be critical. Two attempts at duplicating his machine have used magnetic fields of 620G and 1,240G.

There does not appear to be any Priore-type machine in use at this time. A machine that appears to be in some ways similar to Priore's has been invented by American physicist, Abraham Liboff of Oakland University, California. His "Method and Apparatus for the Treatment of Cancer" (US Patent #5,211,622) produces an alternating magnetic field superimposed on a static magnetic field. Again, as with the Prioré machine, this appears to have caused cancer tumours to die. Again, while the machine has been patented, I have no information as to whether it is in use.

Contemporary Electrical Approaches

I am not suggesting that you go out to deliberately to get struck by lightning, but an early report of lightning and its effects on cancer were reported in *The Lancet* (Hanuary 10, 1880) by a surgeon named Allison. He reported that 30 years previously he had known of a case of a farm labourer suffering from a mouth cancer who had been struck by lightning. This had nearly killed him but he recovered and the tumour also disappeared. It may be relevant that shock therapy of a similar kind is commonly used in the Amazon basin of Brazil – and is known to be very effective in dealing with poisonous snake-bites. Five or six hits with a standard stun gun have not only neutralized the poison but also eliminated the pain of the bite. No one knows how it manages this feat yet it is well attested to. Could this be the answer to cancer?

The idea that electricity can be curative was developed in Germany and Austria under the name galvanotherapy.

Dr. Rudolph Pekar and Galvanotherapy

Dr. Rudolph Pekar (1912–2004), an Austrian medical doctor and inventor, originated a way of treating cancer using an electrical current which he called Galvanotherapy and which is now widely used in Germany and in China where it is, apparently, producing an overall cure rate of 30-40 percent for all types of cancer including advanced cases of malignant cancer - and much higher cure rates with less advanced cancers. Galvanotherapy is sometimes also known as Percutaneous Bio-Electrotherapy

In this treatment electrodes are clipped to needles inserted in the skin near the malignant tumor. A low current is passed through the electrodes. This creates an electromagnetic field in which charged ions cause the inside of the cancer cells to 'melt' and then implode. The resulting waste material is eliminated through detoxification.

Only very weak DC currents not exceeding 10 volts are used. There is little pain involved in the procedure which is done under local anaesthetic. More than 70,000 people have undergone the procedure which is done at a number of European clinics and Chinese hospitals.

For further information contact the International Association for Electromedicine at Onkologische Schwerpunktpraxis, Frauengasse 4 (Villa Gisela), zip code A-4820 Bad Ischl, Austria. An internet search will also find clinics that offer this therapy.

Bob Beck's Blood Purifier and Magnetic Pulse Generator

Bob Beck was an American inventor who played an important role in promoting the use of inexpensive electro-therapy machines. He invented two machines that are relatively inexpensive but claim to eliminate all harmful microbes from the body.

The first machine he called a blood purifier. This is an electronic device that uses two small electrodes that are placed over major blood arteries (not veins) on the wrists or ankles, and held in place with a strap. Both electrodes are placed on the same wrist or ankle about an inch apart. With most models it is possible to modify the strength of the electrical charge.

This small electric current electrifies the blood as it circulates past the electrodes. It takes about ten minutes for blood to circulate throughout the body. It is recommended to use the machine anywhere from 20 minutes to 2 hours a day.

The basic premise of the blood purifier is that microbes and other disease causing organisms have a far lower tolerance to electrical currents than normal cells. However, it is important to note that one side effect of this procedure is to make cells highly porous and so any chemicals - such as alcohol - in the bloodstream are absorbed at a far greater rate. It is recommended that no drugs or alcohol be taken into the body at least 48 hours prior to using the blood purifier.

Bob Beck was also a strong advocate of colloidal silver and most Beck Blood Purifiers double up as cheap colloidal silver makers. In my experience these machines are better than most in the quality of the silver rods they use.

Bob Beck also invented a Magnetic Pulse Generator that uses a high intensity, short duration magnetic pulse of approximately 43,000 Gauss (current normal background magnetic fields are approximately 0.5 gauss) as its means of killing or immobilizing parasites. The coil produces pulses every 5-8 seconds and can be placed anywhere on the body including the head. There are many suppliers of this machine on the internet.

A number of research institutes are experimenting with 'nanopulses' of electricity with cancer cells in Petri dishes with exciting results (as reported by the BBC (5th Feb, 2004). This seems to support the use of machines such as Bob Beck's. Interestingly, these researchers say the same effect of promoting cell death is also seen in cells associated with obesity. It is worth noting that Bob Beck himself lost an immense amount of weight through the use of his machine.

Hulda Clark's Zapper

This is a small, inexpensive, hand held device that operates on the same principles as the Rife Ultrasound Frequency Generator but is limited in the range of frequencies that it addresses. It is also limited in its ability to penetrate deep into the body. It appears to be beneficial for the muscle tissues. One recent experiment into its effectiveness compared the spoiling rate of a chicken leg with and without being exposed to a zapper. This informal experiment found that it takes about three days for normal fresh chicken legs to spoil. After "zapping" for an hour each day the chicken legs will last up to seventeen days before spoiling.

All three devices – Beck's blood purifier, his magnetic pulse generator and Clark's zapper - are attempting to do the same thing, namely, to use either small electrical currents or high intensity magnetic pulses to kill living organisms that are in your body that shouldn't be there. This includes organisms such as viruses, bacteria, mold, fungi, and the larger parasites such as tapeworms, ringworms, roundworms, flukes, etc.

GEIPE

GEIPE is a very specific anti-cancer device that has as its aim the de-activation of an enzyme by means of an electric current. The American independent cancer researcher, Jay Kulsh believes the answer to curing cancer lies in deactivating the enzyme Ribonucleotide Reductase (RR) Without this enzyme the cancer tumour simply cannot grow. Concentrations of the enzyme are much higher in cancer tumours than in normal tissue. There have been previous attempts to deactivate the enzyme using chemotherapeutic drugs - so far without success. Kulsh took the view that the best way of de-activating it was to focus on the fact that at the "core" of this enzyme is a lone electron (free radical) which is essential for its activity. As he writes "Such free radicals can be neutralized or disabled by passing [a] mild direct electric current through the tissue. Since the concentration of the target enzyme RR is much higher in cancerous cells, as compared to healthy resting cells, the gentle DC electrotherapy would act selectively on malignant growth."

Kulsh was not the first to make this suggestion. He reports that a previous experiment using this approach reported 98 percent reduction in the tumour mass of lab animals – representing, in his words, 'a virtual cure'.

Kulsh has two devices that he is willing to sell. One is an invasive device that requires an electrode to be inserted surgically into a tumour. However, he has another non-invasive device that he says can easily be used at home. It needs to be used at least 8 hours a day for up to 8 weeks.

Kulsh claims that the cancers most likely to respond to his approach are solid tumour cancers of bladder, bone, brain, breast, cervix, colon, esophagus, kidney, liver, lung, ovary, pancreas, prostate, rectum, skin, stomach, testicles, throat & uterus.

GEIPE stands for Gentle Electrotherapy to Inhibit Pivotal Enzyme (Ribonucleotide Reductase).

For further information: www.cancer-treatment.net

Contemporary Magnetic Approaches

We all know that the very basic building tool of matter, the atom, already has built into it an electrical component in which negatively charged electrons orbit a positively charged nucleus. This atom is in constant motion. The vitality of the atom motion depends on the strength of the magnetic field within which it exists.

For our body there are only two natural sources of magnetism—the brain and the Earth. The brain is composed very largely (80 percent) of astrocyte cells which have the capacity to generate electricity. They generate a very efficient pulsed, EM field which is the source of our bodies' energies. The Earth is our other source of magnetism and it provides a steady-state magnetic field, which supports the body and enhances molecular reactions. When these two magnetic fields are working together in a strong and healthy way, all the chemical reactions of the body - enzyme activity, hormone production, pH levels and cellular energy production - are positively influenced.

Once we understand this, we can suddenly see how it is that meditation, sleep and even laughter can have such a positive effect on our health. Any activity that helps the brain to regenerate its own electromagnetic generating capacities will have life-enhancing qualities.

Simple Magnet-based Therapy

Some doctors are experimenting with magnets as a healing device in cases of cancer. Dr. William Philpott of Choctaw, Oaklahoma treated a 20-year-old patient with an inoperable glioblastoma - a form of brain cancer. He placed the north-pole of a ceramic magnet on the back of the patient's head at the point where the tumour had initially started to grow, The magnet was left in this position 24 hours a day.

At the beginning of the treatment at the American Biologics (now International BioCare) hospital in Tijuana, Mexico, this patient was incapable of making any response to his environment. After three days of continuous treatment, he was able to wiggle his fingers in response to questions. Three weeks later, he walked out of the hospital with the assistance of only a walker. The patient continued magnetic-field exposure of the brain five hours a day and was reported to be well six months later except for a residual imbalance problem.

Obviously a normal bar magnet is of no use for this kind of treatment as both north and south poles appear on the same side. What is needed is a flat magnet, magnetised so that opposite poles are on opposing flat sides.

It is also possible to buy magnetic beds to sleep on. However, one needs to distinguish between beds that are based on normal magnets that have alternating current force field. These can give temporary benefits but for long-term benefits a bed that gives a steady state magnetic field is required. One, developed by Dr. Dean Bronlie, marketed by Magnetico, has a force field nearly ten times stronger than that we currently experience emanating from the earth. See www.magneticosleep.com for further information.

The flow of this magnetic energy through the body for the eight hours of sleep has, Bronlie claims, a remarkable effect on healing. He focuses particularly on its benefits for people with arthritis, but more interestingly for our purposes, it has a demonstrable and powerful effect on the oxygen levels in the blood and the efficiency of the body's biochemical reactions. What is the evidence? Most athletes find it very difficult to improve their VO2 max readings - this is a measure of the maximum amount of oxygen they can use. However, over a matter of months, Canadian athletes lying on his magnetic bed were able to improve this by 30 percent - an amazing finding. Also the amount of oxygen in the bloodstream increased. This ability to hyper-oxygenate the body suggests that the magnetic bed could have a powerful beneficial effect against cancer.

Gary Null is an American writer whose website at www.garynull.com contains a lot of valuable information on the subject of magnets, the research behind their use, controversies and sources for magnets. He notes that strong magnetic fields can help the body protect itself against viruses, bacteria, and fungi by hyper-oxygenating the blood. Magnetic fields also reduce the acidity of the body's tissues making them more alkaline and therefore healthier and less attractive to these invading microbes.

In relation to cancer he notes that cells depolarise (i.e., they lose their magnetic character) before becoming metastatic. He gives the following advice: "When using magnets for cancer, remember the following rules of thumb: The magnetic pole used must be negative. The field should be larger than the primary lesion and the gauss greater than 25. Success rate increases if both the gauss and duration are increased. A minimal duration of 20 hours per day for no less than three months is required in most cases."

Experiments with cancer cells in Petri dishes have shown clear evidence that north (negative) polarity fields retard growth while there is some slight evidence that positive polarity may have the opposite effect and promote cellular growth. Because of these impacts pregnant women should avoid strong magnetic fields for any length of time.

Null notes also that the use of magnets both improved success when used as an adjuvant therapy by those opting for radiotherapy and/or chemotherapy while at the same time reducing the side effects. Null also takes the view that magnets are more effective when used with herbs and supplements.

Complex Electromagnetic Therapy Machines
Ion Magnetic Induction Therapy Machine

The Ion Magnetic Induction Therapy Machine, developed by Professor Panos T. Pappas, also claims to kill cancer cells. The following website contains specifications for the building of this machine. www.portalmarket.com/specifications.html

Here the general theory behind all these machines, restated time and time again by each new inventor is expressed simply: "All of the many types of living cells that make up the tissues and organs of the body are tiny electrochemical units. They are powered by a "battery" that is continually recharged by the cells' metabolic chemistry in a closed loop of biological energy. When a cell is poisoned, damaged, deprived of nutrients or infected, energy is lost in fighting the problem and the [electrical charge] falls to a level where the cell loses its vitality and either struggles to heal itself or dies...[T]he induction of tiny currents of electricity is remarkably effective in healing, regenerating and revitalizing cells damaged by trauma."

This machine produces continuous harmonic radiation of between 0.3 to 250 MHz. For further information see www.papimi.gr and www.papimi.com

A number of clinics offer this therapy but the machine itself does not appear to be commercially available to the general public.

Magnetic Field Therapy

Swedish engineer Ivan Troeng developed a magnetic bench which has a static electromagnetic field of 650 gauss. Patients lie on the bench for 1-2 hours per day. This treatment appears to be only aavailable at one of Europe's leading alternative cancer centres, the Humlegaarden Clinic in Denmark–see: www.humlegaarden.com

As with all forms of magnetic therapy, the therapy is not focused on producing a cure, rather, it focuses on putting the body into a state where it heals itself.

Quantronic Resonance System

This is the name of a machine developed in Germany. It consists of a pad that you lie on and a pillow for the head. These are plugged into a normal socket. The result is a very low level pulsed (saw-tooth wave) magnetic field. In fact, the EM field is so weak that it is lower than the prevailing background magnetic field of the earth. Originally it was thought that such a low field would have zero impact on the body but it has been demonstrated that even a very short period of time (5 minutes say) spent lying on this pad will have an impact in improving blood flow. The normal recommended treatment, however, is to lie on the machine for two sessions a day, each lasting only eight minutes and to persist for at least 6 weeks. This has for many people with a wide range of severe symptoms been effective in about 40 percent of cases of providing a 'complete relief of symptoms' (a rather euphemistic way of saying 'cure').

This machine has been intensively studied by university researchers and was even used by the Russians in the MIR space station to enhance the magnetic background for their astronauts. Dr. William Pawluk, co-author of the book *Magnetic Therapy in Eastern Europe*, described his experience of the machine: "I was very surprised the first time I laid on it that I could actually feel it. I could feel changes in my body. I could feel heat, the sensation of a vibration and deep relaxation. Physical aches improved on the large pad as the treatment progressed."

His extremely interesting article on this machine can be found at www.quantronmedicine.com.

With cancer, it is known that the cell membrane tension voltage is only 20 mVolts compared with 50 mVolts for a sick cell and 70-110 mVolts for a healthy cell. Background EM fields can help push the cancerous cell's membrane tension voltage up–but if the EM field is too strong this may damage the cell. This explains why a very weak field–a gentle breeze rather than a storm, as Pawluk describes it - may be better.

Pawluk also notes that the level of the QRS radiation is on the same level as the delta brain waves and that part of its benefits may be that it simulates a short period of deep sleep.

Testimonials covering a very wide spectrum of ailments - including cancer - can be read at www.hightechhealth.net/QRS/testimonials.htm Many have commented on its powerful overall healing help for those undergoing surgery and radiation along with pain relief. It is also seen as a powerful anti-ageing tool. Many note that increased blood oxygenation levels have resulted.

The machine is commercially available at around US$2,600

SCENAR

This is a device developed by the Russians and is now widely used in Russia. It looks somewhat like a TV remote control. It is placed on the body where it picks up electromagnetic signals. It processes and responds to these signals–so it is engaging in a kind of energetic conversation with the body. It is claimed to be very successful in treating a wide range of ailments including circulatory, muscular-skeletal, and those relating to the digestive or genitor-urinary systems. Whether or not it can itself cure cancer no one is saying. Such a claim would get it banned in short order. But, nevertheless, for the person with cancer, SCENAR can support and help the healing processes.

Zoetron System

The war against 'quacks' and 'charlatans' resulted (February 2003) in the US Federal Trade Commission (FTC) suing the promoters of a magnetic pulse system for curing cancer called the Zoetron System. The case never came to court as the originators of the Zoetron System mounted a fierce defence. The case has now been settled out of court and the Zoetron system, renamed Nanopulse Therapy, is seeking to establish its scientific credibility through small scale double-blind clinical trials.

The basic theory behind the Zoetron system is as follows: Cancer cells are known have many more receptors for iron on their external surfaces than normal cells do. Cancer cells have a great need for iron (the reason why supplements containing iron should not be taken by cancer patients). In the Zoetron approach, very small particles – nanoparticles – of iron are introduced to the body. The iron particles will then tend to accumulate disproportionately on the surface of cancerous cells compared to non-cancerous cells. The body is then exposed to an externally generated pulsed magnetic field strong enough to reach the area of the tumor. The nanoparticles of iron are excited   by the magnetic fiels and this agitation creates heat. This is really a form of hyperthermia as the objective is to raise the intracellular temperature of cancer cells to 110 degrees (F), which is the temperature at which they die. This system, the creators said, has no effect on normal cells which have low levels of iron.

Until it can prove its value, the therapy is not currently available but, in a personal email to me, Michael Reynolds, one of the developers, said he fervently hopes that one day it will be widely available at a cost of about US$3,000 per course of treatment (including all the associated tests) – but when that will be no one knows.

The V.I.B.E. Machine

The V.I.B.E. (Vibrational Integration Bio-Photonic Energizer) is a machine developed by Gene Koonce,   an electronics technician. This machine is clearly a direct descendent of the Tesla Coil and Lakhovsky's Multi-wave   oscillator.

Koonce believes that "disease is a state of non-vibrating, non-charged or non-energized cells." The V.I.B.E. machine puts out an electromagnetic field with a high voltage pulse. This recharges the cells bringing about a state of high cellular energy. People stand or sit a few feet away from the machine for only a few minutes at a time. People have said they experience a great energizing effect from this. This energizing effect does seem to lessen with time. One suggestion is that you don't feel it so much when your cells are charged up. There is also anecdotal evidence that people with high PSA scores suggesting prostate cancer have experienced sharp drops in this cancer marker. One other anecdote told by Bill Henderson in one of his cancer newsletters testified to a man with lung cancer expelling cancerous matter after having been exposed to a VIBE machine's rays.

For more information go to www.vibemachine.com where you will find testimonials. At the time of writing the machine costs US$17,500.

Essentially identical but rather cheaper   machines can be obtained from a number of other companies. It seems that the founders of these various companies once worked together. Something happened along the way and they each ended up developing their own equipment based on the same concepts.. Compare the Evenstar and SEAD machines at www.bels-tech.com, www.energizeforhealth.com/sead-units-products.html and www.evenstar-tech.com

Miscellaneous Healing Machines and Therapies
The Light Beam Generator

This is a newly developed piece of equipment manufactured by ELF Laboratories, Inc. (www.lightbeamgenerator.com) which claims to have a wide range of healing potentials. Cancer is not listed on their website but there are anecdotal claims that it is beneficial. The company literature says this about the machine: "The LBG® works by helping to rebalance the charge of the cells' electromagnetic fields. Using cold-gas light photons and extremely low-energy electromagnetic frequency patterns, the LBG® helps separate these cells from each other and their accumulated inflammation, swelling, abnormal growths, and other lymph blockages."

Of course anything that works against inflammation is likely to work against cancer cells.

Microwave Resonance Therapy (MRT)

This is a high intensity, low frequency treatment applied to acupuncture points to treat entire acupuncture meridians and in this way to encourage the body to return to physiological equilibrium - known as homeostasis. This has been developed by Professor Sergei Sitko in Russia. He has used this on over 8,000 patients suffering from a wide range of illnesses. Unfortunately, outside Russia, it is difficult to find anyone offering access to this approach so it remains at this stage theoretical.

Light Therapy

A machine called an Eichoterm Solarium is in use at the Humlegaarden Clinic (www.humlegaarden.com) in Denmark. It radiates light combining UVB and UVC rays (but not the cancer-causing UVA rays) with an intensity typical of a nice hot day in the tropics along with 'orange colored heat rays'. Typically a patient will receive the therapy for up to an hour, equivalent to a whole day sunbathing in the tropics. According to the clinic's brochure: "This causes photo chemical processes to be activated in the skin, the result being a strong detoxification of the body. Excellent results have been seen for cancer, disseminated sclerosis, skin diseases, arthritic diseases, circulatory diseases and many other chronic diseases."

Dr. Gorgun's GEMM Therapy

Dr. Seckiner Gorgun is a Turkish medical researcher who has developed a radio-wave generator, which he refers to as a GEMM device. This sends "precisely calculated therapeutic radio waves" that interfere with the ATP production which cancers need to fuel their rapid cell division. When the ATP production is halted the cancer cells are killed. He has apparently had good success treating terminally ill patients with brain tumours, bone cancers, breast cancers and others. For more information email info@gemm-therapy.com.

Subtle Energy Therapies

Most of the machines/therapies discussed so far have made use of electricity or magnetism in an easy to conceptualise manner. There is an enemy – a microbe or parasite - that is attacked by a weapon – or there is a cell whose vibrational frequencies is enhanced.

However, to consider 'energy medicine' to be simply an additional area of medicine on the fringes of other areas of medicine is a misunderstanding. The truth is, energy medicine is a new paradigm, a new way of understanding the body and healing processes that includes all other medicines, including the allopathic tradition that in this book I have referred to as orthodox medicine.

The idea that the body is a pulsing energy system is one familiar to anyone interested in Eastern healing traditions. The Chinese have long used the concept of qi (pronounced 'chee') energy, which they see as a life force that flows through certain 'meridians' or vertical channels. Indian ayurvedic medicine similarly is based on a concept of prana energy that relates to certain energy centres they call chakras. However, in this chapter, we are going to look far beyond these traditional ideas.

Underlying all the therapies that will be discussed below is the idea that the universe, the world and our bodies are systems of energy that interconnect: light, electricity, magnetism and other subtle energies are all at play within these interconnecting systems. The science that underlies this understanding of the world is described by Einsteinian quantum physics rather than classical, Newtonian, mechanical physics. It should also be noted that most of what we call orthodox medicine is virulently hostile to this new concept. This is a major battleground. Readers are invited to make up their own minds.

The old way of looking at the universe and our bodies is to see them as a system of solid physical parts that relate to each other in a way governed by fixed mechanical laws. Our bodies are therefore machines.

The new way of looking at our bodies is to see them as intercommunicating systems of energy – and there are many different forms of energy.

One of these forms of energy is electromagnetic energy. It is present in and around everything. To say that we are wrapped in an envelope of electromagnetic energy, however, seriously understates the complexity of what is going on in our bodies. Every part of our body – and every micro-part of each and every part (down to the level of electrons and beyond) is pulsing and vibrating and so creating micro-electromagnetic fields The interplay of all these myriads of vibrating patterns helps both to establish coherence within the whole system and at the same time is a network of communication from one part to another (or rather between each part and every other part). When there are injuries or imbalances in a specific location within the system this will have an effect on the local vibration which will communicate itself to the rest of the system.

And interestingly, when we look at the body as a system (or systems) of energy, we see that our individuality does not stop at the physical boundary of our skin but flows into the space around the physical body and therefore comes into contact with the energy systems of other living beings around us.

Many, probably most, medical doctors and scientists are extremely uneasy with this kind of talk – but research has established without a shadow of doubt that strange things are going on that simply cannot be explained by a molecular-chemical concept of the body. Acupuncture is one therapy, for example, that has clearly demonstrable and repeatable effects. It is commonly used even in hospitals as a pain-relieving procedure. Yet, to the scientist who cannot escape the confines of the old, mechanical view of the body, the theory of acupuncture is bizarre and indeed meaningless. It is simply 'wrong'. And yet it works. One doctor has suggested that the reason therapies like acupuncture work is that patients are experiencing a placebo effect. Either that 'or the whole of physics and chemistry as we know them are wrong,' as more than one scientist has put it.

It is not possible to even begin a summary of some of the complex ideas suggested by this new paradigm of medicine. For further discussion of the science behind energy medicine you should consult the following books: *Vibrational Medicine* by Richard Gerber, M.D.; *Energy Medicine: the Scientific Basis* by James L. Oschman, *The Body Electric* by Robert O Becker and *Perfect Health* by Deepak Chopra

However, extremely exciting results have been reported from the use of therapies or equipment that interface with the body's bio-energetic system.

Acupuncture

Acupuncturists seek to promote the flow of healing energy through vertical channels that run down the body. They make use of needles to stimulate positive energy or to retard negative energy flows. No one has claimed that acupuncture on its own is effective against cancer (but then again it would be illegal for any non-qualified doctor to make such a claim!). One British veterinary surgeon, John Carter, has used acupuncture successfully as part of a general protocol against cancer in animals. Acupuncture has also been used to help reduce the side effects of chemotherapy and radiation.

AIM (All Inclusive Method) Program

The AIM Program is at the forefront of energy medicine. The starting point is simple enough. We are all energy systems and our health is impacted by energy disharmonies – but these disharmonies are detectable and by focusing a balancing energy to counter the disharmony, the original disharmony can be eliminated. Particular disharmonies have been associated with specific diseases – though the AIM Program makes it very clear that they don't try to 'cure cancer', instead they seek to eliminate the disharmonic energy pattern that they have learnt to associate with cancer.

So far so good. However, to understand where the AIM people are coming from we need to have some understanding of hologram theory. Holograms are three dimensional images created by a complex interaction of lasers. The interesting thing about a hologram is that you can't cut it in two. If you try, you do not end up with two halves but with two wholes. Each part of a hologram contains the whole. This has got some scientists excited because the universe as a whole appears to share some of the characteristics of a hologram. One of these characteristics is that information can be shared instantaneously by two particles irrespective of the distance between them. This has been demonstrated by a French physicist, Alain Aspect. There are many websites dedicated to discussing this issue far beyond my own ability to follow them and for those of you who wish to learn more may I suggest you do a Google search of 'hologram theory'.

But the key point we need to keep in mind is that if something impacts one part of a hologram, the effects are instantly felt by all parts of the hologram. Now, each living entity is a system of energy and is surrounded by an invisible energy matrix. The next conceptual leap that we must make is to accept that the energy matrix that surrounds each person is also present in any photograph of that person.

Following hologram theory, we can surmise that the photograph can be the recipient of balancing energy therapy and the person in the photograph will benefit from this energetic input – even though they may be thousands of miles away. This is precisely what the AIM program does.

The promoters of the AIM Program make a big point of calling their approach 'spiritual healing'. Their website explains their concept: "Our Spiritual Technology delivers thousands of balancing energies for both gross and subtle (e.g., karmic) energetic imbalances. Among the additional energies are special activating frequencies that enable your higher self to select automatically, via your photograph, those frequencies you need at any given time. In addition, there are enhancing energies that help increase your Life Force and ability to respond to energetic crises. The AIM energies cover a wide range of issues for realizing wholeness in living beings"

In practice, those taking part in the AIM Program submit a whole-body photograph which is placed on a tray that is permanently irradiated with subtle energies. Currently, a year's therapy costs US$1,000 per person (US$2,000 per family group of 5). For further information see www.energeticmatrix.com

Is this science or is it a scam? Those who argue that it is science say that the science that underlies the AIM Program is quantum physics and as even Nobel prize winner Richard Feynman commented:"I think I can safely say that nobody understands quantum mechanics." Lynne McTaggart's recent book, *The Field*, is as good an introduction as any to some of the concepts. However, since this technology does seem to be fantastical - almost in the realm of the magical - it is worth pondering a few thoughts:

"Miracles happen, not in opposition to nature, but in opposition to what we know of nature." - St. Augustine

"Any technology which is sufficiently advanced is indistinguishable from magic" - Robert Heinlein

"Those who are not shocked when they first come across quantum theory cannot possibly have understood it." - Niels Bohr

Nevertheless, choosing this approach does involve a huge leap of faith – and I, like anyone with a rational, scientific bent, would dearly love to see a double blind controlled trial. But I do see the problem: who could we trust to carry out this trial? Until then how can we choose this approach without the fear that we are being taken advantage of? Perhaps it comes down to money. If you have the cash and you're prepared to take the risk (who knows, maybe it does everything they say it does). Then why not?

Bio-energetic Healing

Some healers appear to have the ability to work in a subtle way with the energy fields of the body. They have differing understandings of what they are doing but the end result is a patient who is demonstrably healthier. This healing can go under a number of names, with differing philosophies. One such school of healing calls itself pranic healing, another is psychic or spiritual healing. I talked to John Eastman, a naturopath and bio-energetic healer. I asked him about his healing work and how he explained it. This was his response:

"Healing is a universal phenomenon. It is not restricted to any one religion, group, country or culture. Sometimes healing takes place instantly after just one session. More often it works gradually and progressively over time. It certainly doesn't require any belief on the part of the person receiving the healing as witnessed by the fact that babies, children and even people who are unconscious have recovered from ill-health as a result of healing energy.

"There are different levels of energy. On one level, the level of the physical body, there is the energy that flows through us. This is often referred to as 'qi' (or chi) energy (East Asia), or prana energy (South Asia). But there is another energy which we can say both precedes and at the same time transcends chi or prana. Whatever name we use to call it we can say that this energy is spiritual or divine energy.

"It is this spiritual energy that we use to heal with. When I am healing, it is this energy that flows through me. I am not using my own qi energy. I am channelling universal divine energy. That is why instead of feeling tired after healing I feel very clear, extremely energized and even, I can say, spiritually uplifted. Spiritual healing, complementary medicine and orthodox medicine are not mutually exclusive. Certainly spiritual healing can support and improve the outcome of other forms of medicine and healing."

John Eastman can be contacted at www.johneastman.co.uk. There are many such healers.

A case of such healing caused quite a stir in Victorian England. Harriet Martineau was an early nineteenth-century novelist, journalist, social reformer, educator, children's writer, philosopher of naturalism, environmentalist, social scientist and pioneering feminist who published over fifty books and almost two thousand articles and newspaper columns. She became a chronic invalid. The best efforts of all the leading doctors did nothing for her. For five years she suffered until, in 1844, a travelling healer – who interestingly referred to himself as a 'magnetizer' – by the name of Pencer Hall treated her. His treatment consisted of giving her 'magnetic passes'. After three days she was able to eat and sleep comfortably for the first time in five years. Thereafter the treatment was continued by her maid.

Interestingly, John Eastman refers to his own healing technique – which he evolved entirely independently - as bio-energetic alignment: this involves moving the hands over the body without physical contact. Such an action might very well be described as a magnetic pass.

The suggestion that electromagnetic fields are involved is supported experimentally. Dr. John Zimmerman (a leading US researcher in the field of magnetic therapy and who works at the Colorado School of Medicine) using sensitive electromagnetic sensing equipment found that healers are capable of producing very strong electromagnetic fields from their hands – so strong it went off the scale of his magnetometer. Clearly if it can be measured then it's real.

Other healers, such as those using the Chinese qigong technique are doing something different. Qigung therapists are able to transmit heating energy from their palms. They are also, for different purposes, able to absorb infrared energy from the environment.

One organisation that provides free energy healing is the Johrei Foundation. For further information go to www.johrei.com

Throughout the world there are energy healers—many of whom have arrived at their calling by circuitous routes. One way to find one near you is to look for spiritualist churches. See also the discussion on Psychic Surgeons below.

Colour Therapy

This therapy involves irradiating the body - or specific parts of the body - with light of a particular, designated colour which is determined by the therapist after diagnosis of the problem.

Colours are, like X-rays and radio band frequencies, forms of electromagnetic radiation. They inhabit a very narrow stretch of the Spectrum of Electromagnetic Radiation. But just as microwaves, X-rays and ultraviolet rays have an effect on the body, so too, it is argued, do the different colours - both combined in the form of full-spectrum white light or separately.

Research has shown that the average light bulb and neon strip, such as provide the lighting in most homes and offices is not healthy as they do not provide full-spectrum white light. Full-spectrum lights are available. John Ott, who is one of the pioneers in the field of light and its affects on health discovered that full-spectrum lighting helped reduce hyperactivity among children. It was his view that conventional lighting and televisions that leak radiation can cause hyperactivity. The beneficial effects of sunlight are dealt with separately. Here we will look at how colour therapy works.

The colour therapist works with a projector which has five coloured plates - red, yellow, green, blue, violet - that can be used separately or in combination to produce any of the following colours: the primary light colours: red, green and violet; the secondary light colours: yellow, blue and magenta; and the tertiary colours: lemon, orange, turquoise, indigo, purple and scarlet.

Green is the colour that harmonizes and maintains the natural physical balance so this is the colour most often used. Disease and illness cause the body to shift to one side or the other. If it moves more to the yellow this means the body will be feverish or inflamed. This needs to be corrected with a dose of blue light. If the movement is the other way, towards the blue, then the patient will feel dull and sedated and will need a dose of yellow, perhaps.

Each colour has a range of qualities and effects on the body. Red, for example, stimulates the liver and helps build haemoglobin; green stimulates the pituitary and acts as a general purifier and disinfectant of the body; scarlet is aphrodisiac and stimulates the kidneys; orange is for those with weak lungs and who need to stimulate the thyroid. The colours are light colours - not pigment colours.

So far, we have been in the realm of the easily understood. But colour therapists make two claims that are less easily accepted. The first is that water poured into a glass of the correct colour will become energised with the qualities of the colour and can then be drunk as medicine. Secondly, the colour need not be applied directly on the individual's body. In fact the person can be absent, as long as some 'witness' of the patient's presence can be used to receive the treatment. The 'witness' can be a drop of blood, a piece of hair or even the person's own handwritten name and address on an envelope. An explanation of these claims is given below under Vibrational Medicine.

And what is it like to receive colour therapy? One patient described her feelings during a session. First the therapist bathed her in a lemon colour. "At first I felt nothing but as time progressed there was a feeling of fullness and tightness in the area. By the end...I was feeling just slightly nauseous." Then the therapist changed the light to a dark red filter. "I was immediately relieved of the slight discomforts and became aware of a new sensation farther down, a fullness and yet somehow a relaxing and soothing vibration [and after 15 minutes] I was on the verge of being asleep." The therapist changed the coloured light to green. "...the moment he did I was wide awake. My whole body started to tingle. My breath came fast and my heart was pounding. ... It was most similar to the excitement that builds up just before orgasm."

In subsequent treatments this women did not respond so strongly to the sensations - in fact called them mild. This woman was, it is claimed, cured of fibroids and cancer.

A course of colour therapy treatments may consist of only 4-6 sessions. In fact few colour therapists use the whole room colour projection described above — instead many use phials of coloured waters. For further information and referral to colour therapists you can contact

The International Association for Colour Therapy at http://www.iac-colour.co.uk

Crystal Therapy

Recently, crystals have been promoted as having healing properties that vary with the material, colour and shape of the crystal. Crystal healers take as their starting point the belief that all matter is made of nothing but vibrating energies which are aligned with the universal energies and that crystals are forms that unify and focus these energies. During a crystal healing any number and variety of crystals may be used and placed on the body - particularly on and around the chakra points which lie on the central line of the head, body and pelvis.

A crystal healer bases all decisions about placement and arrangement of stones on his/her intuition. In fact, as with many other vibrational practices, the psychic sensitivity of the therapists is considered to be an important healing element in itself. Since the universe is a single energy field, it is argued, then each and every person is a locus for this universal energy. By aligning the healer's energies with the patient's, healing is aided.

Crystals are believed to have the ability to magnify energies and they are generally placed on chakra points. Crystals can also be placed in water to create an energised gem elixir which works along the same principles as the flower essence elixirs - though the latter are generally considered to be more wide-ranging in their effects. Crystals help to align mental and emotional energies.

Crystal healing devotee, Katrina Raphael strongly recommends the crystal Luvulite. "Luvulite is the pressure release valve that can bring peace and understanding to a mind and body that have lost their source of strength..." It helps the mind focus its own healing energies. "This healing force if properly used, has the power to heal any dis-ease and restore complete mental and physical health."

Unfortunately, Luvulite is a fairly rare and expensive stone. However, all quartz stones have healing qualities.

Is this airy-fairy new age nonsense? James Oschman, author of *Energy Medicine: the Scientific Basis* (2003), is not willing to dismiss crystal healing. He notes that all living tissues are essentially crystalline in nature: "Crystalline arrangements are the rule and not the exception in living systems"– but the crystals that comprise muscles, connective tissue and the other organs consist of soft, flexible, liquid crystals. Oschman hypothesises that these crystals enhance the energy exchange between two individuals – that the crystals function not so much on their own but as a vehicle for the healer's own healing energies. "Crystalline molecular arrays found throughout the body are exceedingly sensitive to energy fields in the environment."

Healing Sounds

Primal sound therapy, as taught by the Maharishi Ayur-Veda Health Centres, is based on the idea that all matters of health originate at the 'quantum level' of the body - which is in tune with the energy web of the universe. Ill-health comes when this energy connection is blocked for some reason. It is therefore necessary to open up the energy channels so that we can get back in touch with the primal energy vibrations, which always work in the direction of health. One method of achieving this is to use vibrating sound.

There are a number of sound therapies. Perhaps the simplest to access is that put forward by Jonathan Goldman in this book *Healing Sounds*. He suggests that an harmonic meditation heals by 'balancing the chakras'. To do this is simple. You place yourself in a comfortable meditation pose and breathe from the abdomen. Then you focus on each of the seven chakras in turn starting from:

1. The base of the spine (close to the anus)
2. A point a few centimetres below the navel
3. The navel
4. The heart: this point is in the centre of the chest between the two nipples
5. The throat
6. The brow: the position of the third eye
7. The crown: the top of the head.

I've read his book - he has some CD's that 'balance the chakras' - never mind Chloe hated it - ~~it might be~~

While focusing on each point make an open throated vowel humming sound as full of vibrations as is possible, starting with a low tone and an 'uh' or 'ooo' sound. At each chakra point the tone should shift up a notch and the vowel sound should change like this: uh-ooo-oh-ah-eye-ih-eee.

The more one does this the more proficient one will become, even without previous experience of singing. One doesn't have to be a 'good singer' to get benefit from this. Jonathan Goldman also claims that healers can use sounds to heal their patients.

There is in fact laboratory based experimental support for the idea that sound can directly kill cancer cells. Researcher, Fabien Maman, played the Ionian scale on a xylophone note by note: C-D-E-F-G-A-B and then C and D of the next octave next to a Petri dish containing a cancer cell (one of the HeLa line). After fourteen minutes of this, the cancer cell exploded. His explanation was this: "Healthy cells seem to breathe in a way that allows them to absorb and integrate the sound without resistance. They did not appear to keep the power of the sound frequency inside of themselves like the cancer cells did. The healthy cells appeared supple and able to freely receive, absorb and return the sound energy. In contrast the cancer cells appeared inflexible and immutable in their structure."

For more information contact:

i. Maharishi Ayur-vedic sound healing: www.theraj.com

ii. Sound Healers Association: www.healingsounds.com

Lakhovsky's Cosmic Energy Cure

Georges Lakhovsky, whose Multi-Wave Oscillator we have already discussed, had come to the conclusion that all life radiates vibrations - these radiations emanate from the oscillation of minute cellular magnetic fields. Every cell is essentially an electrical circuit with its own electromagnetic field. Ill-health occurs, then, when there is a disequillibrium caused by a war of radiations between the natural healthy cells and the radiations emanating from viruses or other invading pathogens. If the invading microbial radiation is stronger, the cells' healthy radiations are affected and are unable to maintain their own proper level of radiation. On the other hand, if the cells' healthy radiations are stronger, the microbe is killed.

From this, it follows, that if the body can be flooded with oscillations of the same frequency as that of a healthy cell, then the cells should be able to return to their healthy frequencies and so be able to fight of the disease. For this purpose he developed his multi-wave oscillator described above.

However, he did not stop there. Thinking about the source of the energy needed to charge the cells in the first place, he came to the conclusion that it was the energy that streams through the cosmos. It should therefore be possible, he thought, to focus this energy without the help of any artificial machinery.

He made a copper circlet, thirty centimetres in diameter, and attached it to a support made of ebonite, a material made of black vulcanised rubber, which he stuck into the flower pot. He then took two groups of geraniums. Half he injected with a bacteria that causes cancer - the other half were his controls. When the cancerous growths had developed, he placed the coil round one cancerous plant. After several weeks he found that all the cancer infected plants had died - with one exception. The plant in the coil was not only alive, it was not only cancer-free, but it had grown twice as large as the normal plants.

Subsequently, a number of experiments have been done both with copper circlets in the form of collars, bracelets and belts. These appear to have a profound normalising effect - so making them beneficial for a wide range of illnesses. Even cancer patients have, it seems, experienced remissions. Any length of copper wire can be used - apparently even standard insulated cable.

Some people swear to the beneficial effects of placing copper circlets round the neck, waist, arms above the elbow and legs above the knee. Secure them in place in any way you can. Since the effect is to normalise the body's natural healthy state by eliminating poisons some early discomfort may be experienced - occasional pains, headaches and even flu-like symptoms - and a lot of water should be drunk to help this elimination. Doctors have used these copper circlets in many countries for many problems and no long-term toxic effects have been noted.

Psychic Surgery

Psychic healing (sometimes in the form of so-called psychic surgery) is practised widely in Brazil and the Philippines. And despite investigations that appear to expose them as frauds, practitioners have a good record of healing.

In Brazil, a healer by the name of John of God (Joao de Deus) has attracted thousands of visitors to his centre in Goias in Brazil. One visitor commented to me: "I visited him twice. On both occasions there was healing but no cure." Others, however, claim to have been cured of all manner of illness. For further information go to www.friendsofthecasa.org

In the Phillipines, psychic surgeons appear to perform surgery with their bare hands or with rusty knives without any anaesthesia and without any pain. The hand appears to delve into the flesh and a bloody lump of flesh appears in the psychic surgeon's palm.

Hocus pocus? Quackery? Some investigators say they are out-and-out frauds who use magic sleight of hand to pluck what appear to be cancerous tumours but which are in fact concealed lumps of chicken or cow flesh. Perhaps. But even so they have a very potent weapon that the modern scientific doctor denies himself. The psychic surgeons are working with the placebo effect and not against it.

Nevertheless, they remain an enigma. The placebo effect cannot explain all that they do. One famous Brazilian healer worked without touching his patients he would write down prescriptions as patients filed past. In one test, 1,000 patients filed past. Later, his diagnoses were, according to the report, found to be phenomenally accurate.

This ability should not be easily dismissed as impossible. In 1985, an American doctor by the name of Norman Shealy began to work with a journalist, Caroline Myss, who claimed she had always had an intuitive ability to 'know' things. They lived more than 1,000 miles apart. He would phone her and ask her to help him diagnose the state of health of the patient in his room. Once she was comfortable with this procedure and was able to relax, she would intuitively enter the patient's body, travelling through it to assess the health of each specific organ. According to Shealy, her diagnoses were 93 percent accurate.

In Britain a psychic surgeon called Stephen Turoff has made a name for himself as a healer and a guide. Stephen Turoff sees people for a modest fee at his Danbury Healing Clinic in Chelmsford, England and also in Coin, near Malaga in Spain. Contact: The Danbury Healing Clinic, The Miami Hotel, Princes Road, Chelmsford, Essex CM2 9AJ, ENGLAND, Telephone +44 (0)1245-348325. However, it is worth reading the readers' reviews of a book about his work Stephen Turoff: Psychic Surgeon on www.amazon.co.uk. Most of the reviewers had personal experience of his healing work - not all the reviewers were positive about their experiences.

Biologist Lyall Watson studied a psychic healer in the Philippines. The man would point his finger about an inch from the patient's skin and an incision would appear. One day Watson got too close and his own hand was caught in the path - he got cut.

A final anecdotal note: My otherwise cynical physiotherapist aunt had a friend who had breast cancer. My aunt accompanied her to the Philippines to visit one of these healers. Shortly after the visit the friend noticed her tumour had disappeared.

Should we consider psychic surgery as a form of placebo medicine or are these psychic surgeons working at the energy levels of the body?

Reflexology

Foot massages have been known to have a beneficial relaxing effect since time began. The present day system of reflexology arose as a result first of Dr. William Fitzgerald in 1913. He came to the view that there were ten vertical energy zones running down the body. After further experimentation, he found that by putting pressure on a specific area of the body he could anaesthetise related areas along the zone. This early work was developed by Eunace Ingham in the 1930s. She found that working on the feet alone was the same as working the whole body. It should be noted that acupuncturists also recognise that the foot, hand, ears and other places are microsystems that mirror the workings of the entire body - as a result, some acupuncturists only work on the ear, no matter what or where the ailment is.

Modern reflexologists have mapped out very precise points on the soles and sides of the feet that correspond to the different organs of the body. If there is any problem in any of the organs small crystaline deposits can be felt in the related areas in the feet. The massage eliminates these crystal deposits and this has a healing effect on the organ concerned. As with acupuncture, one way to find areas where there might be a health concern is to test for sensitivity. Any sensitivity is a sign that attention is needed (i.e., rub the spot that hurts or is sensitive)–later you will find it is not so sensitive.

Reflexologists will never diagnose specific illnesses though they will say which tissues or organs are in need of attention.

Clearly, reflexology, while not being an anti-cancer therapy specifically, can play a useful role as part of a bundle of therapies aimed at improving overall health.

Reiki and Therapeutic Touch

Reiki is both a contact and a non-contact therapy in which the Reiki healer focuses healing energy from the palms of his/her hands to the area of an illness or to places on the meridians of the body. As with all Chinese-based healing systems, the body is viewed as being filled with channels, known as meridians, of living energy, qi [pronounced 'chee']. It is the healer's job to invigorate the flow of this energy and to remove blockages in the meridians.

The positions of these meridians is very precisely known to Chinese healers but Western doctors are bemused by them as there is nothing in their knowledge that conforms to these meridians - they do not follow the circulatory or nervous system. However, recently, French researchers injecting radioactive isotopes into human subjects found that they travelled along the lines of the meridians. Also, researchers in bio-magnetism say that the energy flow along the meridians is the way in which the bodily magnetic system completes its cycle. The brain pulses a negative magnetic impulse which travels down the spine and then returns to the brain, along the meridians, through the flesh and organs of the body, in order to complete the circuit.

Reiki is not the only name given to this form of healing: qigong masters also use it and in America there is a technique known as Therapeutic Touch, which despite its name does not involve physical contact.

One clinical test to assess the effectiveness of Therapeutic Touch was conducted by New York University researcher, Daniel Wirth. In a double blind study involving 44 patients with full-skin-thickness surgical wounds cut deliberately for the purposes of the study. The subjects inserted the arm with the wound through a hole in a wall. They could not see what was happening on the other side. They were told that their bio-potential was being measured by a non-contact device, a procedure lasting five minutes each time. Half the patients received non-contact therapeutic touch treatment and half the patients held their arm into an empty room. A doctor who did not know which patients were receiving the treatment was delegated to measure the wounds with a special digital and highly accurate device. There was no placebo effect involved because there was no suggestion that any healing was taking place. By day 16, more than half of the treated group had completely healed (wound-size zero) while none of the untreated group had healed. Something clearly is going on.

In another case demonstrating the healing powers of what is known as 'laying on of hands', a Lutheran nun in Darmstadt, Germany was helping to build a chapel when she had a bad fall which resulted in a compound pelvic fracture. The nuns maintained an all night all day vigil for two days and then, against the doctors advice took her out. They prayed and performed laying on of hands. Immediately after the laying on of hands she stood up and announced that she was free of pain. After two weeks the nun presented herself back at the hospital and the doctors had to agree that she was cured.

It is known that healers appear to have developed an ability to radiate electromagnetic energy, these forms of healing appear to be other manifestations of the same effect.

nd Sunbathing *lots of naturopathic websites advise a few mins. of sun a day to help cancer*

...as been getting a very bad press in recent years. Certainly, there is some evidence to suggest that excess sunlight causes non-fatal forms of skin cancer (but only, some say, in those whose skin is fair and whose diet contains too much animal fat). But to conclude from this that the best thing to do is to stay indoors would be counter-productive. The fact is that there is also a very good correlation between high exposure to sunlight and low incidence of internal cancers. This beneficial effect is far more important than any negative effect.

In one study, rabbits were exposed to different levels of natural light. The rabbits exposed to the most light, developed the fewest tumours, had fewer metastases and fewer deaths. In a Russian study, animals exposed to sunlight had only half the number of malignant growths compared with controls not exposed to sunlight. A US Navy study of cancer incidence amongst sailors found that there was a relatively high incidence of skin cancer, but a substantially reduced incidence of all other cancers (two and a half times lower than the average). The incidence of breast cancer in mice has been cut in half by exposing them to ultraviolet light.

In one anecdotal case described by Dr. Kime, author of a book entitled simply, *Sunlight*, a 41-year-old patient of his had a breast removed because of cancer and had been given chemotherapy treatments, because the cancer had moved into her lungs and bones. However, the doctors treating her were not hopeful of success. She approached Kime who felt there was nothing he could do for her cancer but that he could perhaps help her improve her overall health. He removed the refined polyunsaturated oils and fats - particularly margerine which is known to lower the immune system - from her diet and asked her to eat only whole foods, nothing refined. He also told her about some of the research that had been done with sunlight and cancer. She acted on his advice and started to spend a great deal of time out of doors in the sunlight.

Before starting the sunbathing she had been losing weight, but after several weeks of sunbathing and good dietary practice, her weight levelled off and she began to notice she had more energy. She eventually went back to see her doctors and they could find no apparent symptoms of her widespread cancer.

It is natural for us to visualise the warm rays of the sun as life-enhancing. We feel better out of doors in the sun. This is not an imaginary effect. The immune system responds positively to sunlight, and sunlight has been shown to increase the amount of oxygen in the body's tissues. High blood pressure is also correlated with high cancer incidence and sunlight has a very strong lowering effect on blood pressure - and so reduces the otherwise higher cancer incidence. So, all in all, a day pottering about on a beach or in a garden on a warm summer's day is a day well spent.

Sunlight of course is very important for vitamin D production. Foods supplemented with vitamin D are a poor substitute. In this context, it should be noted that sun creams and sunblocks are to be avoided, as they prevent the intake of vitamin D. The suggestion that sunscreens should not be used is highly controversial and appears to fly in the face of good sense. However, in relation to cancer, the evidence in favour of the protective effects of sunscreens has not been clearly demonstrated in epidemiological studies. For example, in 1998, Dr. Marianne Berwick, an epidemiologist at Memorial Sloan-Kettering Cancer Center in New York, presented an analysis of sunscreen use and skin cancer at the annual meeting of the American Association for the Advancement of Science (AAAS). Her conclusion: "We don't really know whether sunscreens prevent skin cancer."

To deal with all these factors, different strategies have been suggested. One is to spend an amount of time unprotected and then, when there is a danger of being burnt, to add a sunscreen. Others suggest using sunscreen only on the most exposed surfaces. Others still suggest that you should gradually increase exposure without using a sunscreen to prevent burning. There are a number of organic sunscreans coming on to the market and green tea is strongly protective – so keep the kettle on and keep pouring it over you (having waited for it to cool down!). Life Extension Foundation offers a Total Sun Protection Cream SPF-30 that helps protect also against free radical damage www.lef.org . Another suggestion is to use coconut oil. This is a healthy oil and it appears to prevent burning.

For those who do suffer non-melanoma skin cancers, BEC5 curaderm cream is reported to be very effective.

Some people are very sensitive to exposure to sunlight. They should increase their intake of carotene by drinking fresh carrot juice. This will help them become more tolerant. Others, particularly those of African extraction, have dark skins that block absorption of vitamin D. The darker your skin naturally is, the longer you need to be out in the sun to get its benefits. Sadly, whether it is lack of sunlight or down to diet, African Americans have a far higher incidence of cancer than people with white skin, and they also succumb faster to the disease.

One of the ways in which sunlight is supposed to work is that it electrically charges the air as it passes through the atmosphere. Negatively charged ions are good for you and positively charged ions are bad. Heating and air-conditioning systems tend to increase the positive ions and take out the negative ions. The result is ill-health. Negatively charged ions increase one's feelings of health and increased energy and mental and emotional exhilaration. Experiments with rats show that cancers grow faster if they breathe common indoor air as opposed to normal outdoor air.

And of course sunlight is relaxing and so makes the body better able to tolerate physical and mental stress. It also helps make the body's tissues alkaline, the importance of which needs no stressing.

Further evidence that sunlight is beneficial comes from a study that shows that New Yorkers who retire to Florida have lower cancer levels than New Yorkers who stay in New York.

In another study, researchers found that the time of year in which a cancer operation took place had a significant influence on the likelihood of the malignancy recurring. Patients who had a high intake of vitamin D in their diet, and who also had their surgery in the summer were more than twice as likely to be alive five years after cancer surgery compared to those patients who had low vitamin D intake and whose operations took place in the winter.

Earlier, we discussed the advisability of avoiding sunscreen as far as possible, you are also advised to avoid sunglasses, or indeed any form of eye wear, while in the sun.

According to Dr. Joseph Meites, an endocrinologist at Michigan State University, light entering the eyes causes nerve impulses which influence the pituitary and the pineal glands to trigger a release of various hormones. "We have no idea how many diseases are linked with hormone problems, but we do know that several diseases such as diabetes, infertility, cancer and thyroid disorders are involved with hormone imbalance". The pineal gland is the source of melatonin.

The man who did most to raise our awareness of the value of natural full-spectrum sunlight was John Ott, author of a number of books, his first being *Health & Light: the effects of natural & artificial light on man & other living things*. He once found himself talking to the daughter of Albert Schweitzer. He asked if they had found much cancer among the local Africans at his Lambarene clinic. She told him there was no cancer when they first arrived but that it had become a significant problem. Ott casually asked whether the local people were wearing sunglasses. She told him that sunglasses had become the latest sign of status. Everyone had to have a pair.

In another case, cancer researcher, Dr. Jane C. Wright, decided to test Ott's ideas. On his advice, Dr. Wright instructed fifteen cancer patients to stay outdoors as much as possible that summer in natural sunlight without wearing their glasses, and particularly without sunglasses. By that autumn, the tumours of 14 of the 15 patients had either stabilised or gone into remission.. But why had the fifteenth person not also benefited? Ott discovered that this woman had not followed his instructions - although she had not worn sunglasses, she had continued to wear her prescription glasses. This blocked the UV light from entering her eyes and so prevented her from getting the full benefit of the sunlight.

In 1961, Ott's attention was drawn to a curious fact. An elementary school in Niles, Illinois, was found to have the highest rate of leukaemia of any school in the USA, with five times the national incidence. Engineer and health activist Barry Groves tells the story: "Because of the intense glare from the sun, in the newly-constructed building in which glass had been used extensively, the teachers in two of the classrooms kept the blinds drawn and the children were exposed all day only to 'warm-white' fluorescent light. All of the children with leukemia were being taught in these two classrooms. After several years of keeping the blinds drawn and the fluorescent lights on, the teachers in these two classrooms left and were replaced with teachers who preferred to let the sunlight in. At the same time, the warm-white fluorescents were replaced with cool-white lights. From 1964, the time of Ott's last visit, there were no further cases of leukemia reported in that school." (www.second-opinions.co.uk)

In addition to getting as much natural sunlight as possible, you should consider replacing all light bulbs in the home with full spectrum light bulbs.

CANCER: THE MIND AND THE EMOTIONS

Introduction

Is there a connection between cancer and the mind, the way we view ourselves and our emotional states, both conscious and unconscious? Are there ways that we can harness the mind to improve our likelihood of recovering from cancer? These are some of the issues I will be looking at in this chapter.

Psychological Impact of Low-Oxygen State

We have, in previous pages, frequently mentioned the fact that a low-oxygen state is held to be the key cause of cancer. It is easy, but a mistake, to see this as simply a fact that relates only to the state of the body's physical tissues. The truth is a state of low oxygenation has an impact on the whole person. Ingrid Naiman, author of *Cancer Salves: A Botanical Approach to Treatment*, describes the following impacts on the person suffering from low oxygenation: "The symptoms of poor oxygenation include pallor and fatigue, poor circulation to the extremities (cold hands and feet), and sometimes dizziness or mental fuzziness. The psychological symptoms are subtle: lack of fortitude, an easy sense of defeat, conviction that the effort needed to do something cannot be made, vulnerability, and perhaps even some disorientation." (www.cancerchecklist.com)

I have a friend, Pauline, who is, as I write this, dying of colon cancer. She refuses to accept any of the suggestions that I send her. She is totally passive in the face of her disease. Not everyone with cancer feels this way but it is clearly a common enough syndrome. Dr. Shultze, the herbalist, believes that only a small percent of the people who start on his 30 day dietary programme will make it to the end. The rest do not want enough to live – or are not convinced enough in the merits of the diet perhaps - and so cannot force themselves to make the effort.

If you, the reader, have cancer yourself, I would like to suggest to you that you form a personal 'Get Well Again Committee' of say one to three friends whose job it is to read this book with you and to discuss and ultimately advise you on what to do. These friends can also facilitate the getting of whatever it is you need to get. They can force you to do, perhaps, what you may not feel you have the energy to do. But that's what friends are for. And not all of the approaches in this book require effort – but they may require hope and a desire to live. You may not even have that: such is the impact of the body on the mind.

Psychotherapy & Cancer-Prone Personalities

One of the first investigators into the field of psychology and cancer was Dr. Lawrence LeShan, an experimental psychologist and therapist. Starting in the 1950s, he undertook research into whether or not there were psychological predisposing characteristics which might make explain why some people got cancer - and whether or not this could be used to help people to recover. This research spanned three decades and his conclusions were 'yes' to both questions.

He quotes the case of 'John' who had a massive, inoperable brain tumour. After working with LeShan using a special form of psychotherapy - which LeShan characterises as 'crisis therapy' - John recovered without medication even though his doctors had told him he had only months to live. John's psychological state before he met LeShan was one of hopelessness. After going through psychotherapy, he developed a much more positive frame of mind. His attitude to life turned around and his terminal cancer disappeared.

In his book *You Can Fight for Your Life*, LeShan described the process by which John and a number of other patients underwent complete remission. He also argued that even those he worked with who didn't undergo remission, who indeed did die from their cancers, nevertheless had the quality of their lives dramatically transformed for the better through his work with them.

LeShan's work started when he and a co-worker discovered that there seemed to be startling similarities in the personality configurations and in the life histories of people who subsequently died of cancer. A personality configuration very similar to that of people with a predisposition to suicide. LeShan believed that if there was such a configuration it should be tracked down.

In the first stage of his research, he interviewed 250 patients - spending between 2 and 8 hours with each one. Another 200 cancer patients were interviewed on the side for specific concerns. Close relatives of over 50 patients were interviewed for between one and three hours and another 40 close relatives were seen from between 20 and 50 hours. This was over a period of 14 years. In addition he undertook intensive psychotherapy with 71 patients.

As a result of his study, he came to the following conclusions:

i) that "there is a general type of personality configuration among the majority of cancer patients", and

ii) that "people whose personality or life history conforms to this pattern of susceptibility can take steps to protect themselves against the possibility of cancer."

What LeShan discovered was that for a significant majority of cancer cases there had been, prior to the onset of cancer, a loss of a crucial relationship. This loss may have been a physical or, more frequently, an emotional loss - for instance, a failure of a marriage, or a marriage from which the heart had gone, or an attachment to a way of life or activity that promised happiness but which was denied to the person involved for some reason. From this perception he predicted that age-corrected cancer rates for women would be highest for widows, next highest for divorced women, then for married women without children, followed by married women with children and lowest for single women. Epidemiological statistics from various sources appear to support this conclusion.

Secondly. he found that for a large majority of cancer patients there is a clear inability to express hostility, anger or resentment. He went on to discover that cancers developed in people who were in despair because they frustrated their own creative potential. They denied themselves. They felt that they had to be other than themselves to be accepted, and conversely that they would be rejected by others if they were themselves.

His patient John had become a lawyer and joined his father's firm as a result of strong parental suggestion and he had married a woman chosen by his parents who enjoyed being the wife of a lawyer. However, he was deeply dissatisfied. As a child John had shown a great deal of interest in music and he had dreamt of being a pianist. As a result of his therapy, John came to accept that it was possible that he could be a pianist if he really wanted to and that he had a right to fight for what he wanted. He quit his job, divorced his wife, took up the piano seriously and eventually became a pianist with a symphony orchestra. His terminal brain cancer disappeared.

While many people feel despair, LeShan discovered, the despair of the cancer patient has unique features:

"The patient in despair is absolutely alone. At the deepest emotional level he cannot relate, since he does not believe himself worthy of love. He does not despair over 'something', as would the usual depressed patient - rather, he despairs over 'nothing'.

"Trapped in this alone-ness, the cancer patient is in an emotional place where it is impossible to be reached by love, where any kind of fulfilling or satisfying relationship becomes impossible. The cancer patient is even divorced from such negative emotions as anger, resentment and jealousy. As one of his patients said to him: "You don't understand doctor. It's not that I've been or done anything. It's that I've done nothing and been nothing."

"the cancer patient's own desires and wishes had been so completely repressed... that when at the start of the therapy I asked the question, "What do you really want out of life?" the response would be a blank and astonished stare. That question had never been seen as valid."

This despair was evident in 68 out of the 71 patients he worked with. LeShan believed strongly that patients feeling this level of despair could be helped, and his case studies showed that he succeeded. He does not give any statistics in his book regarding the number of remissions that resulted among the 71 patients - but in addition to John, he mentions four other patients who recovered, without medication, from terminal cancer.

Spontaneous remission of cancer among terminal cases is considered to be extremely rare. One in 100,000 has been one estimate. Yet LeShan is implicitly claiming to have achieved an inconceivably higher success rate. One of the reasons LeShan gives no statistics is because he does not want remission of cancer to be the only yardstick of value. Indeed LeShan believes that many of those he worked with rediscovered themselves and led lives that were worth living - after decades of failing to do that. As one of his patients said: "Death is nothing. It is inevitable. Everyone has to die. What matters is how you live and die."

And it wasn't just the patient who was affected by the course of the patient's psychotherapy. The daughter of one patient wrote to LeShan after her mother had died "I know that everyday she grew in courage and understanding... and was learning to fight the fears that surrounded her... My father and I are changed...and I think it influenced her friends who visited her....Mother's last months were filled with hope and thoughts of the future..."

For this reason LeShan is not concerned to boast about success rates on a simple cure-death ratio. Success can be measured qualitatively. It was the objective of his therapy to 'reawaken the inner life of the individual, and to liberate those forces which can enable the person to experience as completely as possible both himself and the meaning of his life and death.'

The crisis therapy that LeShan developed is very different from orthodox psychotherapy. First it dispenses with the view that unconscious forces rigidly control a helpless ego. He believes that the individual can be freed from constrictions to create his or her own world and to express his or her own true feelings. He also believes that this demands absolute honesty and openness from the therapist - the therapist does not allow him/herself to have an unexpressed commentary flowing in parallel to the therapy session. Everything must be made explicit. The therapist is not kind or careful. Time is short and the past needs to be confronted if the therapy is to succeed. This honesty must permeate the relationship and it precludes kindness - which LeShan sees as being a protective device for the therapist and implies a superior position. The crisis therapist must be in full personal contact with the patient, otherwise he is simply conspiring to avoid the key issues that underlie the cancer. "Death, the figure in the background, asks the questions, and the therapist must join in the search for answers that are meaningful to the patient."

The crisis therapist also talks to the family to prepare them for change - because they are certainly a constraining factor whether or not they intend to be. This requires a great deal of support and cooperation from the family.

And what is the goal of this therapy? To make patients confront their true selves, to become aware of their true desires and to make them feel important to themselves. In the mirror of death, some patients feel free to explore this question.

Anyone seeking psychotherapy because of cancer should discuss LeShan's ideas with the therapist at the first meeting. This will establish the foundations of the relationship.

LeShan favours the idea of psychological self-help and suggests two useful techniques: one to confront the past, the other the future.

To confront the past, LeShan suggests the following technique. In the darkness of the imagination, we can enter a time machine and return as adults to the critical times in our pasts, the times that can still cause us pain, the times when the seeds of the present - perhaps the self's self-denial - were sown, and to face the child that was ourselves then. And when we are there, adult and child, face to face, we should think what we would like to say to that child.

This kind of self-confronting journey has a very powerful potential to heal psychic wounds.

For those who feel helpless in the face of the future, LeShan suggests a second technique: the person should focus on the impossible ambition and then to ask himself: "What is the first thing that has to be done, the very first thing, to achieve this goal?" Every journey starts with a single step. If that first step is taken, there is a good chance the journey will be completed. Without that step, there is no journey.

People who are self-determining, LeShan argues, do not get cancer (or are very much less likely to). People who discover and embrace a purpose can cure themselves of cancer, even when medical science has done everything it can do and failed. If they aren't cured, at least every minute of life left to them is enhanced in value.

Key Text: Lawrence LeShan, *You Can Fight for Your Life*, M.Evans and Company, New York, 1976. See also his website at www.cancerasaturningpoint.org

A self-help approach called Emotional Freedom Technique (EFT) claims to be beneficial for a wide range of health concerns. A free 79-page booklet explaining the approach can be obtained at: www.emofree.com/downloadeftmanual.htm.

LeShan's approach has been mirrored in Germany by Dr. Ryke Geerd Hamer. Both Hamer and his wife were diagnosed with cancer shortly after their son was murdered. Hamer subsequently developed a complex understanding of cancer. In his view, cancer is a natural process which gets triggered by an overwhelming emotional shock for which the body is totally unprepared. This shock registers itself physically in the brain. Healing, in his view, cannot occur until there is first an emotional healing. Bizarrely, Hamer has been imprisoned in France for his cancer views. In earlier centuries, heretics got tortured and burned, today non-mainstream cancer researchers get pilloried in the press and arrested. For further details of Hamer's complex views on cancer go to the official English-language website of Dr. Hamer is at www.newmedicine.ca.

Emotional Healing

Pattie, whose story is at the end of this book, tells of how cancer made her re-evaluate her life: "I changed my diet, quit my stressful job, sold my too-big house, rid myself of all negative friends, and divorced my alcoholic hubby." The result? "I had no idea what real happiness was until 2002." Another woman writing in a cancer chat group wrote: "It was not until I got away from him that I really realized how stressed I have been, especially the last two years since the diagnosis."

Emotional healing is important. It almost always involves making hard decisions but the result can be liberating. The body has enough obstacles to healing as it is. It can do without the stress of unhappy relationships. It is also about letting go of anger.

As another cancer patient wrote: "I had lung cancer plus metastasis to the intestines and brain. Once there was metastasis my doctor gave up giving me medicine...I decided to forgive many people because I believed I was heading for an early death. Forgiving is a very strong factor in why I am still alive today."

Mind-Body Interaction

One of the imponderable facts of cancer is that some are aggressive, developing very quickly, while others are slow and steady in their development. LeShan believes the aggressiveness is a direct reflection of the speed at which the cancer occurs after the loss of life's meaning as embodied in a central relationship. That is to say, the cause of an aggressive cancer is to be found shortly before the cancer develops, while the cause of a slow growing cancer is to be found further back in the past. The psychologist, Dr. Bruno Klopfer, claimed to be able to predict with 80 percent accuracy which patients had slow growing cancers, and which fast growing, on the basis of personality tests alone. Those with the more acutely felt despair had the more aggressive cancers.

LeShan and Klopfer seem to be saying that cancer is an accurate measure of despair. This can be true only if the mind and body are inextricably entwined as entities - or indeed if there is no separation of mind and body.

This question is a very contentious one. Traditional Western philosophy and science are based on the assumption that mind and body are distinct and separate. The mind is seen as distinct from the brain, the physical organ that is associated with it. If they are distinct and separate how can one affect the other? If a doctor says, "It's psychosomatic. It's all in the mind," he is saying it isn't real, it isn't true, it exists only as a thought, not as a fact. Against this view is the one - widely accepted in ancient times - and also today by many other non-Western cultures - that mind and body are one inextricable whole. What affects the body affects the mind and vice versa.

The idea that emotions can cause cancer is a common one and indeed for most of the last two thousand years - with the sole exception of the twentieth century - it was the standard view. At the end of the nineteenth century, Sir James Paget, one of the leading medical figures of his time reflected the orthodox view when he wrote: "The cases are so frequent in which deep anxiety, deferred hope and disappointment are quickly followed by the growth and increase of cancer that we can hardly doubt that mental depression is a weighty additive to the other influences favouring the development of the cancerous constitution."

It is only in this century with its over-emphasis on the mechanical features of the body, that the individual's self and his values, beliefs and feelings have been more or less totally ignored. Modern medicine deals with the body as if it were a machine. Each bit and piece can be taken out, replaced, tinkered with and so on. People don't die of broken hearts or despair any more; they die of cerebral haemorrhage or cancer of the cervix. The result is that doctors believe it is for them – the mechanics of the body - to decide what repair is needed. And if excision of the rectum appears to be necessary for the further functioning of the body-machine so be it - out with the rectum.

There is little concern for whether the patient wishes to live with the continuing pain, in convenience and indignity that such an operation bequeaths.

But the great things in life: love, laughter, beauty, courage as well as the negative things such as fear, worry, danger and so on belong as much to the mind as to the chemistry of the body. If mind and body are so separate then why do we cry when we are sad or in pain, why do we feel a physical thrill at the sight of great beauty? Why do we jump immediately we sense danger? Laugh when something is funny? In each of these cases the physical response does not wait for the conscious message, it occurs absolutely in synch with the mental message. Mental and physical responses are two sides of a coin that cannot be separated from each other.

We can conclude from this that all thoughts are facts. If our mind and body are one then our body is intelligent and our thoughts are physical. Similarly, if the body is diseased in some way, then we cannot say that we have the disease but rather that the disease is part us, part of our identity. We are the disease.

This at least is the position of Deepak Chopra. The point of contact between the mind and body are the neuro-peptide transmitters - the body's 'messenger molecules' as Chopra calls them.

"A neuro-peptide springs into existence at the touch of a thought, but where does it spring from? A thought of fear and the neuro-chemical that it turns into are somehow connected to a hidden process, a transformation of non-matter into matter."

Chopra calls the zone where this occurs the "? zone". This question mark zone is a place below the visible. It is a world where quantum rules dictate reality - and one of the rules is that things can happen suddenly, absolutely and inexplicably - the so called quantum leap where A can become B instantaneously. He gives an example of such a quantum cure taking place. A patient of his, a woman in her fifties went to see him complaining of severe abdominal pains and jaundice. He thought at first that she was suffering from gallstones and arranged for surgery, but when she was opened up, it was found that she had a large malignant tumour that had spread to her liver, with scattered pockets of cancer throughout her abdominal cavity. The surgeons considered the cancer to be inoperable and closed the incision without taking further action. Chopra spoke to the woman's daughter first. She pleaded with him not to tell her mother the truth and Chopra agreed to go along with this deceit. He informed the woman that the gallstone operation had been completely successful. He expected her to die within a few months but some time later she appeared before him for a routine examination that revealed no signs of cancer. Much later the woman said to him: "Doctor, I was so sure I had cancer two years ago that when it turned out to be just gallstones, I told myself I would never be sick another day in my life."

We can call an event like this a miracle, a spontaneous remission, a placebo cure. But the fact is, whatever words we give it, it happens.

Placebos

"They can conquer who believe they can." Dryden

A three-year-old boy with a severe case of whooping cough was seen by the doctor. The doctor appeared before the boy in great robes. He sat on the boy's bed and peeled a peach. Then he sugared it and cut it into small pieces. He fed each piece slowly to the boy. As he did so he told the boy that he was going to be fine, as the peaches would make him well again. He made the boy feel his health was inevitable. However, on leaving the room he told the father that he did not hold out much hope for the boy. The whooping cough was so serious it was almost certain to be fatal. However, the next day the boy was still alive and the doctor came again. As before he made sure he was wearing his impressive medical robes. As before, he fed the boy personally with some fruit. After 40 days and 40 visits the boy was well again. The doctor was the famous Sir William Osler and the boy was the brother of Dr. Patrick Mallam who published the story in the *Journal of the American Medical Association* (December 22, 1969). Osler, incidentally, is famous for his comment: "In today's system of medicine a patient has to recover twice: once from the disease and once from the treatment."

Just believing that a pill is a powerful pain-reliever can be enough to get rid of the pain in 30-60 percent of the people given the placebo. We can therefore conclude that the level of faith in a therapy helps to determine how successful that therapy is. Curiously, it is not the least educated and those who are of lower intelligence who are most susceptible to this effect, rather the reverse. Placebos have a higher tendency to work with the more intelligent and educated. And it doesn't appear to be a conscious decision, placebos don't work because we consciously want them to work. The basis of the placebo's action lies deeper in the mind.

One study showed placebos to be 35 percent effective. Other studies support the view that 30-40 percent of people respond to placebos. That the placebo effect may be even stronger is indicated by a number of studies. One showed that valium was more effective than a placebo for the first week of therapy only. After that they had equal effectiveness. This contradicts the prevalent view that placebo cures are short-lasting. Another study substituted saline solution for morphine with morphine-addicted patients who were being withdrawn from their addiction. No withdrawal symptoms appeared until the saline injections were stopped. The placebo effect is clearly reinforced when the attitude of the doctor is positive.

If we can believe a disease or a pain away, then we can believe it into existence - not consciously perhaps, but at some level of awareness. If the body is intelligent then it is intelligent in every part of the body, every organ is intelligent, every cell is intelligent.

Is this really true - or is it just poetic over-statement? Consider the famous case of a child named Timmy, whose story is quoted by Deepak Chopra. Timmy suffers from multiple personality disorder. Nearly a dozen personalities contend within his physical frame. One of these personalities is allergic to orange juice but the allergic reaction stops as soon as another personality takes over.

For this fact to make sense we have to accept that the cells of the antibodies that trigger the allergic reaction have to make a choice as to whether to react or not. This choice is dependent on the choice the mind has made about which personality it is at any moment. This means the mind is capable of choosing to be allergic or not allergic. If it can choose to have an allergy it can also choose to have cancer. If the disease is something we have unconsciously chosen, then the cure too is capable of being chosen.

Given the obvious benefits of placebos, one would think that more would be done with them. But most hospitals seem more concerned to make patients feel depressed and dissociated. Cold bare white corridors; the smell of antiseptic floor wash; cold, plastic tiled floors. Let's face it, hospitals seem to be creating problems for themselves before they even start. Hospitals and doctors seem to be working against placebos rather than with them. The wise patient will create his or her own placebo enhancing mental environment.

The reverse process is true. Many patients told their cancer is incurable promptly fulfil their doctor's expectations by dying. But the case of TB is instructive. 100 years ago, TB had the same fearful prognosis as cancer today - but then a cure was found and suddenly death rates from TB dropped sharply - even though most of those who recovered had not yet received the new antibiotic..

The power of expectations is so strong that there are good reasons for not pursuing any form of treatment towards which you have a negative attitude: The Simontons, a husband and wife team, conducted an 18 month study with 152 patients into the importance of attitude in determining the outcome of treatment with radiation. The results were clear. Patients with positive attitudes had a better response to the radiation treatment than those with negative attitudes. In fact, of the 152 patients only two who had shown a negative attitude had a good response to treatment. Patients who had a good attitude and a more developed cancer generally did better than patients with a negative attitude but less advanced cancer. This leads to a very important conclusion. Cancer patients should only undertake treatments that they have positive attitudes about. If you feel that the best place to deal with cancer is the hospital and that the best weapons are radiation and chemo therapy, then concentrate positive thoughts towards these forms of treatment. If you feel they will not help then don't do them.

One of the classic cases of placebo cure was reported by Dr. Bruno Klopfer. One of his patients took a drug called Krebiozen and his growths "melted like snowballs". A few months later, newspapers reported that the drug was worthless and the patient's tumours promptly recurred. Suspecting that the patient had a powerful belief system, Klopfer announced that he would give him a more active form of the drug. In fact he injected his patient with nothing more than distilled water, yet once again the tumors melted away. After a few more months, there were further reports announcing that Krebiozen was worthless. The patient accepted the truth of these reports, his tumors soon reappeared, and he quickly died.

A Fighting Attitude

A study at King's College Hospital looked at the impact of a fighting spirit on the survival of women who had mastectomies for early stage breast cancer. Ten years later 55 percent of the group who had the strongest fighting spirit - or whose levels of denial were so strong that they refused to believe they had the disease - had survived, compared with only twenty-two percent of the group who felt hopeless and helpless or who stoically accepted their fate.

What is a 'fighting attitude'? This is complex and sometimes controversial question. Possibly the best way of defining it is to say it is having a positive acceptance of the disease and its implications combined with an active desire to get well again.

In another study, having a 'hopeful attitude' was the key that allowed researchers to predict which women out of 68 who came to a hospital for a cervical biopsy had cancer and who did not. Before the results of the biopsy were known the women were interviewed and assessed for personality factors. The researchers then predicted who would have and who would not have cancer. Of the 68 women, 28 had cancer. The researchers correctly predicted 68 percent of the cancer victims and 77 percent of the cancer-free women simply on the basis of their relative hopefulness   or hopelessness.

In other studies, the degree of hope, faith and trust in a surgeon has been shown to correlate highly with speedier recovery. Curiously, people who avoid thinking about the outcome of an operation recover faster than those who are eternally vigilant. This is further demonstration, perhaps, of a simple truth: that the unconscious is more powerful than the conscious.

Clearly the mind is capable of unleashing very powerful forces that can lead to both health and illness. People can will themselves to death and they can will themselves to health. How can we harness these powers? Some methods will already have suggested themselves. Hypnosis, visualisation, and meditation are some of the ways people have recommended. These approaches have been treated separately in the last section of this book.

Spiritual Consciousness

Some cancer patients go beyond an earth-bound mind-body nexus. For them the disease is the key they needed to unlock the secret of themselves. They embrace their disease and take responsibility for their response to it. Like a smack over the head from a Zen master, the diagnosis of cancer has changed their awareness of - and attitude to - life. One such ex-cancer patient is Petrea King.

"Clearly I didn't sit down consciously to figure out ways of making my body sick to achieve some underlying aim. Later in my life, I didn't think, ' Ah yes, a good dose of leukemia with a short prognosis is just what I need right now.' Yet I firmly believe, at some more subtle level, that the particular disease and prognosis were precisely tailor made for me...It's often said 'People don't change.' I believe that statement is made only by people who don't welcome change in themselves...When we make a firm commitment to life and to experiencing our connection with the flow of power and love in the universe, extraordinary and unexpected events begin to unfold. Greater peace, equanimity and joy are experienced even in the midst of disease, and the experience of these states creates the perfect environment for physical healing to take place...Leukemia was the best thing that ever came my way because I learned much more about myself much more quickly than I ever could have without it." (Petrea King, *Quest for Life*, 1992)

The spiritually awakened patient may in the end die of the cancer, but nevertheless, they may be grateful - even in the face of their own self-extinction - that they have woken to a more profound consciousness of existence and of their own lives.

It may seem strange that anyone could love their disease or feel   immense gratitude to something that is seeking their own extinction. But this surprise derives ultimately from a refusal to see something very obvious and very simple: we are all going to die. The spiritually awakened person sees this. Quite simply, he or she no longer fears death. What is there to fear? Death is natural and it is inevitable. It cannot be run away from. Those men and women who embrace the inevitability of death are freed and this freedom feels like a cosmic joke. They can thrill with the streaming energy of the universe and thrill to their awareness of the cosmic dance when the atoms of their physical bodies are dispersed to the universe - then where does the mind's energy go? Die now or die later. What does it matter?

And the curious thing is this: the energy released by this awareness can put the cancer into remission. And it makes the remaining life that is given a life that is more intensely felt and so more profoundly lived.

It is also true that this acceptance of illness is one way in which the patient demonstrates that they have accepted themselves. This acceptance can transform the patient's entire subjective world and this in turn can lead to the healing of disease.

A Japanese study into patients who went home to die from cancer and instead got well showed that a complete acceptance of God's will - or the will of fate - was a constant theme through all their stories. We can see what this means in more personal terms when we consider the following words of an AIDS patient.

"I deal with this disease by looking at it as one of the best teachers I've ever had. I treat it with respect. I try to love it. I talk to it. I'll say: "You are safe with me. Do not worry. I do not hate you." (Young person with AIDS, quoted by Dr. Larry Dossey, 1993)

And another patient, the actor Mandy Patinkin, had this to say: "The greatest thing in my life was getting cancer because it taught me how much I love my life, my family, my friends and my work. And it taught me that I must find some peace and calm every day. I never could sit still long enough to meditate, but I do it every day. I'm like a little baby Zen Buddhist."

Body-Mind Therapies

There are a number of healing activities, behaviours and therapies that make sense once we understand there is a dynamic of interaction between mind and body—that mind is an aspect of body and the body is an aspect of mind.

Bodywork and Posture Therapies

There are hundreds of schools of practitioners who offer some form of bodywork. Kinesiology, Alexander Technique, Chiropractic and Osteopathy, Yoga, Rolfing, Lowen Bioenergetics, Structural Integration, and many other forms of working with the body to promote health, share a basic understanding: mens sana in corpore sano as the Latin motto on many coats of arms expresses it: a healthy mind in a healthy body. You can't have one without the other. And rather than start with the mind, they propose that it makes sense to start with the body.

If we accept that mind and body are one then it makes sense to see the body as a memory system of the mind. Negative thoughts affect the way the muscles are used, the more the muscles are used in a certain way, certain postures result that can lead to postural imbalances which themselves will have other negative effects on the health of the person. Physical traumas too are, it seems, retained in the body long after the original 'insult' (to use the medical term) appears to have been healed.

It is helpful to understand that the entire interiors of our bodies – stomach, heart, liver, intestine and all the rest of it – are interlinked by a sheath of connective tissue -- the fascia – which interconnects with every part of the body. An important element of this fascia is the diaphragm. This is not just useful for breathing but also for massaging all the internal organs. Imbalances in one area of the fascia are therefore felt throughout the system. A slight negative pull in one area can have major long-term impacts elsewhere in the body. If these, as is likely, negatively affect our breathing,   this will in turn affect the amount of oxygen in our blood and tissues.

All the schools of bodywork take this as their starting point and all seek to correct any problems that they identify. Tai Chi and qigong exercises may also be beneficial for the same reason – that they correct imbalances, even though this is not their primary objective.

Kinesiotherapy is one of a number of postural retraining therapies. It involves training the patient in the proper use of the body in posture movement and repose in order to achieve healing.

The principle behind kinesiotherapy is that mental as well as physical energy is tied up in wrong postures and actions.

Poor posture and lack of proper exercise puts a strain on the body. However, by using the body properly we can relieve this stress. Swinging and swaying can loosen up the joints. Jarring and jolting movements need to be avoided. To straighten the spine using simple traction, you can hang your head over the end of your bed. Movements should, where possible, be slow and harmonious.

The Alexander Technique was developed by the Australian Frederick Alexander. According to him 'use affects function' ill-use distorts and misshapes the body and interferes with free functioning. When Professor Tinbergen gave his Nobel prize speech in 1973 (he won the prize for medicine) he used this forum to praise Alexander's work.

American Ida Rolf developed a system known today as 'Rolfing'. Her system is more concerned with structure and bodily mechanics than with posture and movement. This is one of many schools that collectively refer to their work as 'Structural Integration'. They work with the fascia, or connective tissue, that holds the internal body together. The objective is to free it up.

"When the body is out of alignment it creates inefficiency and imbalance resulting in stiffness, discomfort and loss of energy. When a body is aligned and balanced it moves with greater ease. It requires less energy to function. Good posture is effortless and breathing is easier. The body becomes more flexible, more coordinated and athletic performance improves." (www.rolfguild.org)

Osteopathy was developed by Dr. Andrew Taylor Still (1828-1917), a physician from Missouri who developed a drugless system of treatment. He believed that ill health was the result of blockages to the circulatory and nervous systems. All the doctor has to do is to make sure these are cleared and Mother Nature will do the rest. Surprisingly, to the modern reader, he was very effective in curing infectious diseases.

Many modern osteopaths have retreated from this sytem so that the fact that a doctor is a Doctor of Osteopathy is no guarantee that he uses a drugless medicine based on manipulation.

Anyone seeking an osteopath should first ascertain whether or not they use cranial therapy. Cranial therapists believe that through cranial manipulation they can release blockages that impede the flow of living energy that is the essential feature of health and life. Dr. Andrew Weil, in his book: *Spontaneous Healing*, described his observations of an osteopath working in this way. Originally sceptical, he came away from the experience with the belief that everyone the man had 'fixed' had indeed been fixed.

The title of Weil's book is interesting and refers to healing that occurs without any treatment having been taken. Some cancers do just disappear and these are referred to as spontaneous healings. For an interesting discussion of this subject with case histories go to www.noetic.org/research/sr/r_biblio.html

Chiropractic is a more muscular and no-nonsense approach to fixing the joints in the spine and neck. Nevertheless it too can claim its share of success in fixing problems arising from physical trauma. It has been shown to help cure cholera.

It seems very clear that manipulating the body is an effective way of dealing with a wide range of ills and the surprise is that it has not been taken up in any way by orthodox practitioners of medicine.

Rebounding is a useful exercise for those who cannot walk far–get a small trampoline and gently bounce up and down. This activity not only gives the internal and external muscles a mild workout but also stimulates the hypothalamus with the up and down movements. This is important for blood pressure, sleep and much else.

Breathing

Since stress is a major cause and stimulator of cancer, it is helpful if we can learn to relax. But breathing exercises are not just stress-busters, they are fundamental to good health and energy.

In his book, *Spontaneous Healing*, Dr. Andrew Weil describes five breathing practices that will lead to improved health and vigour if practised everyday.

1. Just observe your inhalations and exhalations for a few minutes. Don't try to influence them. Do this while in a comfortable position with your eyes closed.

2. Repeat the above but mentally view the cycle of breath as starting with the exhalation. This actually increases the amount of air inhaled.

3. While seated, or better while lying down, imagine that the breaths that go out and in do not start with you but originate with the universe itself. You are in the way of the cosmic breath. The universe is breathing itself through you. Feel this universal breath permeating every part of your body.

4. Stimulating breath: Sit comfortably with back straight and eyes closed. Place the tip of the tongue on the flesh just above the back of the top teeth: the so-called yogic position. Now breathe in and out rapidly through the nose, keeping the mouth lightly closed. The rhythm of in and out breaths should be rapid, even and audible. Increase duration from 15 seconds to start with to a minute. This is an energy booster if done regularly and can be done whenever you feel sleepy and want to wake up (i.e., in the morning or in the evening while driving).

5. Relaxing breath: This can be done sitting or lying down with the tongue in the yogic position as with the previous exercise. Breathe out with an audible sound completely emptying the lungs to a count of eight. Then close the mouth and inhale quietly for a count of four. Then hold the breath for a count of seven. Do this for four building up to eight cycles after a month. Speed is not important but slow is better than fast.

Weil emphasises that these breathing exercises are genuine spiritual practices aimed at bringing mind and body to a single focus - a focus of energy. Going on from breathing one can, in the mind's eye, let the breath escape from the nostril and follow it up the nose the face, follow it as it explores the cheeks, the skull and the locus of nerves at the back of the neck. Let it flow down the arms, down the back, round the buttocks, the legs, the feet, the toes, then back up the leg, the thighs the pelvic area. Let it rest in the solar plexus for a while then let it move up over the belly and chest and back up the neck to the nose. While your mind is following this route, let it sift the impressions that arise: was there a twinge or pain anywhere. This is a way of listening to the body.

The quality of breathing has a direct influence on the levels of oxygen in the blood and tissues - and this has a direct influence on whether the body's tissues are a good seedbed for the development of cancer tumours.

Good breathing practices also exercise the entire connective tissue of the body to which all the organs are connected. Good breathing therefore moves the diaphragm and in so doing massages the lungs, stomach and heart all of which are necessary for good health.

Exercise

Studies have shown that a 1-2 mile walk 3-4 times a week helps enormously in stabilizing the disease process - and sometimes reversing it. A walk like this helps the appetite, sleep cycle and energy level. Exercise is always helpful and immune enhancing - as long as one doesn't go past the point of being tired - and you allow sufficient time for recovery between sessions.

And how can exercise help? By increasing the blood's oxygen levels, releasing tension from the muscles and the spine and improving the sense of mental well-being.

One study published in the May 2005 *Journal of the American Medical Association* followed 3,000 women who had previously been diagnosed with breast cancer. They found that exercise had an enormous impact on their health and longevity. Even as little as three to five hours per week of normal walking exercise reduced their risk of dying by half.

Qigong (Chi Kung)

Qigong is a traditional form of Chinese health exercise which combines breathing, movement and meditation. There are many different schools and they may all have some benefit for cancer patients – but there is a form of qigong that was specifically developed to benefit people with cancer.

Ms. Guo Lin, a Chinese traditional painter, was originally diagnosed with cancer of the uterus in 1949 and she had it removed by surgery in Shanghai. However, the cancer recurred in 1960 and despite further treatment she was eventually told that her condition was terminal. At this point she remembered that her grandfather had taught her as a child to practice qigong. She studied his books and created her own system of qigong exercise. She practiced this form of qigong for two hours every day, and six months later tests showed that her cancer had shrunk.

She continued her practice and eventually, in 1970, she started giving lessons in a Beijing park in what she called New Qigong Therapy. By 1977 she felt she had demonstrated clearly that qigong had been beneficial for many cancer patients and she announced publicly that Qigong could cure cancer. Her fame spread and soon, everyday, she was leading three to four hundred people through their qigong paces. She became a national celebrity, travelling around China to demonstrate her system. Although she died in 1984, her system of qigong is still widely practised.

Guo Lin Qigong combines the following:

1. Deep and forceful breathing. Two inhalations followed by one exhalation. This is based on the idea of taking in more qi (pronounced 'chee') and releasing less to nourish the practitioner's own inner qi reserves.

2. A brisk walk to increase the blood circulation to generate more qi.

3. Producing a high pitch healing sound to attack the tumor and to stop it from spreading

According to Traditional Chinese Medicine, when qi (vital energy) and blood are flowing freely, the body will maintain the balance of yin and yang and disease will disappear. By practicing qi gong, qi-energy and blood circulation are improved, the balance of yin and yang is restored. From a Western point of view it can be seen that practicing qigong in such an intensive way the oxygenation of the tissues will be enhanced—and cancers do not like surrounding tissues to be highly oxygenated. In fact the need a low oxygen level to thrive.

Another important benefit is the impact on the emotions. By working out so intensively, the body is brought into a state of relaxation and the mental and emotional strength of the practitioner is enhanced.

There is also the potential healing benefit from doing these exercises in groups with other cancer patients. The diagnosis of cancer has great power to create a feeling of psychological isolation. By joining a qigong group, one can overcome this sense of aloneness. This in turn can help transform the feeling that you are a victim of circumstance to one where you are in charge. This is itself immensely energising.

There are many anecdotal reports of people who have been cured of their cancer through qigong, and a number of research studies show that in addition to reported cures there is evidence of increased longevity, improved quality of life and better pain management.

Classes continue to run in a number of Beijing parks but you may be able to find a teacher closer to home. Alternatively a form of Qigong – 'Spring Forest Qigong' – can be self taught using a DVD and CD package obtainable from www.learningstrategies.com/qigong

Mind-Body Therapies

Enthusiasm & Eccentricity

The idea of healing through healthy mindedness is of ancient origin. In modern times it was systemetised as a system of healing by a self-taught healer by the name of Phineas Quimby (1802-66). Among his followers was Mrs. Mary Baker Eddy, the founder of Christian Science.

Quimby preached that the universe was filled with the divine, infinite God. We are part of that infinite universe and so have a divine element in us. Wrong thinking can shut this flow of divine healing influence. Disease is therefore the result of evil or bad thinking. A good thought is worth a dozen drugs. The mind is our very basis. We must therefore fill our mind with good, generous thoughts and shut out mean, evil thoughts. We are who we think we are. Similarly we need to banish unhealthy emotions: fear, anxiety, worry, hatred, anger, lack of faith, complaint, contempt and so on...yes, and lust. We should even wipe these words from our vocabulary. We should fill our hearts with curative thoughts: love, courage, confidence, generosity. We need to relax and let God take over and flow through us (even if we don't believe in God).

And enthusiasm can be developed. Here is a true story. Many years ago a woman was diagnosed as having incurable TB. One doctor she consulted said that he could remove the left lung but he could in any case only give her another six months of life. A second opinion was sought and this second doctor more or less agreed. He might remove the right lung but he could only give her six more months of life. Left lung? Right lung? She lay in the hospital bed in despair. A friend of hers charged into the ward and got her out of bed. "Don't listen to this nonsense. What do doctors know? You're coming with me." Her friend took her to a Christian Science meeting. The woman became a Christian Scientist and lived another twenty years - and indeed lived to go to the funeral of her doctor. This is a true story. That woman was my grandmother. I put this story here because I believe my grandmother's survival depended on a shift in thinking away from the disease towards health - on finding some basis for feeling, once again enthusiastic about life.

Hypnosis

Hypnosis isn't a 'state' of mind like dream-sleep. It is a condition of mind in which all other mental states can be suggested externally.

It is well-known that people in a hypnotic trance can turn their hands warm and cold simply by focusing their attention to achieving these changes. Hypnotic suggestion can create even blisters and rashes on the skin.

The mind's brain waves have different frequencies while it is occupying different states. During wakefulness the brain waves are in the beta range (14 cycles per second or more). In sleep they are in the alpha range (7-14 cycles per second) occasionally dipping into the delta and theta ranges. Through hypnosis, we are taken into the alpha range while still in a state of wakefulness.

In the alpha state, the subconscious mind is open to suggestive input. Hypnotist, William Hewitt refers to the subconscious as 'an obedient slave' that doesn't think or reason.

"It just responds to what it is told. Herein lies the value and power of hypnosis. By hypnosis you can pump powerful suggestions directly into your subconscious. Your subconscious accepts them and causes them to become reality...it is extremely important that all suggestions given are positive, constructive and beneficial." (William Hewitt, 1994)

In his book, *Hypnosis*, Hewitt discounts some myths. He says that people cannot be hypnotised against their will because one of the preconditions is 100 percent cooperation. Secondly, the hypnotised person is always aware of what suggestions are being made and any suggestion that was upsetting would cause the subject to come out of the hypnotic state immediately of their own choice. According to Hewitt, almost everybody can be hypnotised. In fact, you don't need to go to a hypnotist to be hypnotised - you can hypnotise yourself. However, he suggests that it is easier to do this once you have first been hypnotised by someone else.

To hypnotise anyone, you must first induce in them a state of deep relaxation. This requires that their eyes be closed and that they focus their complete attention on a story or a set of actions. It is important to remove possible distractions such as telephones. Once in a comfortable position and in a quiet place, Hewitt advises that you slowly begin to relax the body progressively by focusing on the feet and telling them to relax, then the calves, the knees, the upper legs. You should breathe evenly using the stomach while slowly taking consciousness up to the neck and the head, telling each part to relax. Finally you tell the mind to relax. At this point the entire body is in a state of deep relaxation. You are in a state where you can start self-hypnosis by making suggestions to your subconscious.

Once the deep state has been reached, the key message can be implanted. The message should be something like: I am getting well; or soon, this cancer will be gone and I will be well again; or everyday, I am getting better and better. This key message needs to be repeated slowly and often so that it can sink into the depths of the subconscious. If stress and tension are the problems then the message should simply be: Relax. I want to relax. The mind should focus entirely on the message and follow it into the depths of the mind.

Richard Feynman, the Nobel-prize winning physicist, once underwent hypnosis to see how it felt. His experience of it was that he felt that nothing was happening, he could simply stop cooperating with the hypnotist at any time he felt like it - but somehow he just didn't feel like it!

However, anyone considering hypnosis should be very aware of the dangers. One girl was seriously injured when told to walk off the edge of a stage by a performing hypnotist. She did so and broke her back. Another girl was told to imagine she had been hit by a 10,000 volt charge. Shortly afterwards she went home, lay down and died. Anyone visiting a hypnotherapist should specify in advance exactly what messages are to be uttered. It may be advisable to take a sympathetic companion along to ensure this.

Hypnosis works, as the BBC discovered. In a test in 1946 a televised professional hypnotist put a number of his viewers into a hypnotic trance. Since then all professional hypnotists have been banned from the screen.

Under hypnosis, people can be made to be insensible to pain and to be induced to carry out tasks that would otherwise be considered impossible. Post-hypnotic suggestions can be implanted so that a person will carry out a task at some time after emerging from the hypnotic state. Hypnotic states will normally be slept off.

In some subjects, hypnosis is so deep that deep tissue surgery can be performed without anaesthetic. This was first demonstrated in the mid-nineteenth century by a surgeon in Calcutta, James Esdaile.

Laughter

Laughter is one means by which the body's entire chemistry can be shifted from a state of ill-health to one of health. This was the view of Norman Cousins, who in 1964 found himself in hospital with a profoundly crippling disease which involved the disintegration of the connective tissue of the body. The doctors weren't sure what it was or what to do about it - all they knew was that it was very serious. They could measure how serious it was by testing the sedimentation rate of the red blood cells. The speed with which these cells settle at the bottom of a test-tube measured in millimetres per hour is a sign of health or ill-health. A minor illness will have a sedimentation rate of 30-40. Over 60 is serious. Norman Cousins had a sedimentation rate of over 80 reaching up to 115.

Being very ill he naturally soon found himself in hospital. But Cousins quickly decided that hospital was not the right place for him. "[A] hospital is no place for a person who is seriously ill. The surprising lack of respect for basic sanitation, the rapidity with which staphylococci and other pathogenic organisms can run around an entire hospital, the extensive and sometimes promiscuous use of X-ray equipment..."

Cousins decided that, in his case, the reason he had fallen ill was that his adrenal glands had become exhausted. It is known that stress and emotional tension, frustration, rage, etc. can reduce the functioning of the adrenal glands and the endocrine system to the point where they cannot effectively deal with the toxins in the body caused by these same negative emotions.

"The inevitable question arose in my mind: what about the positive emotions? If negative emotions produce negative chemical changes in the body, wouldn't the positive emotions produce positive chemical changes? Is it possible that love, hope, faith, laughter, confidence, and the will to live have therapeutic value?"

So Cousins took the brave step of refusing any more pain-killing injections and booking himself out of hospital into a hotel where he arranged for a movie projector to be installed. He then set about watching every comic film and television programme he could lay his hands on. When he wasn't watching films he was reading cartoons.

Although his pain was initially all but crippling, he found that laughter gave him real relief. Ten minutes of laughter allowed him two hours of pain-free sleep. It also led to a drop of five points on the sedimentation scale - and this improvement was cumulative.

He supplemented the programme of laughter with large doses of vitamin C, which he took by intravenous drip. He started at 10 grams and deided to build up from there to 25 grams. Again, it had a measurable effect on the sedimentation rate.

Cousins went on to recover, though the after-effects of his illness stayed with him for years. He wrote up the full story in his book: *An Anatomy of an Illness as Perceived by the Patient.*

Although Cousins did not have cancer, we should note that the very factors that led to his illness are the very same ones that are implicated in cancer: stress, anxiety and so on leading to a state of adrenal exhaustion. Also, the blood sedimentation rate is a measure of general health - and general health in Cousins case led to specific improvements relating to a specific disease. If it can work with one disease it can work with all diseases.

Maharishi Ayurvedic Therapy

Maharishi Mahesh Yogi gained instant fame in the West from his association with the Beatles and other pop icons of the sixties. He was already famous in India having launched the Transcendental

Meditation movement. He has also established a number of Maharishi Ayurvedic Health Centers. Anyone seeking help from these centres will be put on a gentle regime involving a change of diet, Ayurvedic herbs, a daily routine of exercises and instruction in Transcendental Meditation.

As Dr. Deepak Chopra, who used to work at the Maharishi Ayurveda Health Center in Lancaster, Massachusetts, says "In Ayurveda, a level of total, deep relaxation is the most important precondition for curing any disorder...the body knows how to maintain balance unless thrown off by disease; therefore, if one wants to restore the body's own healing ability, everything should be done to bring it back into balance."

The Ayurvedic approach to healing also includes two other techniques which Chopra reports but does not describe. One is primordial sound therapy and the other is the bliss technique.

The primordial sound therapy assumes that underlying all matter there are vibrations of energy which can be heard when the meditating person is still and the mind is quiet.

"The theory behind primordial sound treatment is that the mind can return to the quantum level, introduce certain sounds that may have become distorted along the way, and thus have a profound healing influence in the body."

The bliss technique is a method for allowing the flow of joyful energy by the use of what he calls a 'faint mental impulse' which helps the mind come into contact with 'the vibrations of bliss that subtly pervade every cell of the body.'

"In and of itself, this feeling is extremely pleasant, but it also indicates that quantum healing is taking place, that disrupted channels of inner intelligence are being repaired. When these channels are closed, bliss cannot flow. When they are open, contact with the quantum mechanical body is restored."

Dr. Chopra is no longer connected with Maharishi Centers. To learn more of these techniques, you should visit www.maharishi.co.uk, www.theraj.com, or www.ayurveda-germany.com

Meditation

Most people think of meditating as a way of relaxing and emptying the mind. Meditation masters laugh at this way of describing meditation. For them it is a way of entering a state of consciousness where other energy fields can be experienced. And these can be experienced only in the silence of the mind.

It is now known that meditation is a state of consciousness that is different from being awake, from being asleep and from dreaming. This fourth state is a measurable one. Machines designed to measure brain waves can distinguish the state of meditation from the other three states.

The tradition of meditation originated in India where it is known as dhyana, a term meaning to bring the mind to rest in the silence of the fourth state. Chopra describes it like this: "The whole phenomenon is an immediate experience, like recognising the fragrance of lilacs or the sound of a friend's voice. It is immediate, nonverbal, and, unlike a flower's fragrance, totally transforming."

In meditation, the meditator feels a heightened sense of awareness and inner silence. Robert Keith Wallace at UCLA found that people who meditate regularly become physiologically younger than those who don't. For the first five years, each year of meditation has the effect of making the meditator grow approximately one year younger. After that the rejuvenating process appears to speed up.

A 1986 study by the Blue Cross Blue Shield insurance company found that people who meditate have less than half the number of tumours than non-meditators. A 1979 Isreali study found that meditation helps people with abnormally high cholesterol levels to lower these levels and so reduce their risk of heart attack.

How can one learn to meditate? There are a number of different forms of meditation of which the most well-known is Transcendental Meditation (TM). People involved in TM insist that it must be learned from an authorised instructor as there are subtleties that need to be explored. However, many people find that they can meditate perfectly well by following a few basic steps. The first principle of all meditation is to sit quietly in a chair with eyes closed. Then the object is to a stillness or state of vacant mental awareness. Some people use a special word or phrase which they repeat silently. In TM the instructor will provide a mantra, but some studies on meditation have found that almost any word will do: eg peace, let go, relax or just mmm. The most famous mantra of all is Om Mani Padme Hum - or simply Om for short. Others focus on certain aspects of the body or breath.

One guide to good meditation practice recommends these steps:

1. Choose a quiet spot where you will not be disturbed. Make sure you will not be disturbed.

2. Sit in a comfortable position with straight back. Some people like to cross their ankles.

3. Close your eyes.

4. Relax your muscles from head to feet by focusing the mind on the tip of the nose. Then let the mind travel up the nose, round the face and skull to the back of the neck. Then slowly round the shoulders and arms, then the back, the buttocks, the legs and the feet. Become aware of any tensions and with the help of the mind induce relaxation in these places.

5. Become aware of the breathing, watching it go in and out without any desire to control it.

6. Repeat the word you have chosen as your focus word or mantra.

7. If you become aware that your thoughts have drifted. Stop the thoughts and return to your mantra.

8. Practise everyday for 15-20 minutes.

9. Do not judge your performance. Do not judge anything about the performance. In meditation things just happen. It is important to be aware of them happening and to accept that they are happening but do not be in any way critical or judgemental about what happened.

Neuro-Linguistic Programming (NLP)

This is a method for helping people who find themselves constrained by depressive or otherwise negative belief systems and behaviours. As we have seen, this is a feature of many people who have cancer. A practitioner who has been trained in the method uses a number of specific techniques to help 're-programme' people's views about themselves and the world and in doing so helps them take more responsibility for their own healing.

For many people this could be a useful, short-term tool to kick start attitudinal change.

Prayer

In one study, investigators asked people who had undergone remarkable recovery which activities they believed had most helped. 68 percent said prayer, followed by meditation and exercise (64 percent), visualisation (59 percent), walking (52 percent) music/singing (50 percent) other forms of stress reduction (50 percent) - prayer came out top.

We can consider prayer's possible effects in a number of ways. It may be effective psychologically for the praying person to pray for himself. By praying, the person can release thoughts and feelings within himself. Or, if faith is great, there may be a conviction that God will intercede and so there may be a placebo effect. Most people will accept that prayer can be very beneficial under these circumstances.

However, according to Dr. Larry Dossey, prayers are more likely to be beneficial if they are undirected and are accompanied by complete acceptance of the situation. Do with me what you will is more likely to be effective than Dear God please cure me of my cancer in my left breast. Certainly, it is a fact that can be immediately subjectively confirmed, that the mind is more deeply and more wholly at peace when it utters the former prayer than when it utters the latter. It seems almost as if a different, deeper, more pleasure-related part of the mind is engaged.

Is prayer at a distance effective? Larry Dossey argues that some studies do seem to indicate that prayer at a distance(i.e., my prayer for your health) may have an effect.

One man known for his healing abilities was approached by a friend to pray for healing as he had an extremely painful condition that required intensive surgery. The healer promised to do the healing and the following day the friend woke up miraculously cured. The doctors were astounded. This apparently clear cut case would have been a powerful demonstration of prayer's potential to heal at a distance. The healer in this case was Dr. Lawrence LeShan, who we have already met in the discussion of cancer personalities. However, there was a problem.

"It would have been the psychic healing case of the century except for one small detail. In the press of overwork, I had forgotten to do the healing. If I had only remembered, it would have been a famous demonstration of what can be accomplished by this method."

Dossey suggests that LeShan may indeed have prayed but unconsciously. This raises another set of questions. Does this mean that our hidden thoughts and feelings about other people have the power to harm or heal unconsciously? Dossey thinks so. If this is the case are patients affected by their doctors' belief systems? If the doctor is thinking: this woman will die in three months time, will that affect the outcome? Again, many people are convinced that the doctor's negative thoughts will have a very negative effect on the prognosis.

And of course, in the above case, it may have been the man's faith that LeShan could indeed work a distance healing that provoked the cure. The man had handed the matter over to someone he trusted and the consequent relief resulted in the cure.

Also, we should consider the fact that if all our prayers were answered the world would be in a sorry state. If every Indian and Chinese father praying for a son was granted his wish the entire Indian and Chinese people would be dead in a generation. That is a good reason for leaving our fates to God. Che sera sera. What will be will be. Amen.

Taking Good Care of Yourself in Times of Trouble

It is known that physical and, more importantly, emotional trauma can lead to cancer. It therefore makes strong sense, if you have experienced a traumatic event: the break up of a marriage, the death of someone close or a business collapse, for example, to consider yourself to be in danger. At times like these it pays to pamper your health needs. Book yourself into a health farm, have those colonics and aromatherapy massages you've always wanted but never plucked up the courage to do. Go to a naturopath and have a general health assessment done. Ease up in other areas. Allow yourself to be taken care of by others. Decide that you are important enough to pay this attention to yourself. Let's face it, as the advertisement says, you're worth it!

Thinking of Three Good Things That Happened Today

One happiness-boosting exercise is this: every evening think of three good things that happened during the day. Think about why they happened. That's it. People who have tried this exercise say that it has a subtle but positive effect on their attitudes (they focus more on the good stuff rather than the bad stuff). Other say that the exercise has improved their sleep – and their happiness.

Visualisation & Suggestion

The purpose of visualisation is to tell the mind what to think and therefore to tell the mind what to do in the body. The idea is to let thoughts and messages filter from the conscious to the subconscious zones of the mind. Many athletes improve their performances through mental gymnastics, or mental tennis, and so on. The mind becomes its thoughts - and so too does the body. By actively guiding the imagination, the body can be led to a state of health. If you want something enough, then simply imagine it over and over again while you are in a deeply relaxed frame of mind.

Some people may find this a difficult idea to accept. The story of psychiatrist Milton Erickson shows what can be achieved through thought alone. Erickson was paralysed by polio as a young boy and forced to spend a lot of time on his front porch in a rocking chair watching the world go by. One day, left at home strapped to a rocking chair he found he was too far from the window to look out. Suddenly he became aware that his obsession with getting to the window was causing his chair to rock. He started to concentrate his thoughts on getting to the window. The more he did so the more the rocking increased. He soon found that he could direct the movement of the chair by working on his thoughts. It took him all afternoon but he managed to reach the window. This experience led him to the idea that he could influence other movements by concentrating his thoughts. He was eventually able to overcome the paralysis completely and begin to walk again.

How can we use this visualisation to help us stay healthy? By letting ourselves dwell inwardly on a healthy positive image. With eyes closed, for example, imagine the following: imagine your very favourite place. Maybe this is near where you live or a place that you remember from your youth or a place that you have visited on your holidays, it may even be a totally imaginary place - wherever it is it is a place where you are happy. Reflect on the happiness you feel being there. Feel the warmth of the sunlight. Feel the glow of the sun on your body. How comfortable you feel with the warm living rays of the sun permeating your whole body. It is filling your body with health and happiness, energy and love. It suffuses through all the limbs and through the whole of your being. With each breath the warmth and the light grow stronger and lighter. You release yourself into the heart of this feeling and you sit and feel this and let your mind sense these sensations. Then, when you're ready, you can return to normal consciousness.

This is just an example of the kind of creative visualisation that can, it is claimed, restore or maintain the body's health.

Some people visualise the cancer and watch as, in their minds, their body's immune defense system attacks it and slowly destroys it. Some people focus their visualisation on the chemotherapy drug or the radiation they are receiving. They imagine the drug eating up the tumor. They imagine the radiation rays like the healing rays of the sun dissolving the tumour. Or, as one patient did, as golden bullets.

This man had a nearly always fatal form of throat cancer at a late stage of development, his weight having dropped from 130 to 98 lb, and he was barely able to swallow. He was given radiation treatment but was not expected to benefit greatly from it - perhaps some short-lived comfort from a temporarily radiation-shrunk tumour. In addition to the radiation treatment he was asked to visualise the radiation as millions of little bullets bombarding the cancer tumour. He also imagined the cancer cells as being weak and unable to repair themselves - while he imagined the normal cells as being strong and repairing themselves quickly. He visualised the white blood cells swarming over the dead and dying cancer cells and carrying them out of the body through the liver and kidney. He did this three or four times a day. The result? He not only recovered but suffered very little associated radiation damage.

His doctor, O. Carl Simonton, had similar success with a large number of patients who were considered incurable. Of a group of 156 people with 'incurable cancers', 63 were still alive four years later, and in 43 of these the cancer had either disappeared, was regressing or had stabilised.

Some visualisation experiments have shown that volunteers can influence the numbers of various types of cell in the blood. This study conducted by Dr. Jean Achterberg found that students who visualised having more neutrophils, did indeed have higher counts of neutrophils by the end of the experiment, while those who focused on increasing the number of T-cells increased T-cell counts but not neutrophils. This shows how powerful belief can be.

On the negative side, we can make ourselves ill by visualising the worst. Joan Borysenko calls this process 'awfulizing': Tthe tendency to imagine the worst possible consequence of any event. This tendency is often obsessive and habitual, a result of past conditioning: "Awareness of our conditioning is the first step toward unlearning attitudes that have outlived their usefulness. Such awareness opens our ability to respond to what is happening now rather than reacting out of a conditioned history that may be archaic." (Borysenko, 1987)

It is very important to dwell on good thoughts and to stop negative thoughts from invading the inner mental space of our minds.

If we see visualisation as the right brain imagination at work, suggestion is the intellectual-verbal partner. By letting them work together we can harness powerful mental forces. Dr. David Sobel, co-author of *The Healing Brain*, recalled how he was plagued by warts on his hand when he was young. The warts had resisted all standard medical treatments. One day his mother passed him an article from the newspaper. The headline was "Warts Cured by Suggestion". His curiousity aroused, he read on. In the article he was told that hypnosis and suggestion could get rid of warts. He decided to try it out but, as they didn't explain in the article how to go about it, he had to invent his own method.

"I decided...that I must concentrate intensely on the warts while repeating ten times (it had to be exactly ten times) the phrase: "Warts go away. Warts go away." I did this faithfully everyday for about four weeks, at the end of which time...[they] had all vanished."

Dr. Bruno Bloch, known as the 'famous wart doctor of Zurich' built a machine that had a noisy motor and flashing lights. He told patients to put their hands in the machine until they were told the warts were dead. He would then add a pink vegetable dye to the wart and tell the patients not   to wash or touch the wart until it was gone. Roughly 30 percent of his patients were cured after one session. The relevance of this to cancer is this: warts are very similar to tumours. They are benign growths caused, like some cancers, by a viral infection. Anything that can work for warts has a good chance of working for cancer tumours.

Visualisation works. Cancer patients should make it work for them. The greater the visual, auditory and sensory involvement of all the senses they can bring to bear in the act of the visualisation the more likely success will follow.

Group Support

It is useful in this context to consider what part, if any, group support should play in the fight against cancer. There appears to be strong evidence that those who live within a network of strong social relationships live longer and healthier lives. Loneliness kills. Group support should therefore help the healing process. But this is a general statement that does not necessarily apply to many particular people.

Almost every new cancer patient is faced with the problem of who to tell and what to say about the disease. Some people bottle it up and keep it to themselves. Generally speaking this is not a good idea as it prevents people from giving support or providing information or other help that may be important: the name of a good naturopath, someone who is happy to do some research on the internet and so on.. If you have good friends, they will rally round and make a point of giving some kind of support. If you are a good friend you will rally round. The best strategy of all is to tell everyone everything. It really does get a lot of nonsense out of the way.

If group therapy is desired, your doctor should be able to point you in the right direction. However, care should be taken to find the right kind of support group. A group of women who have all had mastectomies, for example, would be very good support for any new member who had also had a mastectomy - but not necessarily for a woman who had refused a mastectomy. It depends on their attitude to not having a mastectomy. If they support the plan, that's good. If they try to get the woman in question to get used to the idea of the necessity of mastectomy, then that woman should find another group - fast.

The emphasis of group support should be on helping people to live as fully as possible, to help communication with family members and friends, to help ease the fears of death and dying and to help, where desired, with the release of emotion.

One possibly negative feature of group therapy may be that it will gradually accustom members to the idea of dying and so place imperceptible obstacles in the way of seeking a cure.

While many people will be able to put together their own support groups made up of friends, others will want to meet and talk to others who have had, or who are undergoing, the same experience. Many forums on the internet are informal support groups of this kind. More formal groups are often organised in such a way that the members can meet up in person.

Annette Crisswell, herself a cancer survivor and who has facilitated a support group for seven years, provided me with the following guidelines on the subject. What follows is her commentary:

"It has been found that people attending a support group do far better in terms of recovery than those who choose not to. However, not everyone flourishes in groups and I believe it is important that they are not made to feel that their chances of recovery are in any way impeded by going it alone. Each person must find the best way back to 'wellness' for themselves, with confidence.

What Is a Support Group?

a) A gathering of people who have experienced a trauma of some kind, either a life threatening illness, a traumatic loss, a situation that is out of control, etc. In fact, an experience which has created chaos in their lives.

b) The group may or may not be run by an experienced counsellor. With a counsellor the group may be based more on actual group therapy, otherwise a support group is exactly what it says: a group that gives support. It is not there to advise people what they should do, condemn what they have done or to criticize or change how they are.

What Are the Purposes of a Support Group?

The purposes of a support group are:

a) To provide as much information about the various and the latest treatments (allopathic, complementary, alternative, etc.) that are available and relevant to the objects of the group. A source of books, articles, etc.

b) To provide a safe place for people to discuss their feelings and fears with people who have, or have had similar experiences, without fear of criticism or negation.

c) To empower people and to revitalize their belief in themselves.

d) To provide specialist speakers who are able to clarify and give information about all types of treatment available, so that people in the group are able to make informed choices for themselves and have their misunderstandings and doubts clarified.

Depending on the needs and desires of its members, a support group can:

a) Be simply a group of people who get together at regular intervals just to chat, exchange information, become friends, etc.

b) Be a regular gathering of people for the purpose of experiencing complementary therapies aimed at empowering the body, mind and spirit. This may include counselling sessions. The underlying principle will be a concern for the whole person of each member of the group.

c) Be a structured series of meetings, say once a week for ten weeks, in which different specialists or practitioners can be invited to give a talk or presentation. This can be combined with counselling and group sharing sessions.

d) Organise themselves - as often, but by no means always, happens with cancer support groups - round the different cancers that the individual members have eg breast cancer group, lung cancer group, etc.

The basic rule of all these groups is to empower people so that each person is helped to define for him/herself positive action and attitude goals.

What a Support Group Is Not.

a) A support group is not there to advise anyone what is the right thing to do. What is right for one person is not necessarily right for another. Whatever someone chooses to do is right for them and they should be supported in their choice and empowered to realize their chosen goals.

b) A support group is not there to counsel people unless there is an experienced, trained counsellor present.

c) A support group is not there to coerce anyone to do or feel anything. Too often empowering people is seen simply as telling people to 'be positive' and in this way attempting to negate fear, anger and sadness. I challenge anyone who has been told that they are going to have a double mastectomy to feel cheerful and positive. There is such loss and fear and pain involved that to be told you must be 'positive' shows a total lack of empathy, bordering on cruelty. If the major focus of a group is on such a rigidly defined attitude then the result will be that members will not admit to their true feelings and so they will feel even more lonely than before. Being positive does not mean blinding oneself to all the negative aspects and possibilities inherent in the situation, replacing them with a thin brittle veneer of grit-your-teeth-and-get-on-with-it cheerfulness. Being positive, in its proper and helpful sense, is having an attitude that recognizes the feelings of sadness and inadequacy, the fears and terrors and all the other complex emotions that are commonly experienced - but knows also that there are options and alternatives - that the future ultimately is not hopeless, that it is not meaningless, that recovery is not impossible, that change for the better will come in its own time and the burdens of the present must be borne until that better time comes.

What People Who Have Attended a Support Group Have Said:

1. I felt so alone until I joined the group. People who have not had this experience just do not understand.

2. It was such a relief to know that how I was reacting was quite normal.

3. It was good to hear what other people had done to come to terms with what had happened to them. It helped me to feel I could once more be in control of my life.

4. I discovered so many ways I could help myself overcome the disease, or the side effects of my treatment in the complementary field. It opened up a whole new fascinating area in my life.

5. It's good to be able to meet people who have been through what I'm going through and have recovered. There is life after cancer.

DECISION TIME

Now it is decision time.

Whether or not you have cancer, NOW is the time to decide what you should do.

    If you have read this book straight through you may be somewhat dazed by the sheer number of options you can choose from. But although you have now reached the end, you still have one more thing to do before laying this book aside. You have to decide what you wish to do. Are you going to:

1. Follow the orthodox regime only. Do what the doctor advises. Avoid anything unorthodox.

2. Follow a regime of a combination of alternative therapies only. Do not consider any of the orthodox regimes.

3. Follow doctor's orders first and if that doesn't work then try the alternative route later.

4. Follow the alternative approaches first and if they don't succeed, fall back on the orthodox treatments

5. Combine orthodox and alternative therapies together from the start.

6. Do nothing.

Each of us is different and so we will make different choices. Some of you will be undeterred by what I have said about surgery, radiation and chemotherapy. You will feel that 'the doctors know best' and will follow their advice come what may. Do so. And good luck to you.

    Some of you may feel confused or weak or you need the approval of someone you feel is in a position to know best. You may find what I have said persuasive but nevertheless you don't feel up to the task of turning your back on your doctor. You will go along with the treatment suggested but you will want to add something from the complementary array of therapies. Do so. And good luck to you.

    Some of you will come to the conclusion that the alternative therapies offer the best chance of surviving cance r– and do so while at the same time impacting positively rather than negatively on our health. You will therefore reject orthodox treatments and select from the array of supplements, herbs and so on, the options that make most sense. Do this and good luck to you.

    And some of you will feel you would rather not know. You don't want to know anything. You don't want to think about it. You don't want to make any decisions. You're just going to pretend it's not there. It's certainly true that some people in denial have continued to live and live and live. Some even find their cancer goes of its own accord. So good luck to you too.

We need to understand that we are all responsible for our own actions and non-actions. We are also all different and we need to respect our differences.

But people with cancer don't live in a vacuum. They are surrounded by partners, lovers, friends, family and so on. It is very important that decisions are discussed. Do not be panicked into rushing to hospital. Your cancer has taken a long time to get to where it is. Unless your cancer is highly aggressive, another week or two, or even month or two, will most likely not make a huge difference. You have time to sit back and consider your options. Take your time. Discuss disagreements. While the partner may have a cooler head, it is the person with cancer who ultimately has to make the decision. Make sure you nurture your close relationships so that they are not adversely affected by serious disagreement as to how to proceed.

For all of you, I have the following suggestion. Ask those friends of yours whose judgement you trust to read this book too and to become your own personal support group. Go through the book chapter by chapter and discuss the information you find there. Note down your choices and decisions. Then follow through. Start the diet, order the herbs, supplements and machines. Embrace the future. Make an adventure of it.

In my view, it is very important that you do what you eventually decide to do not because the 'doctor knows best' or 'that's what mummy (hubby) says I should do.' It is you – the person with cancer - who has to make the decisions that sit comfortably with you. By doing so you will have a greater chance of accessing the placebo effect.

Ignore doctors who dismiss placebo cures as short term in their effects. They are not. They are as powerful and as permanent as any other therapy – actually, likely as not, they will be more so.

Also we must beware of the opposite – the negative, often self-fulfilling 'nocebo' effect. Do not allow negative thoughts about the future to take up residence in your mind.

And, finally, I wish you luck. For whatever else we need, we also need luck.

Choosing Specific Therapies

If you think some of the alternative therapies discussed in this book make sense for you, now is a good time to go back and make a note below of the five therapies you yourself feel most attracted to. Make a note of them:

1.

2.

3.

4.

5.

SOME STORIES TO INSPIRE YOU

The following people beat cancer using alternative therapies either alone or alongside orthodox therapies.

1: Beata Bishop

Beata Bishop was panic stricken when a mole on her leg was diagnosed as malignant melanoma, one of the fastest-spreading and most lethal of all cancers. She underwent painful and disfiguring surgery but within a year it was found that the cancer had spread into the lymphatic system. Rather than undergo further extensive surgery she chose instead to follow the diet developed by an eminent German physician, Dr. Max Gerson. Taking her fate in her hands, she spent two months at the world's only Gerson clinic in Mexico where she learnt the theory and practice of the intensive therapy which she then pursued for a further eighteen months in London.

After two years on the Gerson Therapy, which transformed her both physically and psychologically, Beata Bishop made a full recovery. Today, in her 70s, she is still alive, extremely active and free of her cancer. She wrote her story in a book, *My Triumph Over Cancer*, first published in 1985.

2: Michael Gearin-Tosh

Michael Gearin-Tosh, was, for 35 years, Tutor in English at St. Catherine's College, Oxford. In 1994 he was diagnosed with myeloma, a cancer of the bone marrow. Although urged to take chemotherapy, he discovered that this would give him only a 4 percent possibility of a cure. His conclusion: "Touch it [chemo], and you're a goner. "

He embarked on a series of alternative treatments consisting of 12 freshly-made vegetable juices a day, high-dose vitamin injections, acupuncture, raw garlic, coffee enemas, Chinese breathing exercises. He also used visualisation techniques in which he imagined his immune cells attacking the tumour. The result was that his cancer went into remission. He was still cancer free 11 years later when he died in 2005 from an untreated blood infection.

Gearin-Tosh described his battle with cancer in his book, *Living Proof - A Medical Mutiny*

3: Christopher Sheppard

In November 1999, Christopher Sheppard, a film producer, was diagnosed with 'locally advanced' rectal cancer and his doctors recommended surgery–as did the homoeopathic doctors and acupuncturist that he approached to help him. However, Sheppard refused surgery and chemo but eventually, after a lot of soul searching, did decide to accept radiation treatment. He also decided to go on what he called a healing journey. It was his view that each cancer victim, not their doctor, should be the authority on what they should do for their cancer. And they should make their decisions on the basis of their own self-knowledge, intuition and sense of the world.

r himself, he selected a modified version of the Gerson diet, developed by his nutritionist, plemented with vitamins, minerals and herbs—at one point he was taking over 100 pills a

He also decided to visit a Brazilian spiritual healer, Joao Texeira, also known to his followers as 'John of God'. He felt strongly that there was a spiritual dimension – that his cancer was a sign of a spiritual malaise. This led him to Tibetan Buddhism, and he studied a special form of meditation at a Buddhist community. Another self-devised therapy was to join an emotional counselling group.

Within a year he was cancer free and remains so to this day. Radiation on its own is not generally considered curative for rectal cancers. Christopher describes his journey in great detail at his website at www.christopher-sheppard.com.

4: Anne Frahm

At the age of 34, Anne Frahm found a tiny lump in her breast but having been assured it was not malignant she did nothing. By the time the cancer was diagnosed a year later, it had spread throughout her body. "I will never forget seeing that light board with my skeleton displayed on it. It had tumors covering my body. The tumors covered my skull, my ribs and shoulders. Quarter-size holes had eaten through all my pelvic bones and the report showed that virtually every vertebrae of my spine had tumors grown right through it. At that point, the doctor said that he thought he could keep me alive for a while. He told me straight out, "I can't cure you.""

Despite a mastectomy, chemotherapy, radiation, hormone therapy and a bone marrow transplant During the bone marrow transplant, she was in isolation for 52 days, during which she very nearly died. "My kidneys shut down, my lungs shut down, I got pneumonia, I was covered with fungus rashes from head to toe, my fingernails and toenails fell off. I was a wreck! [Then] toward the end of the 52 days, they did tests and came in and said, "they were very sorry but it just didn't work for you." I found out that I still had a lot of cancer still growing in my body so they basically sent me home to die."

But Anne refused to give up. She decided to follow a strict nutrition plan and five weeks later her astounded doctors could find no trace of the cancer at all.

Anne Frahm, with the help of her husband Dave, wrote her story up in a book called *The Cancer Battle Plan.* Sadly, Anne did eventually die ten years later from cancer. But to live nearly ten years cancer free after being given weeks to live is surely a great achievement.

5: Felicity Corbin-Wheeler

Felicity Corbin Wheeler is a Reader in the Church of England and also has an international biblical-based Health Ministry. She is currently based in Portugal.

Having lost a daughter to cancer, despite what she refers to as "the 'best' of orthodox medicine", she began to research the importance of nutrition in cancer. She eventually came to the conclusion that the answer to nutritional therapy is firmly based on "what God tells us to eat in Genesis 1:29 and 30." In September 2003 she herself was diagnosed with terminal pancreatic cancer. Of all cancers this has one of the worst prognoses. Death usually follows quickly. However she did not give up hope but put her faith in the "the living enzymes in the seeds that God tells us to eat when He creates us, and the seed of the apricot has natural cancer cure qualities of hydrocyanic acid. This is also known as amygdalin, or laetrile, which has been given vitamin status as B17 because the seeds are vital for health." Her source for laetrile was www.cytopharma.com She not only ate the seeds but in order to get the maximum dose of laetrile, she undertook a series of thirteen intravenous laetrile treatments given by a doctor followed by a daily intake of laetrile tablets. She went to Dr Contreras' clinic, Oasis of Hope Hospital in Tijuana and he supervised the laetrile dose levels. Believing God's Word about the importance of the seeds, and having complete faith in the course she was following, she expected to be healed. Within four months scans showed the tumour shrinking, and within a year there was only a scar left. Felicity has told her story in her book *God's Healing Word* and she has a website at www.felicitycorbinwheeler.org . Her case was publicised in a BBC interview published on 25th August 2004

6: Glynn Williams

In 1995, at the age of 28, Glynn Williams was diagnosed with Hodgkin's type Lymphoma. "I went to see the doctor because of swelling on both sides of the groin area which came on within about a week…I was totally exhausted, lethargic, did not have the energy to get up, had no appetite and was losing weight and I was having chills."

He started taking Essiac tea (brand name Flor-Essence)–two ounces in the morning before eating and two ounces at night. The swelling grew larger and then hardened up and the discomfort went away. By this time test results confirmed that he had advanced stage Hodgkin's. He was put on a course of 16 chemotherapy treatments but after experiencing severe side effects he quit the course of treatments after the fifth chemo session. Throughout this treatment he had continued with the Essiac tea, which he supplemented with vitamins and herbs, one 400 IU vitamin E, one 10,000 IU beta carotene, 2 ginseng, one shark cartilage, one 1000 mg. Vitamin C, drops of liquid echinacea on the tongue every 3 hours, and then capsules of echinacea 380 mg. He also took a parasite elimination programme using black walnut tinctures, and wormwood capsules. He drank Kombucha mushroom tea three times a day. Finally he did yoga, with a strong focus on diaphragm breathing.

His doctors were amazed when he was eventually found to be cancer-free, as five doses of chemo was not considered curative. In December 2005, he confirmed that he is still cancer free ten years later.

Contact Glynn's website at www.north.island.net/~glynnw.

7: Elonna McKibben's story

In 1989, having taken fertility treatment, Elonna found herself pregnant with quintuplets. However, as the pregnancy progressed, Elonna began feeling deep-seated pains. It was eventually discovered, after the birth of her children, that the pains were not a side effect of her pregnancy—the exceptional nature of which had camouflaged the fact that she had a tumour on her spine.

This was diagnosed as stage 4 Glioblastoma Multiforme (GBM), a very rare and always fatal cancer. "As mine was in the spinal cord," Elonna wrote later, "it made it even more rare, more aggressive and faster killing. I was told I would not survive long enough to see my children's first birthday."

If that was not bad enough the combined effect of the surgery and cancer had left her paralysed from the waist down. The doctors recommended radiation but were not hopeful that it would do more than delay the inevitable.

Fortunately, someone who read about her situation in the newspaper contacted her husband, Rob, and told him about CanCell (also known as Protocel). Elonna was naturally very sceptical: "If there was a cure for cancer, don't you think they would be using it instead of letting thousands of people die."

However, she started taking it on the basis that she had nothing to lose and everything to gain. Its effects were quickly obvious. "I began to eliminate the cancer waste product about 18 hours after my first dose. It literally poured out of me: I threw it up; my bowel movements were extremely loose, stringy and frequent throughout the day; I lost it in my urine; my nose ran so much I had to keep a tissue with me at all times; I sweated it out profusely; I had hot/cold flashes and night sweats. When the nurses would give me a sponge bath after a night sweat, the water would be a golden brown colour with what they referred to as "tapioca balls" floating in it."

Believing these effects to be a clear sign that CanCell was working, she persevered with it. After several weeks she found she was feeling much better. Christmas came and went and she started to do physical therapy to help her mobility. Then, in February 1990 she went and had scans to see what was happening. The radiologist was stunned to find no trace of the cancer. Although cancer free, Elonna continued the CanCell treatment for a further two years.

As of January 2006, Elonna Mc Kibben is still alive and her full story can be read on her website at www.elonnamckibben.com.

8. Mark Olsztyn's story

In March 1991, Mark experienced a major epileptic seizure which led to him being hospitalized. There, a CAT scan revealed a darkened area in the right frontal lobe of his brain. He was operated on and the tumour removed. It was found to be a low-grade astrocytoma. No further treatment was recommended though frequent repeat scans would, he was told, be necessary.

Mark ignored this recommendation and for the next six years led a normal, hectic life. 'This was my denial phase,' he recalls. When he eventually did go for a scan in 1997, he was shocked to learn that the tumour had returned and was now stage 4. In addition to surgery he would require chemotherapy and radiation. He was also told by one of his doctors that he had better settle his affairs. But Mark insisted in thinking positively that a cure was possible.

He followed doctors orders and underwent all these treatments even though he knew that at best they would be palliative. Fortunately, his father was a doctor of alternative medicine. "My father immediately sent me a case of a foul-tasting liquid called Poly-MVA, which a colleague of his was using successfully on brain tumor patients. Because Poly-MVA can be used as an adjunct to conventional therapy I embraced it. I felt then that any nonconventional therapy that came my way, so long as it didn't interfere with what the doctors wanted me to do, was what God wanted me to do and would give me the edge that I needed to survive.

Among many other things, I became an ascetic, practiced Qi Gong, drank Essiac and Chinese herbs, joined various support groups, received acupuncture, ohmed and prayed and was prayed for, drank shark cartilage, ate macrobiotic, practiced visualization and, after four out of six rounds, quit chemotherapy. That last one was not what the doctors wanted me to do; however, I felt I had enough poisoning.

Over the years I gradually let go of each of the aforementioned life-saving practices except for Poly-MVA and eating organic. Doctors now tell me to keep on doing whatever it is that I'm doing because it seems to be working."

In January 2006, Mark is still very much alive and cancer free. He can be contacted at mark.olsztyn@googlemail.com.

9: Shirley Lipschutz-Robinson

In 1982, doctors recommended a mastectomy on Shirley's left breast. She had suffered recurring cyst lumps which no medication could control. Up until this time Shirley was, as she calls herself, a prescription drug junkie - she was depressed, overweight and suffering from a seemingly endless parade of ailments - and the drugs seemed to only make matters worse. Her overall health was steadily declining.

But Shirley baulked at having her breast removed. She decided she needed to change her approach. She consulted a naturopathic/homoeopathic doctor who put her on a dietary regime - "a wholesome diet of fresh, organically grown fruits, vegetables, and nuts, mostly in their raw form" - supplemented with homoeopathic remedies. The results were, in her own words, 'dramatic'.

Within 6 weeks the lumps were gone. Within 12 weeks she had lost 60lb;. "my energy level and stamina improved dramatically. I was able to function better overall. I became calmer, centered and focused, and generally I felt happier. My overall resistance to infections became excellent."

In the 1990s, she experienced a lump the size of a pea in her left nipple. It grew to be the size of a small grape. She refused to see the doctor, instead self-treating it with extra flaxseed oil, herbal extracts and homoeopathy. Within 2 weeks, her body had reabsorbed the lump, and it never came back.

These experiences sparked her to study a wide range of alternative therapies. Her full story, and the story of how she treated her husband through a series of heart attacks, is told on her excellent website: www.shirleys-wellness-cafe.com

10. Pattie McDonald

In May 2002, Pattie, 58, was diagnosed with breast cancer 'the size of a quarter'. She believes now that contributing factors included being on HRT (Premarin) for six years, long-term antibiotic use and a very poor diet ('I was a fast food freak') coupled with a negative outlook on life. Her doctors recommended surgery and radiation.

However, Pattie had a close and trusted friend who had survived ovarian cancer by using bloodroot. She used both bloodroot paste and tonic. The effects of bloodroot quickly revealed that the cancer had already spread to the neck and three lymph nodes.

The Cansema bloodroot paste was applied to the biopsy site on her breast. It took ten days to expel the tumour from her body. As the neck tumours also began to be expelled, Pattie took the tonic and applied paste against the neck. The whole process of treatment took about a month. She experienced excruciating pain and two days of no sleep. (She found out later you should take pain killers.)

In August 2002, she had an MRI that confirmed that she was cancer free and four years later she has remained cancer free.

"This experience changed my entire life - body, soul and spirit. I am a new woman. I changed my diet, quit my stressful job, sold my too-big house, rid myself of all negative friends, and divorced my alcoholic hubby. I had no idea what real happiness was until 2002." Pattie can be contacted at pjmacblondie@yahoo.com

11. Bruce Guilmette

In November 2004, Bruce discovered that both his kidneys had large cancerous masses inside them. Kidney cancer is known to be highly resistant to treatment and he was given only a matter of months to live unless he had both kidneys removed. Bruce refused this option, turned to a combination of diet, supplements and the use of a Rife machine. Bruce's research led him to the conclusion that cancer needs to be attacked from many different angles to be successfully put into remission. He eventually put together a complex regimen which he followed rigorously. Much of his food intake is in the form of juiced fresh vegetables. He reduced his meat consumption to no more than 10 percent of his total intake and eliminated pork altogether. He has come to accept that the dietary changes he made to defeat cancer will become a lifelong practice. Nearly two years later, as this book was going to press, he was not only still alive but all his blood tests indicate he is in full health and that the cancer is no longer active. His full story is told at www.survivecancerfoundation.org

Postscript: Bruce died in November 2007 – but he did not die of cancer.

12. Bob Davis

In April 1996, Bob Davis discovered he had a massive cancer tumour - a foot wide and several inches thick – in his abdomen and several other tumours in his chest, some "the size of soft balls". The cancer had also spread to his bone marrow.

He was immediately started on a very heavy chemotherapy program over the next three months. This had very little effect: "It [the tumour] seemed to thrive on the stuff." Eventually, his doctor told him that the chemo wasn't working. "He later told me that another treatment would kill me. I knew that this was true because my body was ravaged by the chemo. I was curled up in a fetal position unable to sleep or eat. I was emaciated and had excruciating pain all through my body."

At this time he received a call from a woman who had been selling his wife pills made of dried green barley leaves for her arthritis. During the conversation he mentioned his fight with cancer. "Don't you know that cancer and arthritis can't grow in an alkaline body?" she said. The same barley leaves that his wife was taking for her arthritis would, she told him, also help him in his fight against cancer. He started taking the pills – 20 tablets of dried barley green (340mgs each) - and "in ten days my cancer was 95 percent gone!" A number of tests including a CAT scan showed that scar tissue remained but the cancer had been killed. "I was incredibly lucky. I know most people wouldn't be cured so simply. In fact I only know one other person who had the same response."

A few years later, even though he had maintained his intake of dried barley leaves, Bob was diagnosed with a probable prostate cancer on the basis of a lump and high PSA levels. Resisting pressure to have surgery, Bob went on the Dr. Schulze's Incurable's programme – involving juice fasting and colon cleansing. Three weeks later he demanded a PSA re-test. His PSA levels were now normal.

In 2006 he was still cancer free. He still takes 20 tablets of dried green barley every day. "It costs me a whopping 95 cents or so." He has adopted a 95 percent vegan diet "I really like it. I feel better than I have in 40 years. People say I look younger. I have "lotsa' energy."

Bob Davis can be contacted through his website at www.cancer-success.com

13. Cliff Beckwith

Cliff Beckwith was a retired educationalist living near Knoxville, Tennessee. He was one of the founders of the health Yahoogroups information resource on flaxseed oil: http://health.groups.yahoo.com/group/FlaxSeedOil2/files/

Here he tells his own story:

"In January 1991 I was diagnosed with Advanced Prostate Cancer. Bone scans and other tests indicated no spread so it was decided to operate. During the operation it was discovered that the cancer had spread to the Lymph glands making it stage four. The operation was not completed as that would not be the answer. The only treatment used was Lupron and Eulexin to cancel the male hormones. I was told the male hormone does not cause cancer, but if cancer is present it is like throwing kerosene on a fire.

At the time of the attempted operation my PSA count was 75. It was six months before I had the second PSA. When the call came from the doctor's office I was told "Mr. Beckwith! Your count is completely normal!" It was 0.1 and 0.1 to 0.4 is normal.

The reason it was normal was because, in addition to the hormone drugs, I had started taking flaxseed oil mixed with cottage cheese. I had read a number of books recommending this approach, which was first formulated by Dr. Johanna Budwig and is commonly known as the Budwig protocol.

I quit Lupron after 4 years and 7 months in October of 1995 as it was no longer useful. I thought I was cured but not so. In roughly two years the PSA was again rising. I began changing the amounts I took of Flaxseed oil/Cottage cheese which led to a series of ups and downs with the PSA results.

I learned that there are 30 strains of Prostate Cancer. They are all different and any man may have any combination of strains. This makes the problem different from individual to individual. Mine is a medium aggressive cancer.

In January 2004 my PSA was 6.7 which is very close to normal for a man of 85. I thought I had it beaten. It had now been 13 years since diagnosis. Most men with Advanced Prostate Cancer do not live nearly that long. The doctor told me after a couple of years that I was one of the lucky ones. Most men with the condition I had did not make it 6 months.

In Jan 2004, I decided to try ellagic acid which has proved effective in many cases. However, my PSA went up instead of further down. Then I added Lycopene. I had been told that it needed to be used heavily to be effective; three 12 ounce glasses of tomato juice a day. I did that for four months.

Then I learned two things a couple of days apart. One was that Dr. Budwig had said in 1956 that if one is using flaxseed oil one must not use heavy amounts of antioxidants as it would neutralize the effect of the flaxseed oil. The other was that both ellagic acid and lycopene are powerful antioxidants.

For over a year I was hurting the effect of the Flaxseed oil/cottage cheese and for 4 months I was canceling it completely.

The result was that the cancer again began to develop and by the time I woke up to this fact, the PSA had gone to 131.

I know that Prostate Cancer in the Prostate does not kill. What kills is the cancer in the tissues to which it spreads. Flaxseed oil pretty much stops the spread. Until I went the antioxidant route it hadn't spread in 13 years. Now there are signs it has spread to the bone.

So I immediately increased the flaxseed oil to 6 tablespoons a day and am using my Rebounder (small trampoline). The result appears to be beneficial. I had been aware of an enlargement in the Prostate Gland and now it is getting smaller and urination is easier. I do not believe I am in danger any more." (February 2006)

Cliff Beckwith died from his cancer, aged 85, in late 2007. *16 years later*

14. Ian Gawler

In 1975, Ian Gawler, a 24-year old Australian veterinarian, was diagnosed with bone cancer. He underwent surgery and had his right leg amputated. He was told that he had only a five percent chance of surviving for five years and that if the tumours returned he would only have a few months. The cancer did return later that year.

Deciding to take a proactive approach, Ian and his wife went to the Philippines, where Ian received treatment from several folk healers. On his return to Australia, he decided to follow a diet, take up meditation and explore a wide range of natural therapies, He believed the secret lay in stimulating the immune system and to letting go of stress and anxiety.

He won his battle and the cancer went away. To this day he remains healthy and cancer free. He wrote a book, *You Can Conquer Cancer*, and set up The Gawler Foundation, based in Melbourne, to provide cancer support programmes for anyone seeking to follow the alternative path.

He attributes his success to the fact that he took responsibility for his condition and recognised that he had been responsible for causing it. By taking responsibility, he felt in control and believed that he had the power to reverse it.

In an interview with the journalist Beryl Rule he said: "Psychologically, the big need is to change. If we recognise that a particular pattern has aided in creating the disease, then obviously a new pattern is required...The disease creates the excuse for change. It produces a new situation or insight that allows the patient the space to change their rigid patterns." For more information go to www.gawler.org

15. Fred Eichhorn

In 1976, Fred was found to have islet cell carcinoma, and was given a maximum life expectancy of three years though most of the doctors he consulted believed he would be dead within a year. He underwent surgery in which 90 percent of his pancreas was removed along with his spleen and part of his stomach. However, this was not expected to provide a cure. Fred decided to define the problem. He felt that in every case ill health follows like a domino effect from a first cause. The solution is to find that first cause in terms of the body's biochemistry and correct it. Then a good domino effect will result in the elimination of the disease.

He decided good nutrition–a return to pre-1900s standards (i.e., completely organic)–along with exercise and a positive mental framework were the key cornerstones of good health.

In 1980 Fred, Fred enrolled in medical college and studied for four years followed by a further three years research.

Fred Eichhorn is cancer free today 30 years later and so committed is he to spreading the word that he has set up the National Cancer Research Foundation (www.ncrf.org) and offers help and information completely free of charge. He provides a number of testimonials on his site of people who have benefited from following his regime.

For further information contact Fred@ncrf.org

16. June Black

June Black was first diagnosed with cancer (stage 1) in November 2000. She eventually had a mastectomy but no radiation or chemotherapy. She was put on Tamoxifan but reacted badly to it and "threw it down the toilet". In 2005, June noticed a lump growing on the mastectomy scar and had it biopsied. The tests came back positive. The cancer had returned. She underwent two further operations but it was clear the cancer had spread. By this time she had read a lot of books and had come round to the natural approach to treating cancer. So, when her third oncologist (she had dumped two) told her: "I recommend the whole gamut; chemo, radiation and adjuvant hormone therapy." She found the courage to refuse, saying: "I am sixty years old, I have lived a good life, and I have other plans."

But at first the natural path did not appear to be doing her any good. "After spending a month of a very strict diet and enough vitamins and supplements to fill a small shop, I realized I was losing the war against this cancer. I was losing weight, I had sweats, I was really weak and it was so bad that I thought death would be a wonderful alternative to the hell I was going through."

Then someone suggested the supplement Poly-MVA. She went on it and within four days felt better. This was in October 2005. In June 2006 she had a full array of tests and they all came back clear. She was cancer-free.

Her regime was 8 teaspoons of Poly-MVA a day for 6 1/2 months. She then went to 6 teaspoons a day for about 2 months and since then has been taking 4 teaspoons a day. She also takes CoQ10, Artemisinin, pancreatic enzymes and IP6.

"This is just the tip of the iceberg of what I am taking. I also take different mushrooms, Epicor, Lugol's Iodine, DIM, Calcium-d-Glucarate. If anyone is interested in my complete list please feel free to contact me at june1@mesquiteweb.com. I just had my 62nd birthday March 1, 2007 in Hawaii and gained more weight and feel fantastic. As of now, no signs of illness. I have excellent health and work full time and care for 11 cats."

June's story is one of many testimonials that can be found at www.polymvasurvivors.com

1. Chris Wark (?) Chrisbeatcancer.com 26 yrs old stage 2 or 3 colon cancer. Had surgery & some lymph nodes removed. Found naturopathic doctor went on vegan diet with vitamin supplements vitamin 'C' infusion by IV, hot/cold showers etc diagnosed in 2003 - still cancer free 2011. see his blog - He did "every other alternative therapy he could find."

2. Courtney Campbell - will find interview w/ her on Chris' website. 3 yrs ago diagnosed w/ lymphoma Read Bill Henderson's book (youthquest?) She said it saved her life. Had baby and still cancer free 3. a third guy also mentioned in that interview

352

SUMMATION

Reading the personal stories and the extensive descriptions of the many different alternative anti-cancer approaches described in this book, it is hard to escape the conclusion that there are literally dozens – if not hundreds – of cures for cancer. And yet the medical establishment and the charities that depend for their funding on the pharmaceutical industry remain adamantly opposed to them. How can we explain this? The novelist Upton Sinclair provides a terse answer: "It is difficult to a get a man to understand something when his salary depends on his not understanding it."

This book has attempted to be both a Guide to Complete Recovery and a Complete Guide to Recovery. I hope it has not fallen too far short of both these goals. However, one book cannot tell you everything. Below I have suggested some follow up reading. Also, time does not stand still and new facts are constantly emerging. It is a good idea to stay abreast of these new ideas as far as one can. I have listed below some resources which may be of help.

Some Resources for Further information in relation to alternative medicine

1. First of all I would recommend that you read my shorter book

Cancer Recovery Guide: 15 Alternative and Complementary Strategies for Restoring Health.

This book gives an overview of the strategies and slices the information in a different way. This may help your decision making.

2. For those who would like some background on the medical context I would like to recommend the following books

Dean Black: *Health at the Crossroads*

Ralph Moss: *The Cancer Industry* (This book is a must!)

Robert Procter: *Cancer Wars: How Politics* shapes what we know and don't know about cancer

3. I recommend the following books giving personal testimony

Karon Beattie: *I Beat Cancer! 2,000 cases of ordinary people getting rid of their cancer with natural and non-toxic treatments*

Karon Beattie: *Natural Cancer Treatments That Work*

Beata Bishop: *My Triumph Over Cancer*

John Boik: *Cancer and Natural Medicine: A Textbook of Basic Science and Clinical Research*

John Boik: *Natural Compounds in Cancer Therapy*

Norman Cousins: *An Anatomy of An Illness as Perceived by the Patient*

Anne Frahm: *The Cancer Battle Plan*

Michael Gearin-Tosh: *Living Proof*

David J. Hess: *Evaluating Alternative Cancer Therapies*

Caryl Hirshberg & Marc Barasch: *Remarkable Recovery*

Ralph W. Moss: *Questioning Chemotherapy*

Patrick Quillin: *Beating Cancer With Nutrition*

There are many other books worth reading – many of them mentioned in the text - but these will provide as good a platform as any for your new life-long interest in cancer. I have dispensed with a bibliography. If you wish to follow up a reference in the text I suggest you do a keyword search in Amazon.com (or other preferred internet store) to find the book you are interested in.

4. Up-to-date information on orthodox treatments

If you wish to get further details of what the most up-to-date orthodox treatments are for your cancer, then go to the following National Cancer Institute website and look for the pdq files at www.cancer.gov/cancertopics/pdq.

5. Useful websites

The following are also useful websites for browsing and for regular newsletters:

> www.AnnieAppleseedProject.org
> www.beating-cancer-gently.com
> www.cancerdecisions.com
> www.cancertutor.com
> www.cancure.org
> www.doctoryourself.com
> www.lef.org
> www.MDanderson.org

www.mnwelldir.org
www.shirleys-wellness-cafe.com
www.whale.to/cancer.html

6. Useful discussion groups

The Yahoo chat groups are also well worth joining (Go to www.Yahoogroups.com) - I would recommend the Cancercured, Cancercure, the Alternative Medicine and the FlaxseedOil2 groups particularly.

About the Author

Jonathan Chamberlain was brought up in Ireland and Hong Kong. After graduating in Social Anthropology from Sussex University, he returned to Hong Kong where he lived for many years as a teacher and writer. He is now a full-time author. In addition to his writing, he has founded two charities: The Hong Kong Down Syndrome Association and Mental Handicap Network China Ltd. These involvements were initiated by the birth of his daughter Stevie. He has written a short book, Wordjazz for Stevie, about Stevie and the impact she had on his life. For further information about this book go to Jonathan's cancer website at www.fightingcancer.com

Jonathan's published books include:

Chinese Gods: An Introduction to Chinese Folk Religion

King Hui: The Man Who Owned All the Opium in Hong Kong

Fighting Cancer: A Survival Guide

Cancer Recovery Guide: 15 Alternative and Complementary Strategies for Restoring Health

Cancer: The Complete Recovery Guide

Index

CPSIA information can be obtained at www.ICGtesting.com
Printed in the USA
239382LV00003B/16/P

9 780954 596019